**CARDIOLOGY RESEARCH AND CLINICAL DEVELOPMENTS**

# VENTRICULAR FIBRILLATION AND ACUTE CORONARY SYNDROME

# CARDIOLOGY RESEARCH AND CLINICAL DEVELOPMENTS

Additional books in this series can be found on Nova's website under the Series tab.

Additional E-books in this series can be found on Nova's website under the E-books tab.

**CARDIOLOGY RESEARCH AND CLINICAL DEVELOPMENTS**

# VENTRICULAR FIBRILLATION AND ACUTE CORONARY SYNDROME

### JOYCE E. MANDELL
#### EDITOR

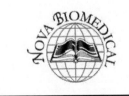

Nova Science Publishers, Inc.
*New York*

Copyright © 2011 by Nova Science Publishers, Inc.

**All rights reserved.** No part of this book may be reproduced, stored in a retrieval system or transmitted in any form or by any means: electronic, electrostatic, magnetic, tape, mechanical photocopying, recording or otherwise without the written permission of the Publisher.

For permission to use material from this book please contact us:
Telephone 631-231-7269; Fax 631-231-8175
Web Site: http://www.novapublishers.com

## NOTICE TO THE READER

The Publisher has taken reasonable care in the preparation of this book, but makes no expressed or implied warranty of any kind and assumes no responsibility for any errors or omissions. No liability is assumed for incidental or consequential damages in connection with or arising out of information contained in this book. The Publisher shall not be liable for any special, consequential, or exemplary damages resulting, in whole or in part, from the readers' use of, or reliance upon, this material. Any parts of this book based on government reports are so indicated and copyright is claimed for those parts to the extent applicable to compilations of such works.

Independent verification should be sought for any data, advice or recommendations contained in this book. In addition, no responsibility is assumed by the publisher for any injury and/or damage to persons or property arising from any methods, products, instructions, ideas or otherwise contained in this publication.

This publication is designed to provide accurate and authoritative information with regard to the subject matter covered herein. It is sold with the clear understanding that the Publisher is not engaged in rendering legal or any other professional services. If legal or any other expert assistance is required, the services of a competent person should be sought. FROM A DECLARATION OF PARTICIPANTS JOINTLY ADOPTED BY A COMMITTEE OF THE AMERICAN BAR ASSOCIATION AND A COMMITTEE OF PUBLISHERS.

Additional color graphics may be available in the e-book version of this book.

**LIBRARY OF CONGRESS CATALOGING-IN-PUBLICATION DATA**
Ventricular fibrillation and acute coronary syndrome / editor, Joyce E. Mandell.
 p. ; cm.
Includes bibliographical references and index.
ISBN 978-1-61728-969-9 (hardcover)
1. Coronary heart disease. 2. Ventricular fibrillation. I. Mandell, Joyce E.
[DNLM: 1. Acute Coronary Syndrome. 2. Ventricular Fibrillation. WG 300]
 RC685.C6V46 2010
 616.1'23--dc22
 2010027149

*Published by Nova Science Publishers, Inc.* ✢ *New York*

# Contents

| | | |
|---|---|---|
| **Preface** | | vii |
| **Chapter I** | Clopidogrel Response in Acute Coronary Syndrome: Clinical Implications and Emerging Therapies<br>*Antonio De Miguel Castro, Alejandro Diego Nieto, Juan Carlos Cuellas Ramón, Armando Pérez de Prado, Javier Gualis Cardona and Felipe Férnandez-Vázquez* | 1 |
| **Chapter II** | Proteomics of Acute Coronary Syndrome<br>*Gloria Alvarez-Llamas, Fernando de la Cuesta, Felix Gil-Dones, Irene Zubiri, Maria Posada, Maria G. Barderas and Fernando Vivanco* | 29 |
| **Chapter III** | Major Bleeding in Acute Coronary Syndrome: Definitions, Magnitude of the Problem, Predictors, Outcomes, Management, and Prevention<br>*Douraid K. Shakir and Jassim Al Suwaidi* | 61 |
| **Chapter IV** | Novel Antiplatelets in Acute Coronary Syndromes<br>*Burak Pamukcu and Huseyin Oflaz* | 89 |
| **Chapter V** | Uncontrolled Immune Response in Acute Myocardial Infarction<br>*Vicente Bodí Peris and María José Forteza de los Reyes* | 115 |
| **Chapter VI** | Tissue Transglutaminase Enzyme and Anti-Tissue Transglutaminase Antibodies: Implication for Acute Coronary Syndrome<br>*Marco Di Tola and Antonio Picarelli* | 139 |
| **Chapter VII** | Electrocardiographic Predictors of Fibrillatory Events in Ventricular Early Repolarization<br>*Xingpeng Liu, Ashok J. Shah, Nicolas Derval, Frederic Sacher, Shinsuke Miyazaki, Amir S. Jadidi, Andrei Forclaz, Isabelle Nault, Lena Rivard, Nick Linton, Olivier Xhaet, Daniel Scherr, Pierre Bordachar, Philippe Ritter, Meleze Hocini, Pierre Jais and Michel Haissaguerre.* | 159 |

| | | |
|---|---|---|
| **Chapter VIII** | Impact of Sodium Channel Dysfunction on Arrhythmogenesis in Brugada Syndrome<br>*Hiroshi Morita, Douglas P. Zipes,*<br>*Satoshi Nagase and Jiashin Wu* | 171 |
| **Chapter IX** | Ventricular Fibrillation: Causes, Symptoms and Treatment<br>*Pasquale Notarstefano, Aureliano Fraticelli,*<br>*Raffaele Guida and Leonardo Bolognese* | 185 |
| **Chapter X** | Primary Ventricular Fibrillation in "Tako-Tsubo" Syndrome<br>*J. Villegas del Ojo, E. Moreno Millán, A.M. García Fernandez,*<br>*F. Bocanegra Martin, and P. Martinez Romero* | 195 |
| **Chapter XI** | Ventricular Fibrillation in the Absence of Apparent Structural Heart Disease: Electrophysiological Mechanisms, Clinical Prognosis and Therapeutic Management.<br>*Osmar Antonio Centurión* | 203 |
| **Index** | | 223 |

# PREFACE

Ventricular fibrillation is a cause of cardiac arrest and sudden cardiac death. The ventricular muscle twitches randomly, rather than contracting in a coordinated fashion (from the apex of the heart to the outflow of the ventricles), and so the ventricles fail to pump blood into the arteries and into systemic circulation. Ventricular fibrillation is a sudden lethal arrhythmia responsible for many deaths mostly brought on by ischaemic heart disease. Acute coronary syndrome (ACS) is a set of signs and symptoms related to the heart. ACS is compatible with a diagnosis of acute myocardial ischemia. This book presents current research from across the globe in the study of ventricular fibrillation and acute coronary syndrome, including clopidogrel response in acute coronary syndrome; primary ventricular fibrillation in "tako-tsubo" syndrome; and ECG predictors of fibrillatory events.

Chapter I - The benefits of clopidogrel on the treatment of acute coronary syndromes are well established. However, not all patients respond in the same way to clopidogrel therapy, and there are patients who suffer major adverse cardiovascular events despite being on treatment, emerging the concept of clopidogrel resistance. This chapter is focused on this topic, mainly in the definition, response assessment, clinical implications, patients' management and emerging therapies (prasugrel, cangrelor and ticagrelor).

There is an interindividual variability in response to clopidogrel therapy, and lower response has been correlated with recurrent adverse cardiovascular events, including late stent thrombosis. Nevertheless, there is not clear and consensual definition of clopidogrel resistance. Clopidogrel response follows a normal distribution, so it would be more appropriate to refer to as variable response to clopidogrel rather than clopidogrel resistance, with its clinical implications: the lower response, the higher probability of suffering thrombotic events. Due to the misleading definition of "resistance" and non-standardized method to assess platelet inhibition, current guidelines do not routinely recommend the use of platelet function assays to monitor the inhibitory effect of antiplatelet drugs and guide therapies. Clopidogrel loading doses higher than 300 mg and daily maintenance doses higher than 75 mg are not routinely recommended by current guidelines, although 600 mg clopidogrel loading dose seems to be safe and effective, and could be used when a faster onset of action is required. Unfortunately, the management of patients with low response to clopidogrel remains uncertain. Strict control of risk factors may improve clopidogrel response. Recently, emerging therapies such as prasugrel and ticagrelor have shown better results than clopidogrel in the prevention of death from cardiovascular cause, nonfatal myocardial infarction, or stroke, but at expenses of a higher rate of bleeding events. It remains uncertain whether patients who suffer a thrombotic event being on clopidogrel treatment would benefit from switching to prasugrel or ticagrelor therapy.

Chapter II - Atherosclerosis is a chronic inflammatory disease of the vascular system. It is a complex multifactorial disease characterized by the accumulation of inflammatory cells (macrophages, lymphocytes), lipoproteins and fibrous tissue in the wall of large arteries. This results in the development of necrotic/lipidic cores within the intima of arteries at particular site in the circulation. These lesions form in the settings of a pre-existing intimal hyperplasia characterized by the proliferation of VSMC within the intima. In advanced lesions, necrosis of macrophages and VSMC results in a lipid-rich core covered by a fibrous cap, which protects the lesions from rupture and consists mainly of collagen and extracellular matrix (ECM) proteins, synthesized by vascular cells. Plaque rupture, resulting from inflammatory activation and MMPs secretion, and the ensuing thrombosis commonly causes the most acute complications of atherosclerosis such as unstable angina or myocardial infarction (acute coronary syndrome) or stroke.

Chapter III - Acute coronary syndrome forms the vast majority of cases seen in daily cardiology clinical practice. It is usually managed using antiplatelet, antithrombotic, and anticoagulation agents, all of which are double-edged swords that also increase the risk of bleeding with an associated increase in morbidity and mortality. Predicting the occurrence of major bleeding and preventing it may help save lives, improve outcomes, and reduce costs. The definition of major bleeding in acute coronary syndrome poses a great challenge when using data from studies and registries around the world to explore the magnitude, predictors, and management of this problem. Different definitions have resulted in inconsistent prevalence and outcomes data. In this chapter, the author explore these issues based on data extracted from a large number of clinical trials and registries, and suggest strategies to address this serious complication of acute coronary syndrome management.

Chapter IV - Atherosclerotic coronary artery disease and acute coronary syndromes are the major cause of death in developed countries and their prevalance are increasing in the developing world. Damaged endothelium, impaired coronary flow and finally almost always rupture in a vulnerable atherosclerotic plaque results with thrombus formation and total luminal occlusion at the atherosclerotic lesion site. Atherothrombosis, the latest phase of the atherosclerotic process, is one of the most studied stages that recent studies provided important evidence for its prevention. In 1980s, aspirin became the first line antiaggregant agent in patients with acute coronary syndromes. However, researchers aimed to discover optimal antiplatelet agents with improved efficacy and reasonable safety profile. Developments in the percutaneous coronary interventions (PCI) and especially the stent technology established requirement for newer antiplatelet agents, which was the beginning of 'age of thienopyridines'. Ticlopidine was the first line thienopyridine, however, serious side effects (neutropenia and severe allergic reactions) limited its clinical use. Then, the ADP $P_2Y_{12}$ receptor antagonist 'clopidogrel' became the most commonly used antiplatelet agent after PCI. Subsequently, new generation and more potent ADP receptor antagonists, prasugrel and ticagrelor were developed. The spectrum of antithrombotics is enlarging by the development of vonWillebrand (eg, ARC1779), thrombin (PAR-1 antagonists, eg, SCH530348) and thromboxane receptor antagonists (eg, terutroban). Novel antiplatelet agents aim to reduce atherothrombosis more efficiently than recent ones but without increasing major or life threathenning bleeding. In this chapter the author aim to focus on recent developments and future therapeutic antithrombotic perspectives in patients with acute coronary syndromes.

Chapter V - Recently, the theory that hyperinflammation is the body's primary response to potent stimulus has been challenged. Indeed, a deregulation of the immune system could be the cause of multiple organ failure. So far, clinicians have focused on the last steps of the inflammatory cascade. However, little attention has been paid to lymphocytes, which play an important role as strategists of the inflammatory response. Experimental evidence suggests a crucial role of T lymphocytes in the pathophysiology of atherosclerosis and acute myocardial infarction (AMI). In summary, from the bottom of an imaginary inverted pyramid, a few regulatory T-cells control the upper parts represented by the wide spectrum of the inflammatory cascade. In AMI, a loss of regulation of the inflammatory system occurs in patients with a decreased activity of regulatory T-cells. As a consequence, aggressive T-cells boost and anti-inflammatory T-cells drop. A pleiotropic proinflammatory imbalance with damaging effects in terms of left ventricular performance and patient outcome is the result of this uncontrolled immune response.

Nowadays, in order to reduce infarct size and microvascular obstruction, a broad range of innovative therapeutic approaches have been proposed, i.e.: cell therapy with regulatory T-cells, inhibition of pro-inflammatory cytokines (TNF-α antagonists), anti-inflammatory cytokines (IL-10 therapy), vaccination with antigens responsables of the immune response in atherosclerosis (vaccination with LDLox or vaccination with Heat Shock Protein 60 HSP60), or the use of gene therapy. The aim of this review is to get an insight into the pathophysiology of the role of the immune system in AMI as well as to describe new therapeutic options on the basis of the regulation of the immune system.

Chapter VI - The type II or tissue transglutaminase (TG2) is an ubiquitous enzyme involved in angiogenesis, fibrogenesis, wound healing, cell adhesion/migration, intracellular signaling pathways, respiratory chain assembly, cell proliferation/differentiation, neurite formation, apoptosis, and inflammation. Some years ago, an increased extracellular localization of TG2 has been demonstrated in damaged or inflamed portions of the small intestine from patients with celiac disease (CD). This antigenic overexpression is able to explain, at least in part, the anti-TG2 antibody induction observable in CD patients. On the other hand, anti-TG2 antibodies have been recently described in patients affected from disorders in which the target organ is located at a distance from the intestine, such as acute coronary syndrome (ACS), dilated cardiomyopathy (DCM), valvular heart disease and other causes of end-stage heart failure. In this regard, a cardiac TG2 overexpression has been described in some experimental models of heart failure and in occurrence of myocardial ischemia/reperfusion injury. In the arteries with or without minimal atherosclerosis, TG2 is detectable only in the medium and along the luminal endothelial border while in the atherosclerotic arteries, especially coronaries and carotid vessels, this enzyme is also evident in the fibrous cup and in shoulder regions of the plaque. Consequently, an anti-TG2 antibody-inducing mechanism similar to those taking part in the intestine of CD patients may also occur in the cardiovascular tissues affected from an acute or chronic disorder. Consistent with this hypothesis, anti-TG2 antibodies seem to be related to severity of the acute coronary event, as well as to extent of the myocardial tissue lesion occurring in ACS patients. Furthermore, since TG2 enzymatic activity may result in myocardial wound healing and stabilization of atherosclerotic plaque, anti-TG2 antibodies could have biological effects able to define a prognostic significance. In this light, vulnerable or ruptured atherosclerotic plaque, as well as injured myocardium (following an infarction, myocarditis, etc.) may be sources of TG2 antigen resulting in formation of anti-TG2 antibodies that in turn, by neutralizing TG2 enzymatic activity, could promote destabilization of the plaque or impaired myocardial wound healing, thereby contributing to a chronic disorder such as DCM. The finding that anti-TG2 antibodies are able to induce proliferation and inhibit differentiation of intestinal epithelial cell, increase epithelial permeability, activate monocytes, and disturb angiogenesis in CD patients suggests that they may have a functional role also in cardiovascular disorders. In the near future, these observations and related hypothesis could to become the subject of interesting researches.

Chapter VII - Early repolarization (ER) pattern is a common electrocardiographic (ECG) variant, characterized by J point elevation manifested either as QRS slurring (at the transition from the QRS segment to the ST segment) or notching (a positive deflection inscribed on terminal S wave), ST-segment elevation with upper concavity and prominent T waves in at least two contiguous leads. The prevalence of ER pattern in normal population varies from 1% to 13%, depending on the age (predominant in young adults), the race (highest amongst black population), and the criterion for J point elevation (0.05 mV vs. 0.1 mV). Since first described by Tomashewski in 1938, ER pattern has been largely considered as an innocent ECG phenomenon for decades. However, this long-held concept has been getting some new momentum by recently published reports. ER pattern has been associated with ventricular fibrillation (VF) in patients with aborted sudden cardiac arrest. It has also emerged as a marker of increased long-term cardiovascular mortality in the general population. Thus, ER pattern is probably not so benign as traditionally believed. Under such a situation, now, the critical clinical question is how to identify the ER subjects who are potentially at risk of arrhythmia. In this chapter, the author review the currently available knowledge on this issue.

Chapter VIII - (Background) Patients with Brugada syndrome (BS) have sodium channel (Na-Ch) SCN5A mutations (20%) as well as calcium channel (Ca-Ch) mutations (8%) that reduce the inward current and affect the action potential (AP). The author investigated the affects of Na-Ch dysfunction on arrhythmogenesis in patients with BS and in experimental models of BS to understand the mechanisms of arrhythmogenesis and the origins of the ECG characteristics of BS.

(Methods) *Clinical study*: the author evaluated 80 BS patients [22 with prior ventricular fibrillation (VF) and implantation of a cardioverter defibrillator], and compared ECG parameters and recurrent VF episodes between the patients with and without SCN5A mutation.

*Experimental study*: The author created 2 experimental models of BS in 18 canine right ventricular preparations: 1) Na-Ch dysfunction model (Na-model) by using pilsicainide and pinacidil (n=11); and 2) Ca-Ch dysfunction model (Ca-model) by using verapamil (n=7). The author then optically mapped multisite APs on the transmural surface of these tissue models, and analyzed the mechanisms of arrhythmogenesis and origins of characteristic BS ECGs.

(Results) *Clinical Study*: Patients with the SCN5A mutation had longer PQ interval (202 ± 31 ms) than patients without the mutation (182 ± 31 ms, $p<0.05$), but no differences in ST elevation. Patients with mutation experienced earlier recurrence of VF (2.0 ± 0.9 months) than patients without mutation (12.7 ± 19 months, $p<0.05$).

*Experimental study*: Transmural activation time (endocardial stimulation to epicardial breakthrough) took longer in the Na-model than in the Ca-model (50 ± 11, vs. 34 ± 10 ms, $p<0.01$). The Na-model also had prominent epicardial AP heterogeneity, which promoted frequent ventricular arrhythmias (VA) via phase 2 reentry (incidence of VAs: Na-model 50% vs. Ca-model 0%, p<0.01).

(Conclusion) Conduction disturbances and AP heterogeneity (especially in the epicardium of the right ventricle) were the underlying causes of frequent VAs and ECG characteristics in Brugada syndrome with Na-Ch dysfunction.

Chapter IX - Ventricular fibrillation (VF) is a disorganised series of very rapid, ineffective contractions of the ventricular muscle caused by several chaotic electrical wavefronts. Its electrocardiographic hallmark is a rapid and grossly irregular ventricular rhythm with marked variability in QRS cycle length, morphology and amplitude. As consequence of poorly synchronized and inadequate myocardial contractions, the heart immediately loses its pump function, with subsequent tissue hypoperfusion and global tissue ischemia. VF very rarely terminates spontaneously. Loss of consciousness occurs in seconds and few minutes are sufficient to cause irreversible brain damage due to cerebral anoxya, followed by death.

Chapter X - Introduction: The "tako-tsubo" syndrome is a recently described process that clinically mimics an acute coronary disease, understanding the association of chest pain with ST-T elevation without coronary artery occlusion, and with a typical and reversible deformation of left ventricle as a result of anteroapical diskinesia with basal hyperkinesia.

Case report: a 64 years old woman without cardiovascular risk factors, featuring presyncope and chest pain and show in the hospital ST segment elevation in inferiorposterolateral area, proceeding to fibrinolysis with tenecteplase, showing 15 minutes after an episode of ventricular fibrillation (VF) that is treated with shock of 360 joules, recovering effective spontaneous circulation. The electrocardiographic ST segment elevation persistence 90 minutes postfibrinolisis, by that an emergency angiography was made showing no signs of coronary arteries occlusion, and finding on ventriculography anteroapical dyskinesia with basal hyperkinesia.

Discussion and Conclusion: Today, there are new diseases, probably undiagnosed, as the "tako-tsubo" syndrome, predominantly female and generated by stress, which simulates an acute coronary syndrome with ST segment elevation and may be responsible for sudden death by primary VF. It is very important to recognize this syndrome, as its management and prognosis are different of the acute myocardial infarction resulting from coronary thrombotic occlusion.

Chapter XI - Up to a third of all cases of unexplained sudden cardiac arrest may be primarily due to cardiac arrhythmias, with ventricular fibrillation (VF) being the culprit arrhythmia in the majority of patients. Sudden cardiac death in the truly normal heart is an uncommon occurrence. The majority of patients without apparent structural heart disease who died suddenly do not actually have "normal" hearts. Idiopathic ventricular fibrillation (IVF) is an uncommon disease of unknown etiology that manifests as syncope, cardiac arrest or seizures caused by rapid polymorphic ventricular tachycardia (VT) or VF in the absence of structural heart disease or identifiable channelopathy. Usually during an arrhythmic storm, it is relatively easy to diagnose IVF in a cardiac arrest survivor when the onset of spontaneous polymorphic VT/VF can be recorded, and this shows initiation of polymorphic VT/VF by very short coupled ventricular ectopy. Conduction block was found responsible for wave front fractionation and reentry, an important mechanism in proliferation of wave fronts and rotors during VF. IVF is essentially a diagnosis by exclusion. However, typical clinical and electrophysiological characteristics present in some patients often allows for a positive diagnosis. Since the rate of recurrence of malignant ventricular arrhythmias in IVF is unacceptably high in the absence of therapy, once a diagnosis of IVF is made, some form of therapy is mandatory. Therapy may include ICD implantation, drug therapy, radiofrequency catheter ablation of the triggering focus or combinations of the above. In this chapter, it will be discussed the electrophysiological mechanisms, clinical prognosis and therapeutic management of VF in the absence of apparent structural heart disease.

*Chapter I*

# CLOPIDOGREL RESPONSE IN ACUTE CORONARY SYNDROME: CLINICAL IMPLICATIONS AND EMERGING THERAPIES

*Antonio De Miguel Castro*[\*][1], *Alejandro Diego Nieto*[1], *Juan Carlos Cuellas Ramón*[1], *Armando Pérez de Prado*[1], *Javier Gualis Cardona*[2] *and Felipe Férnandez-Vázquez*[1]

[1]Department of Interventional Cardiology. Cardiology Division
Hospital Universitario de León, León. Spain
[2]Department of Cardiac Surgery. Hospital Universitario de León, León. Spain

## ABSTRACT

The benefits of clopidogrel on the treatment of acute coronary syndromes are well established. However, not all patients respond in the same way to clopidogrel therapy, and there are patients who suffer major adverse cardiovascular events despite being on treatment, emerging the concept of clopidogrel resistance. This chapter is focused on this topic, mainly in the definition, response assessment, clinical implications, patients' management and emerging therapies (prasugrel, cangrelor and ticagrelor).

There is an interindividual variability in response to clopidogrel therapy, and lower response has been correlated with recurrent adverse cardiovascular events, including late stent thrombosis. Nevertheless, there is not clear and consensual definition of clopidogrel resistance. Clopidogrel response follows a normal distribution, so it would be more appropriate to refer to as variable response to clopidogrel rather than clopidogrel resistance, with its clinical implications: the lower response, the higher probability of suffering thrombotic events. Due to the misleading definition of "resistance" and non-standardized method to assess platelet inhibition, current guidelines do not routinely recommend the use of platelet function assays to monitor the inhibitory effect of antiplatelet drugs and guide therapies. Clopidogrel loading doses higher than 300 mg and

---

[\*] Corresponding author: Antonio Alejandro De Miguel Castro, MD, Department of Interventional Cardiology, Cardiology Division, Hospital Universitario de León, Altos de Nava SN, 24080 León, Spain, Phone & Fax: (+34) 987 237683, E-mail: aademiguel@gmail.com

daily maintenance doses higher than 75 mg are not routinely recommended by current guidelines, although 600 mg clopidogrel loading dose seems to be safe and effective, and could be used when a faster onset of action is required. Unfortunately, the management of patients with low response to clopidogrel remains uncertain. Strict control of risk factors may improve clopidogrel response. Recently, emerging therapies such as prasugrel and ticagrelor have shown better results than clopidogrel in the prevention of death from cardiovascular cause, nonfatal myocardial infarction, or stroke, but at expenses of a higher rate of bleeding events. It remains uncertain whether patients who suffer a thrombotic event being on clopidogrel treatment would benefit from switching to prasugrel or ticagrelor therapy.

## ABBREVIATIONS LIST

| ACS | Acute Coronary Syndrome |
|---|---|
| ADP | Adenosine Diphosphate |
| AMI | Acute Myocardial Infarction |
| DES | Drug Eluting Stents |
| MACE | Major Adverse Cardiovascular Event |
| IPA | Inhibition of Platelet Aggregation |
| NSTE-ACS | Non-ST-segment Elevation Acute Coronary Syndrome |
| PCI | Percutaneous Coronary Intervention |
| PRU | Platelet Reaction Unit |
| STEMI | ST Elevation Myocardial Infarction |
| VASP | Vasodilator Stimulated Phosphoprotein |

## INTRODUCTION

Platelets play a central role in the pathogenesis of acute coronary syndromes (ACS) and complications after percutaneous coronary interventions (PCI). Rupture or erosion of atherosclerotic lesions facilitates the interaction of flowing blood with the inner components of the atherosclerotic lesions. Tissue factor in the plaque activates the clotting cascade leading to acute thrombus formation with its clinical manifestations: unstable angina, non-ST segment elevation acute coronary syndrome (NSTE-ACS), ST elevation myocardial infarction (STEMI) and sudden cardiac death [1, 2].

The benefits of antiplatelet therapy for the treatment and prevention of acute coronary events clinically support the role of platelets in the pathogenesis of atherothrombotic process. The most commonly used antiplatelet drugs are aspirin and clopidogrel, alone or in combination.

Clopidogrel is a second-generation thienopyridine that selective and irreversibly blocks the P2Y12-adenosine diphosphate (ADP) receptor[3, 4]. Despite their platelet inhibitory effects, both aspirin and clopidogrel monotherapy are considered a safe although weak therapy. Given their different mechanisms of action, coadministration of both antiplatelet agents attains higher platelet inhibition [5]. Several clinical trials have demonstrated the additional beneficial role of clopidogrel in addition to aspirin to prevent stent thrombosis after PCI [6-8] and the reduction in the incidence of major adverse cardiovascular events (MACE) in patients with NSTE-ACS [9] and STEMI [10-12]. Nevertheless, dual antiplatelet therapy is not recommended for the prevention of atherothrombotic events in patients with stable cardiovascular disease or multiple cardiovascular risk factors [13].

However, not all individuals show the same response to clopidogrel treatment, and there are patients who suffer adverse events despite being on treatment. Variable response to clopidogrel treatment has been described extensively in different clinical settings and the term of clopidogrel resistance has arisen, but this term is misleading and a standard definition is still lacking; in addition, regardless of the different mechanisms of platelet inhibition, poor responsiveness to aspirin has also been associated with lower response to clopidogrel [14].

This chapter is focused on this topic, mainly in the definition, response assessment, clinical implications, patients' management and emerging therapies (prasugrel, cangrelor and ticagrelor).

## RESISTANCE/VARIABLE RESPONSE TO CLOPIDOGREL. DOES IT EXIST?

There is no standardized definition of clopidogrel resistance, and the exact prevalence remains uncertain; ranges from 5 to 44% [14-22] have been reported in different studies. Resistance definition can be based on a clinical or biochemical approach.

The clinical definition of resistance is based on the failure to prevent adverse events in patients "on treatment". There is large evidence supporting that low response to antiplatelet agents correlates with adverse events, but given the multifactorial etiopathogenesis of atherothrombotic events, results inaccurate to define clopidogrel resistance based on the recurrence of adverse events. Under these clinical criteria, the term "clinical resistance" should be avoided and it would more appropriate to use the term "treatment failure".

The biochemical definition of resistance is based on the failure to achieve "adequate" inhibitory standards on laboratory tests of platelet function. The inhibitory effect has been determined as absolute difference between pre- and post-treatment platelet reactivity (PPR) or percent reduction in aggregation parameters obtained at baseline and after treatment; the latter methodology is also termed IPA (inhibition of platelet aggregation). Patients' response to clopidogrel follows a typical normal distribution (something common to almost all drugs). Therefore, response to clopidogrel therapy shouldn't be considered in a dichotomic way (YES/NO response), but a continuous variable. According to the normal (bell-shaped) curve of response to clopidogrel treatment, it is expectable to find ≈5% of hyper- and hypo-responders, as it is expectable with any other drug [23]. The magnitude of (low) response to clopidogrel treatment might be dynamic, varying even over time during long-term treatments. More importantly, the cut-off values are arbitrary and vary among studies, so it would be more appropriate to refer to as variable response rather than resistance to clopidogrel.

Some studies [24-30] support that *post-treatment platelet reactivity* is a better estimate of thrombotic risk than the degree of IPA, since IPA (percent decrease in platelet aggregation values) does not take into account the absolute level of platelet reactivity. This becomes even more confusing when Gurbel et al [15] showed that there are patients with low post-treatment platelet reactivity who are clopidogrel non-responders (defined as a percent decrease in aggregation values) and some patients who are clopidogrel responders continue to have high post-treatment platelet reactivity.

The biochemical definition of resistance or variable response to clopidogrel (according to laboratory test) has several limitations: different assays used for platelet function assessment (every one with its own limitations), usage of diverse agonist (and doses) to induce and measure platelet aggregation, variable cut-off values, and different time window chosen to measure the platelet aggregation.

Furthermore, the impact of laboratory estimation of response to any antiplatelet therapy is not completely understood, since the relationship between resistance/variable response and adverse clinical events is very heterogeneous. Similarly to clopidogrel resistance, the term aspirin resistance has also arisen, and the results of a recent meta-analysis [31] are very illustrative because stand out the significant different aspirin resistance prevalence depending on the platelet function assay used: 6% vs 26% with optical aggregometry and point-of-care tests, respectively, showing the difficulty to establish a standardized definition of resistance and method to assess platelet inhibition. The correlation between platelet function test and adverse events have been established in different clinical settings with diverse inclusion criteria, clinical end points and follow-up, different clopidogrel loading/maintenance dosage and, more importantly, in small size clinical trials with limited number of cardiovascular events.

The optimal level of inhibition of platelet aggregation to prevent cardiovascular events may vary upon the clinical situation and, to date, there are no universally accepted IPA and/or post-treatment platelet reactivity thresholds identifying patients at higher risk for adverse events in specific clinical settings. Ongoing trials are currently evaluating whether targeting a particular degree of platelet inhibition, either with novel antiplatelet agents or higher doses of current drugs, will prove to be safe and efficacious. These studies will provide the critical missing information about the capability of these methods for monitoring antiplatelet therapies in cardiac patients and other clinical scenarios. Due to the misleading definition of "resistance" and non-standardized method to assess platelet inhibition, current guidelines do not routinely recommend the use of platelet function assays to monitor the inhibitory effect of antiplatelet drugs and guide therapies [32-34].

Another important factor to take into account when analyzing the degree of PPR and IPA achieved with any antiplatelet treatment, is the practical impossibility of obtaining the real baseline values (pre-treatment) of platelet reactivity in some specific clinical settings, since certain pathological conditions such as ACS are characterized by ongoing thrombosis resulting in increased platelet reactivity, leading to unknow the baseline platelet reactivity prior to the ongoing ACS.

## MECHANISMS OF VARIABLE RESPONSE TO CLOPIDOGREL

Interindividual variable response to clopidogrel is multifactorial and the mechanisms have not been fully elucidated; these mechanism can be divided into pharmacokinetic (failure to achieve/maintain adequate levels of the active drug) or pharmacodynamic factors (despite adequate levels there is a failure to inhibit the specific receptors). Also the clinical, environmental, cellular and genetic factors play a role in this regard. Potential mechanisms of variable response to clopidogrel are summarized in table 1.

## Table 1. Potential Mechanism of Variable Response to Clopidogrel

| |
|---|
| 1. Reduced clopidogrel bioavailability |
| - Non-compliance to clopidogrel therapy |
| - Under-dosing or inappropriate dosing of clopidogrel |
| - Poor absorption |
| - Drug-drug interactions involving cytochrome P450 |
| 2. Genetic variables: |
| - Polymorphism of $P2Y_{12}$ |
| - Polymorphism of cytochrome P450 |
| - Polymorphism of multidrug resistance transporter |
| - Polymorphism of GP Ia |
| - Polymorphism of GP IIb/IIIa |
| 3. Increased release of ADP |
| 4. Increased $P2Y_{12}$ receptors |
| 5. Clinical factors leading to high pre-treatment platelet reactivity: |
| - Acute coronary syndrome |
| - Diabetes mellitus/Insulin resistance |
| - Elevated body mass index |
| 6. Up-regulation of $P2Y_{12}$ independent pathways |
| 7. Up-regulation of P2Y independent pathways: |
| - Thrombin |
| - Thromboxane $A_2$ |
| - Collagen |
| - Epinephrine |
| 8. Increased turn-over of platelets |

ADP= Adenosine Diphosphate; GP= Glycoprotein

Increased (baseline) platelet activity and thrombotic burden in specific clinical settings (ACS, diabetes, dyslipemia, heart failure, PCI, and obesity) may also contribute to "lower response" to antiplatelet therapies. Clopidogrel exerts their inhibitory effect via one of the several pathways triggering platelet activation and aggregation. In addition, clopidogrel does not abolish platelet response to stronger agonist such as thrombin, epinephrine and collagen. In high-risk clinical situations, such as ACS, characterized by a high thrombin generation environment, a higher platelet inhibition might be required to protect against atherothrombotic events. However, there are clinical trials involving non-STEMI [35] and STEMI patients [36] that have shown that a dramatically higher inhibition of platelet aggregation achieved with glycoprotein IIb/IIIa inhibitors is not always followed by clinical benefits.

## Genetic Polymorphism

After intestinal absorption, clopidogrel is a prodrug that needs hepatic metabolism to the generation of its active metabolite (85% is hydrolyzed by esterases in the blood). Specifically, 2 sequential oxidative steps through the cytochrome P450 (CYP) system are needed. A variety of P450 enzymes contribute to clopidogrel metabolism. The first metabolic step, which leads to 2-oxo-clopidogrel, is dependent on 3 enzymes (CYP1A2, CYP2B6, and

CYP2C19), whereas the second step, which culminates in the active metabolite, involves 4 enzymes (CYP2B6, CYP2C9, CYP2C19, and CYP3A4). Pharmacogenetic studies have studied different genes polymorphisms implicated in the pharmacokinetics and pharmacodynamics of clopidogrel. Among these, genes included encode proteins and enzymes involved in intestinal absorption, hepatic metabolism, and platelet membrane receptors.

There are consistent data that relate clopidogrel variability response to hepatic CYP polymorphisms, mainly, the CYP2C19 loss of function polymorphism [37]. Importantly, in addition to modulation of pharmacodynamic and pharmacokinetic profiles, this polymorphism has also been associated with greater ischemic event rates [38], including stent thrombosis [39]. These findings have led to suggest genetic testing for this polymorphism as a screening measure for clopidogrel response. Point-of-care assays are currently under development to allow rapid genetic testing for this polymorphism.

## Drug-Drug Interactions

Another factor affecting response to clopidogrel is the possibility of drug-drug interactions (cardiac patients are being prescribed with multiple drugs). As previously described, clopidogrel is an inactive prodrug that requires two-step oxidation by the hepatic CYP system to generate its active compound. Drugs that are substrates or inhibit the CYP system can potentially interfere with the conversion of clopidogrel into its active metabolite, leading to reduce its antiplatelet effects. Among these drugs, there has been special focus on statins, proton pump inhibitors (PPIs) and calcium channel blockers, common concomitant drugs prescribed with clopidogrel in cardiac patients.

### *Statins*

Preliminary studies have shown that lipophilic statins, such as atorvastatin, lovastatin and simvastatin, which require CYP3A4 metabolization, hamper clopidogrel-induced antiplatelet effects [40, 41]. However, recent reports have denied this interaction [42, 43].

### *Proton Pump Inhibitors*

Patients receiving dual antiplatelet treatment with aspirin and clopidogrel are commonly treated with PPIs with the objective of minimising the risk of gastrointestinal (GI) bleeding complications. Current guidelines recommend prescription of a PPI in all patients under dual antiplatelet treatment [44]. Hepatic metabolization of PPIs is CYP-dependent and it has been hypothesized that a potential drug-drug interaction at the level of the hepatic CYP system exists causing an attenuated response to clopidogrel under concomitant omeprazole treatment due to diminished CYP-dependent metabolization of clopidogrel into its active thiol metabolite.

In a double-blind, placebo-controlled trial [45], 124 consecutive patients undergoing PCI treated with aspirin (75 mg/day) and clopidogrel (300 mg loading dose, followed by 75 mg/day) were randomized to receive omeprazole (20 mg/day) or placebo for 7 days. Clopidogrel effect was tested on days 1 and 7 in both groups by measuring vasodilator stimulated phosphoprotein (VASP) phosphorylation, expressed as platelet reactivity index

(PRI). On Day 7, 16 patients (26.7%) were poor responders in the placebo group compared with 39 patients (60.9%) in the omeprazole group (p < 0.0001). The odds ratio of being a poor responder to clopidogrel when concomitantly treated with omeprazole was 4.31 (95%, CI 2.0 to 9.2). The clinical impact of these results was not assessed.

Different studies [46, 47] have confirmed the attenuating effects on clopidogrel response reported in the OCLA trial for the PPI omeprazole, but not for pantoprazole and esomeprazole, which do not attenuate the antiplatelet action of clopidogrel, supporting that the attenuating effects of PPI treatment on clopidogrel response are not a phenomenon observed for all PPIs in general. However, the results of the Clopidogrel Medco Outcomes study including 16.690 patients presented in the SCAI 2009 Annual Scientific Sessions (Las Vegas, Nevada, USA) defended a possible "class effect" for PPIs on top of clopidogrel therapy.

Several retrospective studies have evaluated the risk of adverse events associated with concomitant use of clopidogrel and PPIs. In patients undergoing PCI with DES, the prescription of a PPI at discharge was associated with a greater rate of MACE at 1 year, with an adjusted hazard ratio of 1.8 (95% confidence interval 1.1 to 2.7, p = 0.01) after multivariate analysis [48]. An additional study [49] has shown in patients after ACS that the use of clopidogrel plus PPIs is associated with an increased risk of death or rehospitalization for ACS compared with the use of clopidogrel without PPI (adjusted OR, 1.25; 95% CI, 1.11-1.41).

Great expectation was focus on the results of the COGENT trial, a large randomized double-blind, clinical trial. The COGENT trial was prematurely stopped with only 3627 patients enrolled out of the roughly 5000 investigators had expected to recruit. Patients requiring clopidogrel for at least 12 months (typically following NSTE-ACS, STEMI, or stent implantation) were included and randomized to receive omeprazole or placebo. The results of the COGENT trial were presented in the TCT 2009 Congress, San Francisco, California, USA, reporting (survival data out to 390 days) 67 cardiovascular events in the placebo group and 69 in the omeprazole group, with similar event curves (a composite of CV death, nonfatal AMI, CABG or PCI, or ischemic stroke). For the end points of MI alone and revascularization procedures alone, event curves once again were identical. In analyses taking into account baseline variables or medical history, there was no signal of increased cardiovascular events for patients treated with omeprazole in any subgroup. By contrast, looking just at GI events (upper-GI bleeding, symptomatic upper-GI bleeding, pain of presumed GI origin with underlying multiple erosive disease), researchers found that event rates were significantly higher in patients randomized to placebo.

Considering all available evidence, experts recommend that PPI use should be limited to situations clearly indicated in patients on clopidogrel treatment after PCI or ACS.

## *Calcium-Channel Blockers*

Calcium-channel blockers (CCBs) inhibit the cytochrome P450-3A4 enzyme, which metabolises clopidogrel to its active form. Two observational prospective studies have described the influence of CCBs on clopidogrel mediated platelet inhibition in vivo [50, 51]. In both studies, concomitant CCB therapy was significantly associated with decreased platelet inhibition by clopidogrel. Moreover, intake of CCBs was associated with adverse clinical outcomes, driven by a higher rate of revascularization procedures. Due to the small sample size, baseline differences between treatment groups and the observational nature instead of interventional of these studies, large randomized clinical trials are required before drawing definitive conclusions.

## IS IT POSSIBLE TO ACCURATELY ASSESS THE INHIBITORY EFFECT OF ANTIPLATELT DRUGS?

When assessing the inhibitory effect of any antiplatelet agent, the mechanism of action of the drug should be fully understood. It has been already noted that clopidogrel blocks the P2Y12-ADP receptor. Therefore, in order to assess the inhibitory effects of clopidogrel, an ADP-dependent technique should be respectively applied.

The different options to assess the inhibitory effect of clopidogrel have been described elsewhere [3, 52]; however, there is not standardized method and none of them evaluate platelet activation as a whole, since platelets can be activated by several different pathways. Table 2 summarizes the advantages and limitations of the more common asssays used to evaluate the response to clopidogrel.

Optical aggregometry is considered the gold standard to assess platelet activity, mainly because the abundance of data generated with this technique rather than its advantage over other techniques. Several circumstances as the time, equipment and training required for mastering it, makes this technique impracticable for the cath lab or private office daily practice. Therefore, several point-of-care devices have been developed to surpass the inconvenients of optical aggregometry. Some of them have been specifically modified for assessing clopidogrel response.

The VerifyNow system (Accumetrics, San Diego, California, USA) is a point-of-care device that uses the same principle than platelet aggregometry but measures agglutination of fibrinogen-coated beads in whole blood in response to ADP and prostaglandin E1 in case of clopidogrel assay.

The Platelet Function Assay-100 (PFA-100) is a point-of-care device that simulates haemostasis by flowing whole blood through a cartridge that contains an aperture coated with collagen, epinephrine or ADP and the time required for aperture closure and cessation of blood flow is used as a measure of platelet activation.

The Multiplate analyzer (Dynabyte, Munich, Germany) is point-of-care device available for rapid and standardised assessment of platelet function parameters in different clinical settings. This device, based on multiple electrode platelet aggregometry, is highly capable of detecting the effect of clopidogrel treatment and the results correlate well with light transmission aggregometry.

Flow cytometry assessment of VASP phosphorilation assay (BioCytex, Marseilles, France) is a specific marker of P2Y12 receptor reactivity and, therefore, clopidogrel-induced inhibition, but this method is expensive and needs sample preparation, requires a flow cytometry and an experienced technician.

There are other laboratory test such as the point-of-care systems Plateletworks (Helena Laboratories, Beaumont, Texas, USA), Thromboelastography platelet mapping system (Haemoscope, Niles, Illinois, USA), and Impact cone and plate analyzer (DiaMed, Cressier, Switzerland) and flow cytometry to measure activation dependent changes in platelet surface P-selectin, platelet surface glycoprotein IIb/IIIa or leukocyte-platelet aggregates; however, these platelet function test are less studied than those described above and have not been tested in clinical settings to predict clinical outcomes; moreover, flow cytometry is too laborious to perform on a patient-to-patient basis.

**Table 2. Platelet Function Asssays to Evaluate Response to Clopidogrel**

| Laboratory Test | Advantages | Limitations |
|---|---|---|
| Optical aggregometry | Widely available<br>Correlated with clinical outcomes<br>Considered gold-standard | Poor reproducibility, operator- and interpreter-dependent<br>Not specfic<br>Uncertain sensitivity<br>High sample volume and sample preparation<br>Requirement for a skilled technician<br>Length of assay time and labour intensive<br>Assesses platelet function in the absence of erythrocytes and blood flow (shear stress) |
| Platelet Function Assay-100 | Point-of-care use<br>Simplicity and rapidity<br>Low sample volume<br>Whole blood and no sample preparation<br>Correlated with clinical outcomes | Uncertain specificity<br>Uncertain sensitivity<br>Expensive<br>Not recommended for monitoring clopidogrel therapy<br>Dependent on von Willebrand factor levels, citrate concentration haematocrit |
| VerifyNow Rapid Platelet Function Assay | Point-of-care use<br>Simplicity and rapidity<br>Low sample volume<br>Whole blood and no sample preparation<br>Correlated with clinical outcomes | Uncertain specificity<br>Uncertain sensitivity<br>Expensive |
| VASP Phosphorylation Assay | $P2Y_{12}$ receptor reactivity specific marker<br>Low sample volume<br>Whole blood | Specific assay for clopidogrel-induced platelet inhibition<br>Flow cytometry requirement<br>Requirement for a skilled technician<br>Sample preparation<br>Expensive<br>Correlation with clinical outcomes less stablished |

VASP= Vasodilatador Stimulated Phosphoprotein.

From the practical point of view, it could be summarized that there are several alternatives for assessing resistance/variable response to clopidogrel. Despite the more friendly-use and speed of the point-of care devices, optical aggregometry and flow cytometry are still considered the best methodologies for accurately assessing platelet reactivity.

## CLINICAL IMPLICATIONS OF VARIABLE RESPONSE TO CLOPIDOGREL

The clinical implications of low inhibition after clopidogrel therapy have been described in several clinical studies. Geisler et al [53] described a higher risk of cardiovascular events among "clopidogrel low-responders" compared to "clopidogrel normo-responders" in patients undergoing elective PCI. Similarly, Matetzky et al [16] showed that, in patients with AMI undergoing primary angioplasty, lower platelet inhibition at days 3 and 6 after PCI was associated with recurrent cardiovascular events at 6 months. Patients with stable angina (n=105) undergoing elective PCI, the only 2 cases of subacute stent thrombosis occurred among clopidogrel non-responders [17].

The prognostic value of post-treatment platelet reactivity has been correlated with clinical outcomes in different clinical trials, most of them involving a reduced number of patients with equally low number of events. In the POPULAR study [54] was evaluated the ability of multiple platelet function tests in predicting atherothrombotic events, including stent thrombosis, in clopidogrel pre-treated patients undergoing PCI with stent implantation. High PPR, when assessed by light transmittance aggregometry (both 5 µmol/L and 20 µmol/L ADP), VerifyNow P2Y12 assay, and Plateletworks, was significantly associated with atherothrombotic events. In contrast, the shear stress-based tests IMPACT-R (with and without ADP prestimulation) and the Dade PFA-100 system (the collagen/ADP and Innovance PFA P2Y) did not show an association with outcome. However, the predictability of these 3 tests was only modest. Cuisset et al [55] described that higher PPR is associated with higher incidence of myonecrosis after stenting for NSTE-ACS. Our group has shown that in patients with NSTEACS undergoing elective early PCI, PPR predicts myocardial damage better than response to clopidogrel [56]. Marcucci et al [57] showed that high PPR affects the severity of myocardial infarction independently of other clinical, procedural, and laboratory parameters in patients with AMI undergoing PCI.

A lot of expectancy was generated by two large clinical studies. Gurbel et al [58] demonstrated that PPR is higher in patients who suffered subacute stent thrombosis compared to those without thrombosis. The difference between both groups was significant, but a careful analysis of the data shows a significant overlapping on the individual data of platelet aggregation and/or thromboelastography from both groups. This overlapping significantly reduces the value of these methodologies when applied to a single patient debilitating their possibilities for individualized medicine. Similar data were reported by Hochholzer et al [24] in patients following elective PCI after 600 mg clopidogrel loading-dose: a 10% increase in ADP-induced platelet aggregation on treatment before PCI was associated with higher risk for 30-days events; in addition to the association between PPR and the risk for 30 days adverse events observed in this study, it should be noticeably marked that the same patients also shared the shortest time from clopidogrel loading dose to PCI (mean 1.8; range 0.8-4.0 hours); this observation is of critical importance on the basis of previous reports suggesting a minimum time of 4 to 6 hours for achieving the maximal antiplatelet effect of clopidogrel.

As previously noticed, PPR is considered a better estimate of thrombotic risk than the degree of IPA, since IPA (percent decrease in platelet aggregation values) does not take into account the absolute level of platelet reactivity. Our group published [30] that in patients with NSTE-ACS undergoing early coronary angiography, the independent predictors of MACE at 1 year were only PPR (10-unit increase in PPR is associated with adjusted OR [AOR], 1.12;

95% CI, 1.01-1.24; P=0.02) and previous antiplatelet therapy (AOR, 4.56; 95% CI, 1.13-23; P=0.033). Cuisset et al [25] described the relationship between PPR before PCI with the subsequent occurrence of MACE at 30-days follow-up in NSTE-ACS patients: irrespective of clopidogrel loading dose (300 mg vs 600 mg), only the persistence of high PPR was significantly associated with cardiovascular events, remarking the importance of the effect of antiplatelet treatment rather than the loading dose. In addition, it is also known that low platelet reactivity at the time of PCI, irrespective of whether this is due to pharmacological inhibition or low baseline platelet reactivity, is beneficial in terms of clinical outcomes [24]. Despite the number of patient enrolled in these studies, the still limited number of events hampers the validity of the conclusions.

## Drug Eluting Stent

Recent meta-analysis have associated drug-eluting stents (DES) with an increased risk of late stent thrombosis and adverse events compared to bare metal stents [59, 60]. A multivariate analysis has identified premature discontinuation of combined antiplatelet therapy as the major independent predictor for late stent thrombosis after DES deployment [61]. In fact, some studies have suggested an increase in the risk of stent thrombosis within drug eluting stents when clopidogrel is discontinued within 6 months after implantation by a factor of more than 30, and an increase by a factor of approximately 6 when clopidogrel is discontinued at 6 months or beyond [61, 62]. Lower response to antiplatelet therapy is also associated with an increased risk of late stent thrombosis in patients receiving DES [63, 64], more evident in patients with dual aspirin and clopidogrel non-responsiveness compared to isolated aspirin or clopidogrel non-responsiveness [65]. Of notice, different observational studies has suggested that early, but not late stent thrombosis, is influenced by residual platelet aggregation in patients treated with dual antiplatelet therapy undergoing PCI [66, 67]. Acute resistance/low response to antiplatelet therapy should not be a key factor since the definition of late stent thrombosis involves a minimum of 1-month post-stenting and very late stent thrombosis 12-months post-stenting. Therefore, DES late and very late stent thrombosis seems to be more correlated with early withdrawal rather to treatment failure. As such, prolonged dual-antiplatelet inhibition therapy for at least 1 year in patients with DES has been recommended. Any elective procedures with significant risk of bleeding should be deferred until appropriate completion of dual antiplatelet therapy [68]. In case of mandatory discontinuation, clopidogrel should be restarted as soon as possible.

A recent study by Park et al has reported that the use of dual antiplatelet therapy for a period longer than 12 months in patients who had received drug-eluting stents was not significantly more effective than aspirin monotherapy in reducing the rate of myocardial infarction or death from cardiac causes [69], but this finding has not been confirmed or refuted yet. Hence, larger, randomized clinical trials evaluating specifically the appropriate duration of dual antiplatelet therapy are needed.

## WHAT TO DO WITH PATIENTS WITH REDUCED RESPONSE TO CLOPIDOGREL THERAPY?

Unfortunately, the management of patients with low response to clopidogrel remains uncertain. In an initial approach, certain factors such as patient compliance and appropriate dosage are assumed to take place. In addition, strict control of risk factors may improve the response to clopidogrel.

Inhibitory effects of clopidogrel are time- and dose-dependent; 600 mg loading dose of clopidogrel causes an earlier, more sustained and stronger inhibition of ADP-induced platelet aggregation than 300 mg loading dose [70, 71]. In addition, there is evidence that 600 mg loading dose of clopidogrel reduces recurrent atherothrombotic events without increasing major bleeding complications in patients undergoing elective PCI compared to 300 mg loading-dose [25, 72]. However, 900 mg clopidogrel loading dose does not result in further suppression of ADP-platelet aggregation, and the clinical impact of clopidogrel loading doses higher than 600 mg is not well established [73, 74]. In patients following elective PCI, at least 6 hours are necessary to achieve full antiplatelet effect after 300 mg clopidogrel loading-dose [74] and 2 hours after 600 mg loading-dose [24]. NSTE-ACS and PCI guidelines [32-34] do not support the routinely use of clopidogrel loading doses higher than 300 mg, and only when is necessary to achieve a more rapid onset of platelet inhibition, 600 mg clopidogrel loading dose may be used in STEMI patients following primary PCI as suggested by STEMI guidelines [75, 76].

The results of the ARMYDA-4 and ARMYDA-5 trials were presented in the TCT 2007 Scientific Sessions (Washington, Washington State, USA). The ARMYDA-4 (ARMYDA-RELOAD) trial assessed the additional clinical benefit of 600 mg clopidogrel loading dose pre-PCI compared to placebo in patients already on chronic clopidogrel treatment undergoing elective PCI in a prospective, randomized, double blind-design study (180 patients received clopidogrel and 180 patients placebo). No clinical benefit (composite end point of death, AMI and target vessel revascularization) was found at 30 days follow-up with the additional 600 mg clopidogrel loading. The ARMYDA-5 (ARMYDA-PRELOAD) trial evaluated the occurrence of clinical events (composite end point of death, AMI and target vessel revascularization) at 30 days follow-up in patients undergoing elective PCI receiving 600 mg clopidogrel loading dose 4-8 hours before PCI compared to 600 mg clopidogrel loading dose immediately before PCI. No clinical benefit was found when clopidogrel loading dose was administered 4-8 hours before PCI.

The CURRENT-OASIS 7 study, was a randomized, 2 x 2 factorial design trial evaluating a clopidogrel high-dose regimen (600 mg loading dose on day 1 followed by 150 mg once daily on days 2 to 7, followed by 75 mg once daily on days 8-30) compared with the standard-dose regimen (300 mg loading dose on day 1, followed by 75 mg once daily on days 2-30) and high-dose aspirin (300-325 mg daily) versus low-dose aspirin (75-100 mg daily) in patients with ST or non-ST-segment-elevation ACS managed with an early invasive strategy no later than 72 hours after randomization. The primary outcome was the composite of death from cardiovascular causes, myocardial (re)-infarction or stroke up to day 30. The primary safety outcome was major bleeding. The results of the CURRENT OASIS-7 presented at the European Society of Cardiology 2009 Congress (Barcelona, Spain) support doubling the loading and maintenance doses of clopidogrel in ACS patients undergoing planned PCI. This strategy significantly reduced stent thrombosis and cardiovascular events in the PCI cohort (17.232 patients), largely driven by reductions in myocardial infarction, with a significant increase in major or severe bleeding according to CURRENT definition. However, the trial failed to meet its primary end point in the overall cohort (25.087 patients) and the absolute effect in the PCI cohort was modest. In addition, there was no difference in the safety or efficacy of higher-dose aspirin when compared with lower-dose aspirin.

Safety and efficacy of clopidogrel daily maintenance dose higher than 75 mg remains uncertain. Angiolillo et al [77] showed that diabetic patients receiving 150 mg clopidogrel daily maintenance dose showed higher platelet inhibition than those receiving 75 mg; however, response to antiplatelet therapy remained highly variable and suboptimal clopidogrel response was still present in 60% of patients receiving 150 mg/day; in addition, this trial was not powered to evaluate clinical outcomes and bleeding events. Von Beckerath et al [78] have shown in stable patients undergoing successful PCI after administration of 600 mg clopidogrel loading dose more intense inhibition of platelet aggregation with 150 mg compared with 75 mg daily maintenance dose, but potential clinical benefits were not explored in this trial. Current guidelines do not recommend clopidogrel daily maintenance dose higher than 75 mg [32-34, 75, 76].

## Optimise Clopidogrel Response According to Platelet Function Tests

With regard to optimise clopidogrel response according to platelet function tests, Neubauer et al [79] had proposed in a observational study with stable patients, pre-treated with 600 mg clopidogrel loading dose followed by 75 mg daily maintenance dose undergoing elective PCI, an algorithm to reduce the incidence of clopidogrel resistance assessed by impedance aggregometry and evaluate therapeutic options: low responders received an additional 600 mg clopidogrel loading dose followed by 75 mg twice a day maintenance dose; in case of persistence of low response to clopidogrel high dose regimen, the antiplatelet therapy was changed to ticlopidine 250 mg twice daily. The incidence of low response to clopidogrel was reduced from 23.6% to 5.0%; nevertheless, this study lacks a clinical follow-up of patients to prove if optimised therapy translates into a reduction of cardiovascular events. Similarly, Bonello et al [80] have shown that in patients scheduled for elective PCI after 600 mg clopidogrel loading dose, adjusting the clopidogrel loading dose according to the results of platelet function assessed with the VASP assay is feasible, safe, and efficacious in reducing post-PCI MACE. In this trial, clopidogrel resistance was defined as a VASP-index >50% after 600 mg clopidogrel loading dose; thus, patients in the assay-guidance group were allowed up to three additional clopidogrel loading dose of 600 mg each, given successively as needed every 24 hours until the VASP-index dropped below 50%, prior PCI. Patients receiving standard clopidogrel loading dose compared to patients receiving VASP index-guided clopidogrel loading dose suffered higher rates of MACE at 30-day follow up (10% vs. 0%, p=0.007), without higher incidence of major or minor bleeding (5% vs. 4%, p=NS). However, due to the small sample size and the lower event rate registered (fewer than expected), these results should be taken into account cautiously before putting then into practice in a clinical basis.

Several PPR cut-off values have been proposed subsequent to platelet function assessed with the VerifyNow P2Y12 assay (Accumetrics Inc, San Diego, California): 175 PRU identified patients with NSTE-ACS undergoing early coronary angiography as being at higher risk for MACE at 1 year follow-up [30]; ≥240 PRU identified patients with ACS (STEMI and NSTEACS patients) who underwent PCI with a significantly higher risk of cardiovascular death and nonfatal myocardial infarction at 1-year follow-up [81]; ≥235 PRU identified patients (>90% with stable angina) following PCI with DES with significantly higher incidence of MACE at 6-months follow-up, including stent thrombosis [82]. The correct treatment, if any, of high PPR remains unknown pending the completion of currently ongoing clinical trials: the GRAVITAS (NCT00645918), the DANTE (NCT00774475), the ARCTIC (NCT00827411), and the TRIGGER-PCI (NCT00910299), which may reveal whether individualized antiplatelet treatment based on platelet function testing improves outcome. Until then, clinical practice should not be guided by (point-of-care) platelet function testing and current guidelines do not support this management. A position paper [83] of the Working Group on Thrombosis of the European Society of Cardiology do not support the routine or even the occasional determination and/or monitoring of platelet function while on therapy with antiplatelet drugs and subsequent therapeutic decisions.

## EMERGING THERAPIES

The same studies that have established the safety and effectiveness of clopidogrel have also indicated the significant variable response associated with this treatment. In a way to improve the benefits of antiplatelet treatment, a new generation of P2Y12-ADP receptor antagonists has been developed. These new agents (Prasugrel, Cangrelor and Ticagrelor) are more potent, with a more rapid onset of action and less inter-individual variability. Table 3 summarizes current P2Y12-ADP receptor inhibitors.

Table 3. P2Y$_{12}$-ADP Receptor Inhibitors

|  | Clopidogrel | Prasugrel | Cangrelor | Tcagrelor |
|---|---|---|---|---|
| Group | Thienopyridine | Thienopyridine | ATP analogue | Cyclopentyl-triazolo-pyrimidine |
| Administration | Oral | Oral | Parenteral | Oral |
| Biodisponibility | Prodrug | Prodrug | Direct-acting | Direct-acting |
| Receptor Inhibition | Irreversible | Irreversible | Reversible | Reversible |
| Dose Frequency | Once daily | Once daily | Bolus and infusion | Twice daily |

### Prasugrel

Prasugrel is a third-generation thienopyridine that selective and irreversibly blocks the P2Y12-ADP receptor, with much more rapid and consistent inhibitory effects on platelet aggregation than clopidogrel. Prasugrel is a prodrug with rapid and almost complete absorption after oral ingestion of a loading dose. Its distinct chemical structure permits conversion to its active metabolite with less dependence on CYP enzymes than clopidogrel.

Prasugrel (60 mg loading dose followed by 10 mg daily maintenance dose), compared to clopidogrel (600 mg loading dose followed by 75 mg [84] or 150 mg [85] daily maintenance dose), provides faster onset, greater inhibition and less variability of P2Y12-ADP receptor-mediated platelet aggregation because of greater and more efficient generation of its active metabolite (in circulating blood within 15 minutes of dosing, which reaches maximal plasma concentration at 30 minutes). Other advantages of prasugrel over clopidogrel are that CYP genotype has no influence on its pharmacokinetics and pharmacodynamics and the much lower interindividual variability in the inhibition of P2Y12 dependent platelet responses leading to an extremely low prevalence of subjects who display resistance to prasugrel.

In the TRITON-TIMI 38 trial, patients with NSTE-ACS or STEMI undergoing PCI were randomly assigned to receive either prasugrel (60 mg loading dose followed by 10 mg daily maintenance dose) or clopidogrel (300 mg loading dose followed by 75 mg daily maintenance dose). A significant decrease in the combined primary end point (death from cardiovascular cause, nonfatal myocardial infarction, or stroke) was found with prasugrel as compared with clopidogrel, but a significant excess of TIMI major bleeding, life-threatening bleeding and fatal bleeding was shown in patients assigned to prasugrel, so that, for each death from cardiovascular causes prevented by the use of prasugrel compared with clopidogrel, approximately one additional episode of fatal bleeding was caused by prasugrel, leading to similar net clinical benefit with no significant differences in death from any cause [86]. In the TRITON-TIMI 38, the loading dose of clopidogrel was 300 mg (the FDA-approved regimen), while in the PRINCIPLE-TIMI 44 [85], prasugrel was compared to 600 mg loading dose of clopidogrel, a regimen increasingly used in patients undergoing PCI. Subsequent analysis has shown that the net clinical benefit with prasugrel was greater for patients with diabetes than for patients without diabetes, including a gradient from no DM to DM without insulin therapy to DM with insulin therapy [87].

In summary, in the TRITON-TIMI 38 studies the main topics to point out are:

1. prasugrel significantly reduces the risks of recurrent myocardial infarction (spontaneous and procedural) and stent thrombosis as compared with clopidogrel.
2. these benefits are particularly sizable among patients with diabetes or ST-segment elevation.
3. the finding of an approximately 50% reduction in the rate of stent thrombosis (for both drug-eluting and bare-metal stents) supports the use of prasugrel after PCI.
4. there is an excess of major bleeding events in prasugrel treated patients, leading to similar net clinical benefit.

Concerning the increase in bleeding events associated to prasugrel therapy, three subgroups appeared to be particularly prone to serious bleeding: the elderly (75 years of age or older), the underweight (weigh less than 60 kg), and patients with a previous stroke or transient ischemic attack. Therefore, it would be the best to avoid prasugrel therapy in such patients. Reduce loading and maintenance dose is an alternative approach, but there is no direct evidence that efficacy would be maintained. However, it should be noticed that older patients in two subgroups at particularly high thrombotic risk (patients with diabetes and patients with a prior myocardial infarction) appeared to benefit substantially from prasugrel. Therefore, choosing a therapy requires balancing the reduction in the risk of thrombotic events against the bleeding risk.

A small number of patients underwent CABG. Among these patients, the rate of major bleeding in the prasugrel group was more than four times that in the clopidogrel group (13.4%

vs. 3.2%). Then, early prasugrel treatment without delineation of the coronary anatomy by cardiac catheterization should not be routine in patients with unstable angina/myocardial infarction without ST-segment elevation.

Finally, on July 10, 2009, after an 18-month review, the Food and Drug Administration (FDA) approved the prasugrel (60 mg loading dose followed by 10 mg daily maintenance dose) for use in patients with unstable angina or myocardial infarction who undergo PCI. The clinical efficacy of prasugrel in patients with NSTE-ACS following medical treatment will be tested in the TRILOGY-SCA trial (Targeted Platelet Inhibition to Clarify the Optimal Strategy to Medically Manage Acute Coronary Syndromes) (NCT00699998).

## Ticagrelor

Ticagrelor, previously known as AZD6140, belongs to the new chemical class cyclopentyl-triazolo-pyrimidines. Ticagrelor is an oral direct-acting P2Y12 inhibitor that changes the conformation of the P2Y12 receptor leading to a reversible inhibition of the receptor without the need for any metabolic activation. The plasma half-life is 6-13 hours and therefore the treatment is given twice daily. Ticagrelor provides faster, greater and more consistent P2Y12 inhibition than clopidogrel [88].

The safety, tolerability, and efficacy of ticagrelor plus aspirin in comparison with clopidogrel plus aspirin were initially evaluated in patients with NSTE-ACS in the DISPERSE-2 study [89] (a randomized, double-blind, double-dummy trial). No difference in major bleeding but an increase in minor bleeding occurred with ticagrelor 90 mg twice daily compared to clopidogrel 75 mg once daily.

In the PLATO trial [90] (a phase III randomized, double-blind, parallel group efficacy and safety study enrolling 18,624 patients), ticagrelor (180-mg loading dose, 90 mg twice daily thereafter) was compared to clopidogrel (300-to-600-mg loading dose, 75 mg daily thereafter) for the prevention of cardiovascular events in patients admitted to the hospital with ACS, with or without ST-segment elevation. After 12 months of follow-up, the primary end point (a composite of vascular death, myocardial infarction, or stroke) occurred in 9.8% of patients receiving ticagrelor compared with 11.7% of patients receiving clopidogrel. There was a higher incidence of TIMI major non-CABG related bleeding in patients who received ticagrelor (2.8%) compared with those treated with clopidogrel (2.2%; P=0.03). However, the incidence of TIMI major CABG related bleeding was similar in the 2 groups. Because of the rather high incidence of CABG-related bleeding in both groups (446 of 931 [47.9%] in ticagrelor-treated patients versus 476 of 968 [49.2%] in clopidogrel-treated patients), the incidence of total bleeding was not significantly different. Therefore, consistent with TRITON-TIMI 38, the PLATO trial showed that a more consistent, adequate inhibition of P2Y12-dependent platelet function is associated with greater antithrombotic efficacy and increased risk of non CABG-related major bleeding. Treatment with ticagrelor was more advantageous than treatment with clopidogrel in patients undergoing CABG; in fact, the 2 treatments were associated with similar incidences of CABG-related bleeding despite the fact that ticagrelor had been withheld for only 24 to 72 hours before surgery compared with clopidogrel, which had been withheld for 5 days. The results of the PLATO-CABG analysis have been reported in the American College of Cardiology 2010 Scientific Sessions (Atlanta, Georgia, USA). This analysis was intended to evaluate the efficacy and safety of ticagrelor in comparison with clopidogrel after CABG, in patients with last intake of study drug within seven days of surgery. There was no difference in the composite primary end point between the two study arms or in the rates of MI or stroke. Cardiovascular death was reduced by 50% in the ticagrelor arm, despite the absence of any difference in bleeding between the clopidogrel and ticagrelor arms.

Like the DISPERSE and DISPERSE-2 trials, the PLATO trial showed an increased incidence of dyspnea in ticagrelor-treated patients (13.8% versus 7.8%; P=0.001), which required discontinuation of the drug in 0.9% of patients (0.1% in the clopidogrel arm). There was a higher incidence of ventricular pauses of greater than or equal to 3 seconds in the first week in the ticagrelor group compared to clopidogrel group, without significant differences in the incidence of syncope or pacemaker implantation. The levels of creatinine and uric acid increased slightly more with ticagrelor than with clopidogrel during the treatment period.

The results of the PLATO trial were confirmed in the subgroup of patients following an invasive management. The PLATO INVASIVE substudy [91] showed that ACS patients undergoing an early invasive strategy (13408 patients -72% of the study population-) have significantly lower rates of cardiovascular death, ischemic events and stent thrombosis at 1 year follow-up with ticagrelor as compared with clopidogrel. This study also clarifies that the overall benefits of ticagrelor versus clopidogrel were identical regardless of the loading dose of clopidogrel. As previously described in the overall study population of the PLATO trial, the rate of major or minor bleeding events non-CABG-related were significantly higher in the ticagrelor group (8.9% in ticagrelor-treated patients versus 7.1% in clopidogrel-treated patients; P=0.0004), with no significant difference in the rates of total major bleeding o severe bleeding according to the GUSTO classification.

In the same way, ticagrelor was superior to clopidogrel in a subset of 8430 STEMI patients undergoing planned PCI. The results of this predefined subanalysis of PLATO were reported during a late-breaking clinical-trial session at the American Heart Association 2009 Scientific Sessions (Orland, Florida, USA) [92]. Definite stent thrombosis, myocardial infarction and all-cause mortality was significantly lower among STEMI patients taking ticagrelor compared with those receiving clopidogrel, with no significant difference in the rates of total major bleeding.

In addition, in patients with stable coronary artery disease who are already taking aspirin therapy [93], ticagrelor compared with clopidogrel, achieves more rapid and greater platelet inhibition, continued during the maintenance phase, and the offset of action is faster with ticagrelor therapy than with clopidogrel. These pharmacodynamic effects may explain why ticagrelor treatment was associated with a lower occurrence of the primary end point (myocardial infarction, stroke, or cardiovascular death), similar coronary artery bypass graft-related bleeding, and no overall difference in major bleeding compared with clopidogrel therapy in the PLATO trial.

The RESPOND study [94] enrolled 98 patients with stable coronary artery disease on aspirin therapy and has shown that ticagrelor therapy overcomes non-responsiveness to clopidogrel and high platelet reactivity during clopidogrel therapy. In addition, the antiplatelet effect of ticagrelor was essentially uniform and high in both clopidogrel responders and non-responders; there was an extremely low prevalence of high platelet reactivity associated with ticagrelor therapy and platelet inhibition was enhanced by switching to ticagrelor therapy in both patients responsive and non-responsive to clopidogrel. These data suggest that ticagrelor may be an important therapeutic alternative in patients who have experienced thrombotic events during clopidogrel therapy. The authors state that all of these findings support the particular utility of ticagrelor in clinical settings associated with high platelet reactivity, such as ACS, PCI and stent thrombosis. However, this study only enrolled patients with stable coronary artery disease, was unpowered to investigate safety end points and these results were not correlated with thrombotic events at follow-up.

In summary, ticagrelor compared to clopidogrel, has a more rapid onset, pronounced and consistent platelet inhibition, with faster offset after cessation. The adverse effects of ticagrelor may require evaluation in a much larger number of patients to establish the overall impact before drawing definitive conclusions. Given the potential adverse effects described, the use of ticagrelor should be done with caution in patients with an excessively high risk of bleeding, and should be avoided in case of chronic obstructive pulmonary disease, hyperuricemia, moderate or severe renal failure, bradyarrhythmias unprotected by pacemakers or a history of syncope.

## Cangrelor

Cangrelor, a nonthienopyridine ATP analogue, is a potent direct-acting, selective, and specific inhibitor of the ADP receptor P2Y12. Cangrelor does not require conversion to an active metabolite, therefore, is immediately active after intravenous infusion with a plasma half-life of 3 to 6 minutes, and is metabolized through dephosphorylation pathways. Platelet function normalizes within 30 to 60 minutes after discontinuation.

A large, 2-part phase II study [95] assessed the safety and pharmacodynamics of cangrelor in patients undergoing PCI. The first part of the study enrolled 200 patients undergoing PCI who were randomized to an 18- to 24-hours intravenous infusion of placebo or to 1, 2, or 4 µg/Kg-min cangrelor in addition to aspirin and heparin before the procedure. In the second part of the study, 199 patients were randomized to receive either cangrelor (4 µg/Kg-min) or the anti-glycoprotein IIb/IIIa inhibitor abciximab before the procedure. The incidence of combined major and minor bleeding was not significantly higher in cangrelor-treated patients compared with placebo- or abciximab-treated patients. Mean inhibition of platelet aggregation in response to 3 µmol/L ADP was complete in both the group of patients treated with cangrelor 4 µg/Kg-min and the group treated with abciximab. However, after termination of drug infusion, platelet aggregation returned to baseline values much faster in the cangrelor-treated group than in the abciximab-treated group. These data suggest that cangrelor may be useful during the periprocedural period in patients undergoing PCI. However, for long-term prevention, these patients should be treated with orally available agents.

Two large, phase 3, randomized clinical trials [96, 97] comparing cangrelor with clopidogrel have been made recently in order to establish the role of cangrelor in patients with acute coronary syndrome undergoing elective PCI. The major difference between the two trials was the timing of the administration of the study drugs. In the CHAMPION PCI [97] (with a double-blind, double-dummy design), cangrelor administered 30 minutes before PCI (30 µg /kg bolus followed by 4µg/Kg/min infusion and continued for 2 hours after PCI) was compared to clopidogrel administered 30 minutes before PCI (600 mg loading dose). Patients in the cangrelor group received received 600 mg clopidogrel loading after the end of the cangrelor infusion. In the CHAMPION PLATFORM [96] (double-blind, placebo controlled sudy), cangrelor was started at the beginning of PCI (30 μg /kg bolus followed by 4μg/Kg/min infusion with a minumum duration time of 2 hours, and a maximum duration time of 4 hours), whereas clopidogrel (600 mg loading dose) was not administered before the end of PCI. Patients in the cangrelor group received received 600 mg of clopidogrel after the end of the cangrelor infusion.

In the two CHAMPION trials, an interim analysis concluded that cangrelor would not show superiority for the composite primary end point and enrollment was stopped. So that, cangrelor was not superior to an oral loading dose of 600 mg of clopidogrel reducing the composite end point of death from any cause, myocardial infarction, or ischemia-driven revascularization at 48 hours. However, in the CHAMPION PLATFORM trial, in the cangrelor group, as compared with the placebo group, two prespecified secondary end points were significantly reduced at 48 hours: the rate of stent thrombosis, from 0.6% to 0.2% (odds ratio, 0.31; 95% CI, 0.11 to 0.85; $P = 0.02$), and the rate of death from any cause, from 0.7% to 0.2% (odds ratio, 0.33; 95% CI, 0.13 to 0.83; $P = 0.02$).

The most important lesson from the two CHAMPION trials is that in patients with ACS in whom the administration of an P2Y12-ADP receptor antagonist was deferred until diagnostic angiography had established the indication for PCI, intravenous cangrelor did not provide additional advantages to those achieved with 600 mg of clopidogrel. However, cangrelor is a potent intravenous P2Y12-ADP receptor inhibitor with a rapid onset and offset of action. These valuable qualities certainly warrant further studies aimed at identifying more suitable clinical scenarios for cangrelor and more appropriate approaches to its use.

## REFERENCES

[1] Ibanez B, Vilahur G, Badimon JJ. Plaque progression and regression in atherothrombosis. *J Thromb Haemost.* 2007;5 Suppl 1:292-299.

[2] Fuster V, Fayad ZA, Moreno PR, Poon M, Corti R, Badimon JJ. Atherothrombosis and high-risk plaque: Part II: approaches by noninvasive computed tomographic/magnetic resonance imaging. *J Am Coll Cardiol.* 2005;46(7):1209-1218.

[3] Cattaneo M. Resistance to antiplatelet drugs: molecular mechanisms and laboratory detection. *J Thromb Haemost.* 2007;5 Suppl 1:230-237.

[4] Gachet C. P2 receptors, platelet function and pharmacological implications. *Thromb Haemost.* 2008;99(3):466-472.

[5] Ibanez BV, G. Badimon, J. Pharmacology of thienopyridines: rationale for dual pathway inhibition. *European Heart Journal* 2006;Suppl 8:G3-G9.

[6] Mehta SR, Yusuf S, Peters RJ, Bertrand ME, Lewis BS, Natarajan MK, Malmberg K, Rupprecht H, Zhao F, Chrolavicius S, Copland I, Fox KA. Effects of pretreatment with clopidogrel and aspirin followed by long-term therapy in patients undergoing percutaneous coronary intervention: the PCI-CURE study. *Lancet.* 2001;358 (9281):527-533.

[7] Sabatine MS, Cannon CP, Gibson CM, Lopez-Sendon JL, Montalescot G, Theroux P, Lewis BS, Murphy SA, McCabe CH, Braunwald E. Effect of clopidogrel pretreatment before percutaneous coronary intervention in patients with ST-elevation myocardial

infarction treated with fibrinolytics: the PCI-CLARITY study. *JAMA.* 2005; 294(10): 1224-1232.

[8] Steinhubl SR, Berger PB, Mann JT, 3rd, Fry ET, DeLago A, Wilmer C, Topol EJ. Early and sustained dual oral antiplatelet therapy following percutaneous coronary intervention: a randomized controlled trial. *JAMA.* 2002;288 (19): 2411-2420.

[9] Yusuf S, Zhao F, Mehta SR, Chrolavicius S, Tognoni G, Fox KK. Effects of clopidogrel in addition to aspirin in patients with acute coronary syndromes without ST-segment elevation. *N Engl J Med.* 2001;345(7):494-502.

[10] Chen ZM, Jiang LX, Chen YP, Xie JX, Pan HC, Peto R, Collins R, Liu LS. Addition of clopidogrel to aspirin in 45,852 patients with acute myocardial infarction: randomised placebo-controlled trial. *Lancet.* 2005;366(9497):1607-1621.

[11] Sabatine MS, Cannon CP, Gibson CM, Lopez-Sendon JL, Montalescot G, Theroux P, Claeys MJ, Cools F, Hill KA, Skene AM, McCabe CH, Braunwald E. Addition of clopidogrel to aspirin and fibrinolytic therapy for myocardial infarction with ST-segment elevation. *N Engl J Med.* 2005; 352(12):1179-1189.

[12] Zeymer U, Gitt A, Junger C, Bauer T, Heer T, Koeth O, Mark B, Zahn R, Senges J, Gottwik M. Clopidogrel in addition to aspirin reduces in-hospital major cardiac and cerebrovascular events in unselected patients with acute ST segment elevation myocardial. *Thromb Haemost.* 2008;99(1):155-160.

[13] Bhatt DL, Fox KA, Hacke W, Berger PB, Black HR, Boden WE, Cacoub P, Cohen EA, Creager MA, Easton JD, Flather MD, Haffner SM, Hamm CW, Hankey GJ, Johnston SC, Mak KH, Mas JL, Montalescot G, Pearson TA, Steg PG, Steinhubl SR, Weber MA, Brennan DM, Fabry-Ribaudo L, Booth J, Topol EJ. Clopidogrel and aspirin versus aspirin alone for the prevention of atherothrombotic events. *N Engl J Med.* 2006;354(16):1706-1717.

[14] Lev EI, Patel RT, Maresh KJ, Guthikonda S, Granada J, DeLao T, Bray PF, Kleiman NS. Aspirin and clopidogrel drug response in patients undergoing percutaneous coronary intervention: the role of dual drug resistance. *J Am Coll Cardiol.* 2006;47(1):27-33.

[15] Gurbel PA, Bliden KP, Hayes KM, Yoho JA, Herzog WR, Tantry US. The relation of dosing to clopidogrel responsiveness and the incidence of high post-treatment platelet aggregation in patients undergoing coronary stenting. *J Am Coll Cardiol.* 2005;45(9):1392-1396.

[16] Matetzky S, Shenkman B, Guetta V, Shechter M, Bienart R, Goldenberg I, Novikov I, Pres H, Savion N, Varon D, Hod H. Clopidogrel resistance is associated with increased risk of recurrent atherothrombotic events in patients with acute myocardial infarction. *Circulation.* 2004;109(25):3171-3175.

[17] Muller I, Besta F, Schulz C, Massberg S, Schonig A, Gawaz M. Prevalence of clopidogrel non-responders among patients with stable angina pectoris scheduled for elective coronary stent placement. *Thromb Haemost.* 2003;89(5):783-787.

[18] Jaremo P, Lindahl TL, Fransson SG, Richter A. Individual variations of platelet inhibition after loading doses of clopidogrel. *J Intern Med.* 2002;252(3):233-238.

[19] Mobley JE, Bresee SJ, Wortham DC, Craft RM, Snider CC, Carroll RC. Frequency of nonresponse antiplatelet activity of clopidogrel during pretreatment for cardiac catheterization. *Am J Cardiol.* 2004;93(4):456-458.

[20] Lepantalo A, Virtanen KS, Heikkila J, Wartiovaara U, Lassila R. Limited early antiplatelet effect of 300 mg clopidogrel in patients with aspirin therapy undergoing percutaneous coronary interventions. *Eur Heart J.* 2004;25(6):476-483.

[21] Angiolillo DJ, Fernandez-Ortiz A, Bernardo E, Ramirez C, Barrera-Ramirez C, Sabate M, Hernandez R, Moreno R, Escaned J, Alfonso F, Banuelos C, Costa MA, Bass TA, Macaya C. Identification of low responders to a 300-mg clopidogrel loading dose in patients undergoing coronary stenting. *Thromb Res.* 2005;115(1-2):101-108.

[22] Dziewierz A, Dudek D, Heba G, Rakowski T, Mielecki W, Dubiel JS. Inter-individual variability in response to clopidogrel in patients with coronary artery disease. *Kardiol Pol.* 2005;62(2):108-117; discussion 118.

[23] Serebruany VL, Steinhubl SR, Berger PB, Malinin AI, Bhatt DL, Topol EJ. Variability in platelet responsiveness to clopidogrel among 544 individuals. *J Am Coll Cardiol.* 2005;45(2):246-251.

[24] Hochholzer W, Trenk D, Bestehorn HP, Fischer B, Valina CM, Ferenc M, Gick M, Caputo A, Buttner HJ, Neumann FJ. Impact of the degree of peri-interventional platelet inhibition after loading with clopidogrel on early clinical outcome of elective coronary stent placement. *J Am Coll Cardiol.* 2006;48(9):1742-1750.

[25] Cuisset T, Frere C, Quilici J, Morange PE, Nait-Saidi L, Carvajal J, Lehmann A, Lambert M, Bonnet JL, Alessi MC. Benefit of a 600-mg loading dose of clopidogrel on platelet reactivity and clinical outcomes in patients with non-ST-segment elevation acute coronary syndrome undergoing coronary stenting. *J Am Coll Cardiol.* 2006;48(7):1339-1345.

[26] Campo G, Valgimigli M, Gemmati D, Percoco G, Tognazzo S, Cicchitelli G, Catozzi L, Malagutti P, Anselmi M, Vassanelli C, Scapoli G, Ferrari R. Value of platelet reactivity in predicting response to treatment and clinical outcome in patients undergoing primary coronary intervention: insights into the STRATEGY Study. *J Am Coll Cardiol.* 2006;48(11):2178-2185.

[27] Gurbel PA, Bliden KP, Guyer K, Cho PW, Zaman KA, Kreutz RP, Bassi AK, Tantry US. Platelet reactivity in patients and recurrent events post-stenting: results of the PREPARE POST-STENTING Study. *J Am Coll Cardiol.* 2005;46(10):1820-1826.

[28] Samara WM, Bliden KP, Tantry US, Gurbel PA. The difference between clopidogrel responsiveness and posttreatment platelet reactivity. *Thromb Res.* 2005;115(1-2):89-94.

[29] Bliden KP, DiChiara J, Tantry US, Bassi AK, Chaganti SK, Gurbel PA. Increased risk in patients with high platelet aggregation receiving chronic clopidogrel therapy undergoing percutaneous coronary intervention: is the current antiplatelet therapy adequate? *J Am Coll Cardiol.* 2007;49(6):657-666.

[30] de Miguel Castro A, Cuellas Ramon C, Diego Nieto A, Samaniego Lampon B, Alonso Rodriguez D, Fernandez Vazquez F, Alonso Orcajo N, Carbonell de Blas R, Pascual Vicente C, Perez de Prado A. Post-treatment platelet reactivity predicts long-term adverse events better than the response to clopidogrel in patients with non-ST-segment elevation acute coronary syndrome. *Rev Esp Cardiol.* 2009;62(2):126-135.

[31] Hovens MM, Snoep JD, Eikenboom JC, van der Bom JG, Mertens BJ, Huisman MV. Prevalence of persistent platelet reactivity despite use of aspirin: a systematic review. *Am Heart J.* 2007;153(2):175-181.

[32] King SB, 3rd, Smith SC, Jr., Hirshfeld JW, Jr., Jacobs AK, Morrison DA, Williams DO, Feldman TE, Kern MJ, O'Neill WW, Schaff HV, Whitlow PL, Adams CD, Anderson JL, Buller CE, Creager MA, Ettinger SM, Halperin JL, Hunt SA, Krumholz HM, Kushner FG, Lytle BW, Nishimura R, Page RL, Riegel B, Tarkington LG, Yancy CW. 2007 focused update of the ACC/AHA/SCAI 2005 guideline update for percutaneous coronary intervention: a report of the American College of Cardiology/American Heart Association Task Force on Practice guidelines. *J Am Coll Cardiol.* 2008;51(2):172-209.

[33] Anderson JL, Adams CD, Antman EM, Bridges CR, Califf RM, Casey DE, Jr., Chavey WE, 2nd, Fesmire FM, Hochman JS, Levin TN, Lincoff AM, Peterson ED, Theroux P, Wenger NK, Wright RS, Smith SC, Jr., Jacobs AK, Halperin JL, Hunt SA, Krumholz HM, Kushner FG, Lytle BW, Nishimura R, Ornato JP, Page RL, Riegel B. ACC/AHA 2007 guidelines for the management of patients with unstable angina/non-ST-Elevation myocardial infarction: a report of the American College of Cardiology/American Heart Association Task Force on Practice Guidelines (Writing Committee to Revise the 2002 Guidelines for the Management of Patients With Unstable Angina/Non-ST-Elevation Myocardial Infarction) developed in collaboration with the American College of Emergency Physicians, the Society for Cardiovascular Angiography and Interventions, and the Society of Thoracic Surgeons endorsed by the American Association of Cardiovascular and Pulmonary Rehabilitation and the Society for Academic Emergency Medicine. *J Am Coll Cardiol.* 2007;50(7):e1-e157.

[34] Bassand JP, Hamm CW, Ardissino D, Boersma E, Budaj A, Fernandez-Aviles F, Fox KA, Hasdai D, Ohman EM, Wallentin L, Wijns W. Guidelines for the diagnosis and treatment of non-ST-segment elevation acute coronary syndromes. *Eur Heart J.* 2007;28(13):1598-1660.

[35] Simoons ML. Effect of glycoprotein IIb/IIIa receptor blocker abciximab on outcome in patients with acute coronary syndromes without early coronary revascularisation: the GUSTO IV-ACS randomised trial. *Lancet.* 2001;357(9272):1915-1924.

[36] Topol EJ. Reperfusion therapy for acute myocardial infarction with fibrinolytic therapy or combination reduced fibrinolytic therapy and platelet glycoprotein IIb/IIIa inhibition: the GUSTO V randomised trial. *Lancet.* 2001;357(9272):1905-1914.

[37] Brandt JT, Close SL, Iturria SJ, Payne CD, Farid NA, Ernest CS, 2nd, Lachno DR, Salazar D, Winters KJ. Common polymorphisms of CYP2C19 and CYP2C9 affect the pharmacokinetic and pharmacodynamic response to clopidogrel but not prasugrel. *J Thromb Haemost.* 2007;5(12):2429-2436.

[38] Trenk D, Hochholzer W, Fromm MF, Chialda LE, Pahl A, Valina CM, Stratz C, Schmiebusch P, Bestehorn HP, Buttner HJ, Neumann FJ. Cytochrome P450 2C19 681G>A polymorphism and high on-clopidogrel platelet reactivity associated with adverse 1-year clinical outcome of elective percutaneous coronary intervention with drug-eluting or bare-metal stents. *J Am Coll Cardiol.* 2008;51(20):1925-1934.

[39] Mega JL, Close SL, Wiviott SD, Shen L, Hockett RD, Brandt JT, Walker JR, Antman EM, Macias W, Braunwald E, Sabatine MS. Cytochrome p-450 polymorphisms and response to clopidogrel. *N Engl J Med.* 2009;360(4):354-362.

[40] Lau WC, Waskell LA, Watkins PB, Neer CJ, Horowitz K, Hopp AS, Tait AR, Carville DG, Guyer KE, Bates ER. Atorvastatin reduces the ability of clopidogrel to inhibit platelet aggregation: a new drug-drug interaction. *Circulation.* 2003;107(1):32-37.

[41] Neubauer H, Gunesdogan B, Hanefeld C, Spiecker M, Mugge A. Lipophilic statins interfere with the inhibitory effects of clopidogrel on platelet function--a flow cytometry study. *Eur Heart J.* 2003;24(19):1744-1749.

[42] Mitsios JV, Papathanasiou AI, Rodis FI, Elisaf M, Goudevenos JA, Tselepis AD. Atorvastatin does not affect the antiplatelet potency of clopidogrel when it is administered concomitantly for 5 weeks in patients with acute coronary syndromes. *Circulation.* 2004;109(11):1335-1338.

[43] Gorchakova O, von Beckerath N, Gawaz M, Mocz A, Joost A, Schomig A, Kastrati A. Antiplatelet effects of a 600 mg loading dose of clopidogrel are not attenuated in patients receiving atorvastatin or simvastatin for at least 4 weeks prior to coronary artery stenting. *Eur Heart J.* 2004;25(21):1898-1902.

[44] Bhatt DL, Scheiman J, Abraham NS, Antman EM, Chan FK, Furberg CD, Johnson DA, Mahaffey KW, Quigley EM, Harrington RA, Bates ER, Bridges CR, Eisenberg MJ, Ferrari VA, Hlatky MA, Kaul S, Lindner JR, Moliterno DJ, Mukherjee D, Schofield RS, Rosenson RS, Stein JH, Weitz HH, Wesley DJ. ACCF/ACG/AHA 2008 expert consensus document on reducing the gastrointestinal risks of antiplatelet therapy and NSAID use. *Am J Gastroenterol.* 2008;103(11):2890-2907.

[45] Gilard M, Arnaud B, Cornily JC, Le Gal G, Lacut K, Le Calvez G, Mansourati J, Mottier D, Abgrall JF, Boschat J. Influence of omeprazole on the antiplatelet action of clopidogrel associated with aspirin: the randomized, double-blind OCLA (Omeprazole CLopidogrel Aspirin) study. *J Am Coll Cardiol.* 2008;51(3):256-260.

[46] Sibbing D, Morath T, Stegherr J, Braun S, Vogt W, Hadamitzky M, Schomig A, Kastrati A, von Beckerath N. Impact of proton pump inhibitors on the antiplatelet effects of clopidogrel. *Thromb Haemost.* 2009;101(4):714-719.

[47] Cuisset T, Frere C, Quilici J, Poyet R, Gaborit B, Bali L, Brissy O, Morange PE, Alessi MC, Bonnet JL. Comparison of omeprazole and pantoprazole influence on a high 150-mg clopidogrel maintenance dose the PACA (Proton Pump Inhibitors And Clopidogrel Association) prospective randomized study. *J Am Coll Cardiol.* 2009;54(13):1149-1153.

[48] Gaglia MA, Jr., Torguson R, Hanna N, Gonzalez MA, Collins SD, Syed AI, Ben-Dor I, Maluenda G, Delhaye C, Wakabayashi K, Xue Z, Suddath WO, Kent KM, Satler LF, Pichard AD, Waksman R. Relation of proton pump inhibitor use after percutaneous coronary intervention with drug-eluting stents to outcomes. *Am J Cardiol.*105(6):833-838.

[49] Ho PM, Maddox TM, Wang L, Fihn SD, Jesse RL, Peterson ED, Rumsfeld JS. Risk of adverse outcomes associated with concomitant use of clopidogrel and proton pump inhibitors following acute coronary syndrome. *JAMA.* 2009;301(9):937-944.

[50] Siller-Matula JM, Lang I, Christ G, Jilma B. Calcium-channel blockers reduce the antiplatelet effect of clopidogrel. *J Am Coll Cardiol.* 2008;52(19):1557-1563.

[51] Gremmel T, Steiner S, Seidinger D, Koppensteiner R, Panzer S, Kopp CW. Calcium-channel blockers decrease clopidogrel-mediated platelet inhibition. *Heart.*96(3):186-189.

[52] Michelson AD, Frelinger AL, 3rd, Furman MI. Current options in platelet function testing. *Am J Cardiol.* 2006;98(10A):4N-10N.

[53] Geisler T, Langer H, Wydymus M, Gohring K, Zurn C, Bigalke B, Stellos K, May AE, Gawaz M. Low response to clopidogrel is associated with cardiovascular outcome after coronary stent implantation. *Eur Heart J.* 2006;27(20):2420-2425.

[54] Breet NJ, van Werkum JW, Bouman HJ, Kelder JC, Ruven HJ, Bal ET, Deneer VH, Harmsze AM, van der Heyden JA, Rensing BJ, Suttorp MJ, Hackeng CM, ten Berg JM. Comparison of platelet function tests in predicting clinical outcome in patients undergoing coronary stent implantation. *JAMA*.303(8):754-762.

[55] Cuisset T, Frere C, Quilici J, Morange PE, Nait-Saidi L, Mielot C, Bali L, Lambert M, Alessi MC, Bonnet JL. High post-treatment platelet reactivity is associated with a high incidence of myonecrosis after stenting for non-ST elevation acute coronary syndromes. *Thromb Haemost.* 2007;97(2):282-287.

[56] Perez de Prado A, Cuellas C, Diego A, de Miguel A, Samaniego B, Alonso-Orcajo N, Carbonell R, Pascual C, Fernandez-Vazquez F, Calabozo RG. Influence of platelet reactivity and response to clopidogrel on myocardial damage following percutaneous coronary intervention in patients with non-ST-segment elevation acute coronary syndrome. *Thromb Res.* 2009;124(6):678-682.

[57] Marcucci R, Paniccia R, Antonucci E, Poli S, Gori AM, Valente S, Giglioli C, Lazzeri C, Prisco D, Abbate R, Gensini GF. Residual platelet reactivity is an independent predictor of myocardial injury in acute myocardial infarction patients on antiaggregant therapy. *Thromb Haemost.* 2007;98(4):844-851.

[58] Gurbel PA, Bliden KP, Samara W, Yoho JA, Hayes K, Fissha MZ, Tantry US. Clopidogrel effect on platelet reactivity in patients with stent thrombosis: results of the CREST Study. *J Am Coll Cardiol.* 2005;46(10):1827-1832.

[59] Stone GW, Moses JW, Ellis SG, Schofer J, Dawkins KD, Morice MC, Colombo A, Schampaert E, Grube E, Kirtane AJ, Cutlip DE, Fahy M, Pocock SJ, Mehran R, Leon MB. Safety and efficacy of sirolimus- and paclitaxel-eluting coronary stents. *N Engl J Med.* 2007;356(10):998-1008.

[60] Lagerqvist B, James SK, Stenestrand U, Lindback J, Nilsson T, Wallentin L. Long-term outcomes with drug-eluting stents versus bare-metal stents in Sweden. *N Engl J Med.* 2007;356(10):1009-1019.

[61] Iakovou I, Schmidt T, Bonizzoni E, Ge L, Sangiorgi GM, Stankovic G, Airoldi F, Chieffo A, Montorfano M, Carlino M, Michev I, Corvaja N, Briguori C, Gerckens U, Grube E, Colombo A. Incidence, predictors, and outcome of thrombosis after successful implantation of drug-eluting stents. *JAMA.* 2005;293(17):2126-2130.

[62] van Werkum JW, Heestermans AA, Zomer AC, Kelder JC, Suttorp MJ, Rensing BJ, Koolen JJ, Brueren BR, Dambrink JH, Hautvast RW, Verheugt FW, ten Berg JM. Predictors of coronary stent thrombosis: the Dutch Stent Thrombosis Registry. *J Am Coll Cardiol.* 2009;53(16):1399-1409.

[63] Buonamici P, Marcucci R, Migliorini A, Gensini GF, Santini A, Paniccia R, Moschi G, Gori AM, Abbate R, Antoniucci D. Impact of platelet reactivity after clopidogrel administration on drug-eluting stent thrombosis. *J Am Coll Cardiol.* 2007;49(24):2312-2317.

[64] Sibbing D, Braun S, Morath T, Mehilli J, Vogt W, Schomig A, Kastrati A, von Beckerath N. Platelet reactivity after clopidogrel treatment assessed with point-of-care analysis and early drug-eluting stent thrombosis. *J Am Coll Cardiol.* 2009;53(10):849-856.

[65] Gori AM, Marcucci R, Migliorini A, Valenti R, Moschi G, Paniccia R, Buonamici P, Gensini GF, Vergara R, Abbate R, Antoniucci D. Incidence and clinical impact of dual nonresponsiveness to aspirin and clopidogrel in patients with drug-eluting stents. *J Am Coll Cardiol.* 2008;52(9):734-739.

[66] Geisler T, Zurn C, Simonenko R, Rapin M, Kraibooj H, Kilias A, Bigalke B, Stellos K, Schwab M, May AE, Herdeg C, Gawaz M. Early but not late stent thrombosis is influenced by residual platelet aggregation in patients undergoing coronary interventions. *Eur Heart J.*31(1):59-66.

[67] Sibbing D, Morath T, Braun S, Stegherr J, Mehilli J, Vogt W, Schomig A, Kastrati A, von Beckerath N. Clopidogrel response status assessed with Multiplate point-of-care analysis and the incidence and timing of stent thrombosis over six months following coronary stenting. *Thromb Haemost.*103(1):151-159.

[68] Grines CL, Bonow RO, Casey DE, Jr., Gardner TJ, Lockhart PB, Moliterno DJ, O'Gara P, Whitlow P. Prevention of premature discontinuation of dual antiplatelet therapy in patients with coronary artery stents: a science advisory from the American Heart Association, American College of Cardiology, Society for Cardiovascular Angiography and Interventions, American College of Surgeons, and American Dental Association, with representation from the American College of Physicians. *Circulation.* 2007;115(6):813-818.

[69] Park SJ, Park DW, Kim YH, Kang SJ, Lee SW, Lee CW, Han KH, Park SW, Yun SC, Lee SG, Rha SW, Seong IW, Jeong MH, Hur SH, Lee NH, Yoon J, Yang JY, Lee BK, Choi YJ, Chung WS, Lim DS, Cheong SS, Kim KS, Chae JK, Nah DY, Jeon DS, Seung KB, Jang JS, Park HS, Lee K. Duration of Dual Antiplatelet Therapy after Implantation of Drug-Eluting Stents. *N Engl J Med.*

[70] Muller I, Seyfarth M, Rudiger S, Wolf B, Pogatsa-Murray G, Schomig A, Gawaz M. Effect of a high loading dose of clopidogrel on platelet function in patients undergoing coronary stent placement. *Heart.* 2001;85(1):92-93.

[71] Kandzari DE, Berger PB, Kastrati A, Steinhubl SR, Mehilli J, Dotzer F, Ten Berg JM, Neumann FJ, Bollwein H, Dirschinger J, Schomig A. Influence of treatment duration with a 600-mg dose of clopidogrel before percutaneous coronary revascularization. *J Am Coll Cardiol.* 2004;44(11):2133-2136.

[72] Patti G, Colonna G, Pasceri V, Pepe LL, Montinaro A, Di Sciascio G. Randomized trial of high loading dose of clopidogrel for reduction of periprocedural myocardial infarction in patients undergoing coronary intervention: results from the ARMYDA-2 (Antiplatelet therapy for Reduction of MYocardial Damage during Angioplasty) study. *Circulation.* 2005;111(16):2099-2106.

[73] von Beckerath N, Taubert D, Pogatsa-Murray G, Schomig E, Kastrati A, Schomig A. Absorption, metabolization, and antiplatelet effects of 300-, 600-, and 900-mg loading doses of clopidogrel: results of the ISAR-CHOICE (Intracoronary Stenting and Antithrombotic Regimen: Choose Between 3 High Oral Doses for Immediate Clopidogrel Effect) Trial. *Circulation.* 2005;112(19):2946-2950.

[74] Montalescot G, Sideris G, Meuleman C, Bal-dit-Sollier C, Lellouche N, Steg PG, Slama M, Milleron O, Collet JP, Henry P, Beygui F, Drouet L. A randomized comparison of high clopidogrel loading doses in patients with non-ST-segment elevation acute coronary syndromes: the ALBION (Assessment of the Best Loading

Dose of Clopidogrel to Blunt Platelet Activation, Inflammation and Ongoing Necrosis) trial. *J Am Coll Cardiol.* 2006;48(5):931-938.

[75] Van de Werf F, Bax J, Betriu A, Blomstrom-Lundqvist C, Crea F, Falk V, Filippatos G, Fox K, Huber K, Kastrati A, Rosengren A, Steg PG, Tubaro M, Verheugt F, Weidinger F, Weis M, Vahanian A, Camm J, De Caterina R, Dean V, Dickstein K, Funck-Brentano C, Hellemans I, Kristensen SD, McGregor K, Sechtem U, Silber S, Tendera M, Widimsky P, Zamorano JL, Aguirre FV, Al-Attar N, Alegria E, Andreotti F, Benzer W, Breithardt O, Danchin N, Di Mario C, Dudek D, Gulba D, Halvorsen S, Kaufmann P, Kornowski R, Lip GY, Rutten F. Management of acute myocardial infarction in patients presenting with persistent ST-segment elevation: the Task Force on the Management of ST-Segment Elevation Acute Myocardial Infarction of the European Society of Cardiology. *Eur Heart J.* 2008;29(23):2909-2945.

[76] Kushner FG, Hand M, Smith SC, Jr., King SB, 3rd, Anderson JL, Antman EM, Bailey SR, Bates ER, Blankenship JC, Casey DE, Jr., Green LA, Hochman JS, Jacobs AK, Krumholz HM, Morrison DA, Ornato JP, Pearle DL, Peterson ED, Sloan MA, Whitlow PL, Williams DO. 2009 Focused Updates: ACC/AHA Guidelines for the Management of Patients With ST-Elevation Myocardial Infarction (updating the 2004 Guideline and 2007 Focused Update) and ACC/AHA/SCAI Guidelines on Percutaneous Coronary Intervention (updating the 2005 Guideline and 2007 Focused Update): a report of the American College of Cardiology Foundation/American Heart Association Task Force on Practice Guidelines. *Circulation.* 2009;120(22):2271-2306.

[77] Angiolillo DJ, Shoemaker SB, Desai B, Yuan H, Charlton RK, Bernardo E, Zenni MM, Guzman LA, Bass TA, Costa MA. Randomized comparison of a high clopidogrel maintenance dose in patients with diabetes mellitus and coronary artery disease: results of the Optimizing Antiplatelet Therapy in Diabetes Mellitus (OPTIMUS) study. *Circulation.* 2007;115(6):708-716.

[78] von Beckerath N, Kastrati A, Wieczorek A, Pogatsa-Murray G, Sibbing D, Graf I, Schomig A. A double-blind, randomized study on platelet aggregation in patients treated with a daily dose of 150 or 75 mg of clopidogrel for 30 days. *Eur Heart J.* 2007;28(15):1814-1819.

[79] Neubauer H, Lask S, Engelhardt A, Mugge A. How to optimise clopidogrel therapy? Reducing the low-response incidence by aggregometry-guided therapy modification. *Thromb Haemost.* 2008;99(2):357-362.

[80] Bonello L, Camoin-Jau L, Arques S, Boyer C, Panagides D, Wittenberg O, Simeoni MC, Barragan P, Dignat-George F, Paganelli F. Adjusted clopidogrel loading doses according to vasodilator-stimulated phosphoprotein phosphorylation index decrease rate of major adverse cardiovascular events in patients with clopidogrel resistance: a multicenter randomized prospective study. *J Am Coll Cardiol.* 2008;51(14):1404-1411.

[81] Marcucci R, Gori AM, Paniccia R, Giusti B, Valente S, Giglioli C, Buonamici P, Antoniucci D, Abbate R, Gensini GF. Cardiovascular death and nonfatal myocardial infarction in acute coronary syndrome patients receiving coronary stenting are predicted by residual platelet reactivity to ADP detected by a point-of-care assay: a 12-month follow-up. *Circulation.* 2009;119(2):237-242.

[82] Price MJ, Endemann S, Gollapudi RR, Valencia R, Stinis CT, Levisay JP, Ernst A, Sawhney NS, Schatz RA, Teirstein PS. Prognostic significance of post-clopidogrel

platelet reactivity assessed by a point-of-care assay on thrombotic events after drug-eluting stent implantation. *Eur Heart J.* 2008;29(8):992-1000.

[83] Kuliczkowski W, Witkowski A, Polonski L, Watala C, Filipiak K, Budaj A, Golanski J, Sitkiewicz D, Pregowski J, Gorski J, Zembala M, Opolski G, Huber K, Arnesen H, Kristensen SD, De Caterina R. Interindividual variability in the response to oral antiplatelet drugs: a position paper of the Working Group on antiplatelet drugs resistance appointed by the Section of Cardiovascular Interventions of the Polish Cardiac Society, endorsed by the Working Group on Thrombosis of the European Society of Cardiology. *Eur Heart J.* 2009;30(4):426-435.

[84] Wallentin L, Varenhorst C, James S, Erlinge D, Braun OO, Jakubowski JA, Sugidachi A, Winters KJ, Siegbahn A. Prasugrel achieves greater and faster P2Y12receptor-mediated platelet inhibition than clopidogrel due to more efficient generation of its active metabolite in aspirin-treated patients with coronary artery disease. *Eur Heart J.* 2008;29(1):21-30.

[85] Wiviott SD, Trenk D, Frelinger AL, O'Donoghue M, Neumann FJ, Michelson AD, Angiolillo DJ, Hod H, Montalescot G, Miller DL, Jakubowski JA, Cairns R, Murphy SA, McCabe CH, Antman EM, Braunwald E. Prasugrel compared with high loading- and maintenance-dose clopidogrel in patients with planned percutaneous coronary intervention: the Prasugrel in Comparison to Clopidogrel for Inhibition of Platelet Activation and Aggregation-Thrombolysis in Myocardial Infarction 44 trial. *Circulation.* 2007;116(25):2923-2932.

[86] Wiviott SD, Braunwald E, McCabe CH, Montalescot G, Ruzyllo W, Gottlieb S, Neumann FJ, Ardissino D, De Servi S, Murphy SA, Riesmeyer J, Weerakkody G, Gibson CM, Antman EM. Prasugrel versus clopidogrel in patients with acute coronary syndromes. *N Engl J Med.* 2007;357(20):2001-2015.

[87] Wiviott SD, Braunwald E, Angiolillo DJ, Meisel S, Dalby AJ, Verheugt FW, Goodman SG, Corbalan R, Purdy DA, Murphy SA, McCabe CH, Antman EM. Greater clinical benefit of more intensive oral antiplatelet therapy with prasugrel in patients with diabetes mellitus in the trial to assess improvement in therapeutic outcomes by optimizing platelet inhibition with prasugrel-Thrombolysis in Myocardial Infarction 38. *Circulation.* 2008;118(16):1626-1636.

[88] Husted S, Emanuelsson H, Heptinstall S, Sandset PM, Wickens M, Peters G. Pharmacodynamics, pharmacokinetics, and safety of the oral reversible P2Y12 antagonist AZD6140 with aspirin in patients with atherosclerosis: a double-blind comparison to clopidogrel with aspirin. *Eur Heart J.* 2006;27(9):1038-1047.

[89] Cannon CP, Husted S, Harrington RA, Scirica BM, Emanuelsson H, Peters G, Storey RF. Safety, tolerability, and initial efficacy of AZD6140, the first reversible oral adenosine diphosphate receptor antagonist, compared with clopidogrel, in patients with non-ST-segment elevation acute coronary syndrome: primary results of the DISPERSE-2 trial. *J Am Coll Cardiol.* 2007;50(19):1844-1851.

[90] Wallentin L, Becker RC, Budaj A, Cannon CP, Emanuelsson H, Held C, Horrow J, Husted S, James S, Katus H, Mahaffey KW, Scirica BM, Skene A, Steg PG, Storey RF, Harrington RA, Freij A, Thorsen M. Ticagrelor versus clopidogrel in patients with acute coronary syndromes. *N Engl J Med.* 2009;361(11):1045-1057.

[91] Cannon CP, Harrington RA, James S, Ardissino D, Becker RC, Emanuelsson H, Husted S, Katus H, Keltai M, Khurmi NS, Kontny F, Lewis BS, Steg PG, Storey RF, Wojdyla

D, Wallentin L. Comparison of ticagrelor with clopidogrel in patients with a planned invasive strategy for acute coronary syndromes (PLATO): a randomised double-blind study. *Lancet.*375(9711):283-293.

[92] Steg PG. STEMI subanalysis of the PLATO trial. Paper presented at: American Heart Association 2009 Scientific Sessions November 15th 2009, 2010; Orland, Florida, USA.

[93] Gurbel PA, Bliden KP, Butler K, Tantry US, Gesheff T, Wei C, Teng R, Antonino MJ, Patil SB, Karunakaran A, Kereiakes DJ, Parris C, Purdy D, Wilson V, Ledley GS, Storey RF. Randomized double-blind assessment of the ONSET and OFFSET of the antiplatelet effects of ticagrelor versus clopidogrel in patients with stable coronary artery disease: the ONSET/OFFSET study. *Circulation.* 2009;120(25):2577-2585.

[94] Gurbel PA, Bliden KP, Butler K, Antonino MJ, Wei C, Teng R, Rasmussen L, Storey RF, Nielsen T, Eikelboom JW, Sabe-Affaki G, Husted S, Kereiakes DJ, Henderson D, Patel DV, Tantry US. Response to Ticagrelor in Clopidogrel Nonresponders and Responders and Effect of Switching Therapies: The RESPOND Study. *Circulation.*121(10):1188-1199.

[95] Greenbaum AB, Grines CL, Bittl JA, Becker RC, Kereiakes DJ, Gilchrist IC, Clegg J, Stankowski JE, Grogan DR, Harrington RA, Emanuelsson H, Weaver WD. Initial experience with an intravenous P2Y12 platelet receptor antagonist in patients undergoing percutaneous coronary intervention: results from a 2-part, phase II, multicenter, randomized, placebo- and active-controlled trial. *Am Heart J.* 2006;151(3):689 e681-689 e610.

[96] Bhatt DL, Lincoff AM, Gibson CM, Stone GW, McNulty S, Montalescot G, Kleiman NS, Goodman SG, White HD, Mahaffey KW, Pollack CV, Jr., Manoukian SV, Widimsky P, Chew DP, Cura F, Manukov I, Tousek F, Jafar MZ, Arneja J, Skerjanec S, Harrington RA. Intravenous platelet blockade with cangrelor during PCI. *N Engl J Med.* 2009;361(24):2330-2341.

[97] Harrington RA, Stone GW, McNulty S, White HD, Lincoff AM, Gibson CM, Pollack CV, Jr., Montalescot G, Mahaffey KW, Kleiman NS, Goodman SG, Amine M, Angiolillo DJ, Becker RC, Chew DP, French WJ, Leisch F, Parikh KH, Skerjanec S, Bhatt DL. Platelet inhibition with cangrelor in patients undergoing PCI. *N Engl J Med.* 2009;361(24):2318-2329.

*Chapter II*

# PROTEOMICS OF ACUTE CORONARY SYNDROME

*Gloria Alvarez-Llamas[a], Fernando de la Cuesta[a], Felix Gil-Dones[b], Irene Zubiri[a], Maria Posada[a], Maria G. Barderas[b] and Fernando Vivanco*[*a,c]

[a]Department of Immunology, Fundación Jimenez Diaz, Madrid.
[b]Department of Vascular Physiopathology,
Hospital Nacional de Parapléjicos (HNP), SESCAM, Toledo.
[c]Department of Biochemistry and Molecular Biology,
Universidad Complutense, Madrid.

## 1. INTRODUCTION

Atherosclerosis is a chronic inflammatory disease of the vascular system. It is a complex multifactorial disease characterized by the accumulation of inflammatory cells (macrophages, lymphocytes), lipoproteins and fibrous tissue in the wall of large arteries. This results in the development of necrotic/lipidic cores within the intima of arteries at particular site in the circulation. These lesions form in the settings of a pre-existing intimal hyperplasia characterized by the proliferation of VSMC within the intima. In advanced lesions, necrosis of macrophages and VSMC results in a lipid-rich core covered by a fibrous cap, which protects the lesions from rupture and consists mainly of collagen and extracellular matrix (ECM) proteins, synthesized by vascular cells. Plaque rupture, resulting from inflammatory activation and MMPs secretion, and the ensuing thrombosis commonly causes the most acute complications of atherosclerosis such as unstable angina or myocardial infarction (acute coronary syndrome) or stroke [1].

---

* Author for correspondence:Dr. Fernando Vivanco. Department of Immunology, Fundación Jiménez Diaz, Avda Reyes Catolicos 2, 28040-Madrid, Spain, E-mail: fvivanco@fjd.es, Tf: +34915498446

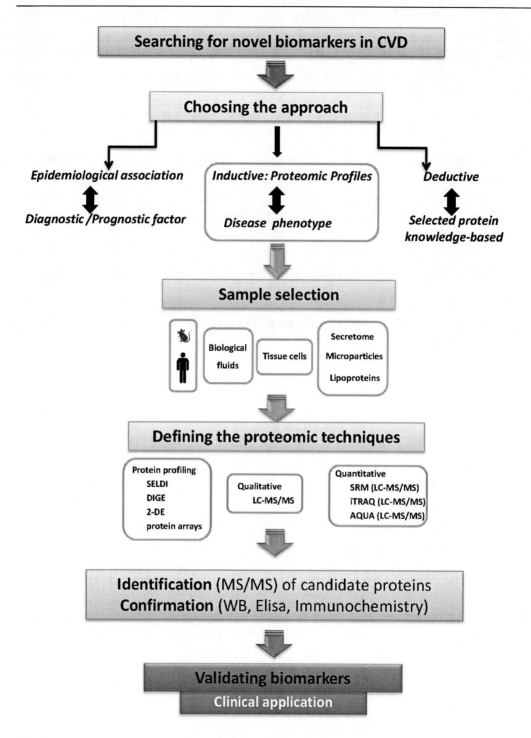

Figure 1. Different alternatives that must be chosen in the search for novel biomarkers in CVD. In a proteomic approach, an inductive strategy (unbiased) is selected and applied to different types of samples using several techniques. If the identification process is successful, a confirmatory step by an independent technique is mandatory. A final validation step must be performed before using the novel biomarker in clinical practice.

## 2. PLASMA

Atherosclerosis is the principal cause of heart disease and a leading cause of stroke, making it the most common cause of death in developed countries. Proteomics is seeking to fully understand the biochemical processes mediated by proteins in atherosclerosis in dealing with the clinical consequences of this prevalent disease and in order to personalize its diagnostic treatment. Classical studies of individual components (gene, protein, and metabolite) are necessary to establish the function of such components, but they are not sufficient to explain complex processes such as atherotrombosis. It is necessary a more global analysis in which the activities of all relevant proteins are integrated and thus could provide a complete view of how they function together. These global approaches, named systems biology, enable the identification of networks of proteins associated with cardiovascular diseases (CVD) in general and with atherosclerosis in particular[2, 3]. The ultimate clinical presentation of CVD results from the interaction of multiple cell types (macrophages, endothelial cells, VSMC, lymphocytes) and organ systems (vascular, endocrine, adipose, liver, kidney, gastrointestinal) in which a myriad of interconnected proteins are expressed. Thus, systems-based approaches are very well suited for elucidating the high-order interactions underlying the process of atherosclerosis and providing a framework for the identification of potential biomarkers[4], novel drugs and personalized treatments[5].

This chapter describes how proteomics is discovering an increasing number of novel proteins and pathways of activation involved in atherotrombosis and how many of them are considered as potential protein candidates with clinical applications as biomarkers in the near future. When approaching a comprehensive biomarker research, several decisions must be adopted beforehand. Such choices may be crucial to the final results (Figure 1). All these data are an essential element to be used by systems biology capable of integrating them into a holistic view of atherosclerosis.

From a viewpoint of clinical application, biological fluids are the most accessible source for the discovery of novel biomarkers. For this reason, proteomic studies in atherosclerosis have traditionally focused on plasma or serum (alternatively in urine), while other proteomic approaches represent a smaller portion of current atherosclerosis research (i.e., tissue proteomics; section 4). Proteins in the plasma are easily accessible and can serve as a surrogate measure of the presence of atherosclerotic disease and its progression. Biomarkers found in the plasma/serum have the great advantage of low-invasive quantification for diagnosis because factors released from lesions areas can accumulate in the general circulation (i.e., initial development of atherome plaque or advanced progress prior to rupture). However, we currently have a total of 205 plasma proteins with utility in the clinical laboratory, which are measured by immunoassays. These assays provide a view of the current clinical plasma proteome, which correspond to about 1% of the estimated total proteome [6]. The most successful test introduced in the last 15 years encompasses 8 immunoassays, from which 3 are from the cardiovascular area (in italics): *Cardiac TnI*, *Lpa*, cancer antigen 15-3, pancreatic amylase, Cystatin C, *NT-proBNP/BNP*, soluble transferrin receptor (sTfR)[7]. Traditional, clinical validation of biomarkers has relied primarily on immunoassays because of their specificity and sensitivity. However, new methods are emerging based on MS to quantify clinically relevant proteins in patient's plasma. Multiple reactions monitoring (MRM) coupled with stable isotope dilution has recently been shown as a quantitative, multiplexed assays for six plasma proteins of clinical relevance to cardiac injury[8]. Although there are several protein candidates in clinical trials, proteomics has not produced to date new biomarkers. Only the recent FDA approval of the use of SELDI-TOF for ovarian cancer [9] is an exception.

The analysis of plasma proteome in the search of novel biomarkers is challenging owing to the protein complexity of plasma, the high dynamic range of protein concentrations (encompassing more than 10 orders of magnitude) and the difficulty of detecting low abundance proteins in the presence of the most abundant ones (a handful of proteins represent more than 95% of total plasma proteins)[10]. The HUPO Plasma Proteome Project identified a total of 3020 proteins in human plasma and a subset of 345 proteins was associated for their relevance to cardiovascular function and diseases[11]. Since then many new proteins have been described in the plasma of patient with cardiovascular diseases. Figure 2 and Table 1 summarize recent novel potential biomarkers measured in plasma and their association with several pathologies. The most representative studies related to ACS and stroke, are described below.

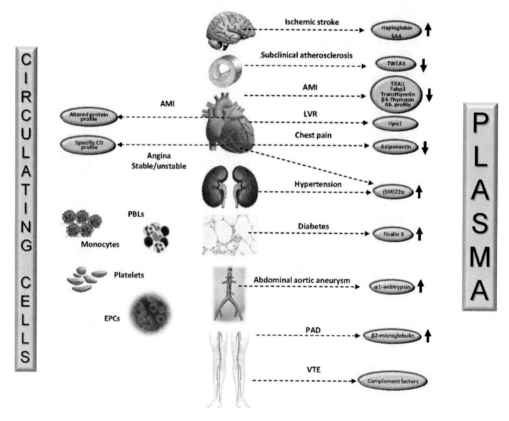

Figure 2. Recent potential novel biomarkers that are associated with different cardiovascular pathologies and have been evaluated in plasma and circulating cells. Altered plasma levels in patients versus controls are shown (↑↓). The proteomic techniques used to detect the proteins are also included (right and left margins).

**Table 1.** Compilation of proteomic studies reported to date in the field of vascular diseases. The most relevant proteins identified in the different pathologies and the sample sources are described.

| Sample source | Pathology | Methodology | Proteins identified | Most relevant | Validation method | Reference |
|---|---|---|---|---|---|---|
| Human Serum/plasma | Ischemic stroke (Atherotrombotic cardioembolic stroke) | 2-DE | 2 | SAA ↑ haptoglobin↑ | - | 11 |
| Human Serum/plasma | Peripheral arterial disease (PAD) | SELDI-TOF-MS | 1 | $\beta_2$-microgobulin↑ | - | 21 |
| Human carotid secretome | Atherosclerosis | SELDI-TOF-MS | 1 | TWEAK↓ | - | 20 |
| Human Serum/plasma | Acute myocardial infarction (AMI) | SELDI-TOF-MS | 1 | Troponin I | | 19 |
| Human Serum/plasma | Venous Thromboembolism (VTE) | Direct MALDI-TOF-MS 2-DE | 12 | Actin, α1-B glycoprotein, CD5 antigen-like, Complement 4A, Haptoglobin, Hemopexin, IgA heavy Chain, Leucine rich-α2 glycoprotein 1, Myosin heavy chain, Platelet coagulation factor XI, Plasma kalikreinB1 precursor, Proapoliprotein | | 18 |
| Human Serum/plasma | Diabetes | Label free proteomic with LC-MS/MS | 68 | Ficolin 3↑ | WB | 23 |
| Human Serum/plasma | AMI | Non proteomic approach | 1 | TRAIL ↓ | --- | 26 |
| Human Serum/plasma | Coronary atherosclerosis | Non proteomic approach (WB) | 2 | Adiponectin↓ | --- | 27 |
| Swine Serum/plasma | Hypercholesterolemia / Diabetes | Non proteomic approach | 1 | Lipoprotein Associated phospholipase A2 | --- | 42 |
| Human Urine | Severe Coronary Artery Disease (CAD) | Capillary Electrophoresis+ ESI-TOF/MS | Peptide profile (15 peptides) | Collagen α 1 (I) Collagen α 1 (III) | --- | 30 |
| Human Circulating monocytes | ACS | 2-DE | 20 | Protein profile | WB | 47,48 |
| Human carotid | Atherosclerosis | 2-DE | 1 | $\alpha_1$-antitrypsin ↑ | WB, 2D-WB | 120 |
| Human carotid | Atherosclerosis | 2-DE | 21 | hsp27 ↓ | WB, IHC | 149 |
| Human carotid | Atherosclerosis | 2-DE | 9 | fibrinogen fragment D ↑, ferritin light subunit ↑, SOD2 ↑, annexin A10 ↓, glutathione transferase P1-1 ↓, hsp20 ↓, hsp27 ↓, Rho GDI ↓, SOD3 ↓ | WB, ---, ---, ---, ---, ---, ---, ---, --- | 105 |
| Human aorta | Atherosclerosis | 2-DE | 27 | annexin A5 ↑, decoy receptor 1 ↑, 14-3-3γ ↓ | WB, WB, WB | 105 |

**Table 1. (continued)**

| Sample source | Pathology | Methodology | Proteins identified | Most relevant | Validation method | Reference |
|---|---|---|---|---|---|---|
| Human carotid | Atherosclerosis | Antibody arrays | 21 | TRAF4 ↑<br>Gads ↑<br>GIT1 ↑<br>Caspase-9 ↑<br>c-src ↑<br>TOPO-I ↑I-α<br>JAM-1 ↑ | WB, IHC<br>WB, IHC<br>WB, IHC<br>WB, IHC<br>WB, IHC<br>WB, IHC<br>WB, IHC | 119 |
| Human coronary | Atherosclerosis | LC-MS/MS<br>LMD (layers)+ LC-MS/MS | 806 | PEDF<br>Periostin<br>MFG-E8<br>Annexin I | IHC<br>IHC<br>IHC<br>IHC | 116 |
| Human carotid | Atherosclerosis | Manual microdissection (intima) + proteoglycan extraction + LC-MS/MS | 8 | Lumican↑ | IHC | 108 |
| Apo E mice aorta | Atherosclerosis | Biotin perfusión (ECs surface proteins) + LC-MS/MS | 454 | Immune and inflammatory response<br>Cell adhesion<br>Lipid metabolism | ---<br>---<br>--- | 110 |
| Human carotid secretome | Atherosclerosis | 2-DE | 2 | HSP27<br>Cathepsin D | WB, IHC,<br>ELISA | 148 |
| Human aorta | Abdominal Aortic aneurysm | SELDI-TOF-MS | 1 | Hemorphin-7 | IHC | 93 |
| Human aorta | Abdominal aortic aneurysm | SELDI-TOF-MS | 13 | Calpain, filamin A fragment | WB | 91 |
| Human aorta | Abdominal aortic aneurysm | 2-DE | 4 | Peroxiredoxin-2, actin, vitronectin, Calreticulin | WB | 92 |
| Plasma | Type 2 diabetes | SELDI-TOF-MS | 4 | Transthyretin, hemoglobin-alpha chain, hemoglobin-beta chain, apolipoprotein H | --- | 22 |
| Plasma | Atherosclerosis | SELDI-TOF-MS | 1 | Lysozyme | IHC | 24 |
| Serum | Coronary stenting | ELISA | 1 | Vitronectin | --- | 25 |
| Plasma/serum | Diabetes | ELISA | 1 | YKL-40 | --- | 28 |
| Serum | Acute ischemic stroke | MALDI-TOF | 2 | Hemoglobin-alpha chain, hemoglobin-beta chain | --- | 13 |

Serum samples immunodepleted of the 12 most abundant proteins from ischemic stroke patients were analyzed by Brea et al[12]. The levels of two proteins, haptoglobin and serum amyloid A (SAA), could distinguish atherotrombotic from cardioembolic stroke. In order to identify potential protein candidates for ischemic stroke diagnosis Huang et al [13], analyzed serum samples (47 patients and 34 controls) by MALDI-TOF. It was found that the peaks of hemoglobin α-chain and β-chain were differentially expressed between stroke patients and controls. In recent years SELDI-TOF analysis has become a very useful approach in the detection and identification of novel protein candidates in cardiovascular diseases and is at present widely used. Zhang et al [14] used this platform as a potential tool for identifying serological biomarkers of AMI at an early stage in a rat model and three specific peaks were detected. However the corresponding proteins were not identified. Few other papers which do not identify the proteins corresponding to the m/z peaks differentially detected have been published and therefore its value is difficult to evaluate. For example Florian-Kugawski et al [15] reported that a cluster of unique peaks between 10 and 12 kDa was specific to the patients with ACS. Similarly, Zhang et al [16] identified 13 m/z peaks that could distinguish acute cerebral infarction from controls. In the same context Hong et al [17] analyzed by SELDI-TOF the presence of potential plasma biomarkers for thromboembolic diseases and several m/z peaks were detected that discriminated DVT (deep venous thromboembolism) from healthy subjects and AMI from DVT, but the corresponding proteins were not identified. Other group have investigated the plasma proteome in DVT by a direct MS method and identified a group of proteins, including CD5 antigen-like, several complement components, haptoglobin, Hemopexin, myosin heavy chain, which add specificity to currently available blood assays[18]. Thrombus formation is a general phenomenon that not only occurs in VTE but also mediates the development of many CVD, including ACS and stroke. Plasma and cellular proteins that contribute to thrombus formation have been analyzed by proteomic approaches and have been recently reviewed[19]. Blanco-Colio et al [20] identified that the soluble tumor necrosis-like weak inducer of apoptosis (sTWEAK), a 18.4 kDa SELDI-TOF peak, could be used as a diagnostic biomarker for subclinical atherosclerosis. Measurements of sTWEAK in plasma showed reduced concentrations in subjects with carotid stenosis compared with healthy controls. In addition, sTWEAK plasma concentrations in a cohort of 106 asymptomatic subjects negatively correlated with the carotid intima-media thickness, an index of subclinical atherosclerosis. SELDI-TOF analysis was also applied to study the plasma proteome of patients with peripheral arterial disease (PAD) and β2-microglobulin was found elevated in comparison with healthy controls; importantly, this elevation correlated with disease severity[21]. Likewise, Sundsten et al [22] studied variations in plasma protein levels in subjects with type 2 diabetes mellitus (T2DM) and differences in β-cell function, characterized by early insulin response (EIR) and to compare these protein levels with those observed in individuals with normal glucose tolerance (NGT). Levels of two forms of transthyretin (TTR), hemoglobin α-chain and hemoglobin β-chain were all decreased in plasma from subjects with T2DM compared with those subjects with NGT. Apo H (β2-glycoprotein I) was decreased in subjects with T2DM+high EIR compared with subjects with NGT. Four additional unidentified plasma proteins also varied in different ways between the three groups. The differences in protein profiles between non-diabetic and diabetic sera were also studied by a label-free proteomic method (LC-MS/MS) and 68 proteins were significantly over-represented in the diabetic sera[23]. Curiously 12 proteins belonged to the Complement System, including ficolin 3, which was elevated in the serum of type-2 diabetic patients. Ficolin 3 is an activator of the lectin pathway of complement activation and the reason of this increased concentration in diabetic sera is unknown.

Very recently Abdul-Salam et al [24] explored the presence of potential plasma protein biomarkers of atheromatous disease in patients presenting with chronic stable angina pectoris by comparing patients with 3-vessels disease(3-VD) with those without any evidence of coronary artery disease (NV). Arterial blood was analyzed by SELDI-TOF and lysozyme was identified at elevated levels (3-fold higher intensity) in 3-VD patients compared with the NV controls. This data were confirmed by ELISA in an independent group of patients and the presence of lysozyme was demonstrated in the atherosclerotic plaques by immunohistochemistry. Other group tested whether vitronectin serum concentration correlate with adverse outcomes in ACS patients [25]. It was found that measuring vitronectin enabled the identification of a group of patients at particularly high risk of suffering a major adverse cardiovascular event after coronary intervention with stenting. The potential relationships between the serum level of TRAIL (TNF-related apoptosis inducing ligand) protein and clinical outcomes in patients with AMI was assessed in 60 patients and 60 controls both during hospitalization and at follow-up of 12 months [26]. A low level of TRAIL was detected in AMI patients at baseline versus healthy controls. Interestingly, low TRAIL levels at the time of patient discharge were associated with increased incidence of cardiac death and heart failure during the follow-up. Another protein whose low serum levels may be an important marker in the pathogenesis of atherosclerosis is adiponectin. Low adiponectin serum levels were predictive of total coronary plaque burden and inversely correlated with the number of mixed and non-calcified plaque [27]. However, in which way adiponectin may contribute to plaque vulnerability is at present unknown. YKL-40 has recently emerged as a putative marker of cardiovascular disease [28]. Different studies support a role of YKL-40 in endothelial dysfunction, atherosclerosis and manifest CVD. Clinical studies have shown that YKL-40 serum levels are associated with the presence and extent of CAD and are even higher in patients with AMI. However further research is necessary in order to assess the value of this protein as a cardiovascular biomarker in clinical practice.

Capillary electrophoresis (CE) has recently begun to be used for the analysis of urine in the search for new biomarkers of CVD [29]. Important advantages of urine in comparison to other body fluids are its stability against proteolytic degradation, contain low concentrations of irrelevant proteins and can be collected noninvasively. When CE was applied to a group of patients with severe coronary artery disease a set of 15 peptides that define a characteristic CAD signature panel was identified [30]. The majority of these peptides are small fragments of collagen α-I (I) chains and collagen α-I (III), the predominant proteins in arterial walls which colocalizes in the intima of atherosclerotic plaques. A subsequent study, using the same approach confirmed these results[31].Recently, the feasibility and utility of saliva as an alternative diagnostic fluid for identifying biomarkers of AMI has been reported[32]. A combination of Luminex and –on-a-chip methods were used to assay 21 proteins in serum and whole saliva obtained from 41 AMI patients and 43 healthy controls. Panels involving CRP, MYO and MPO, when used as companion tests for EGC were found to yield excellent diagnostic accuracies. Although further studies are needed, saliva-based tests within lab-on-a-chip systems may provide a rapid screening method for cardiac events for AMI patients in the near future.

## 3. BLOOD CELLS IN ACUTE CORONARY SYNDROME

The plasma, platelet and peripheral mononuclear cells (PBMC) are subject to rapid changes in response to external signals, for example, diurnal rhythm, postprandial metabolism pathological process and inflammatory state. PBMC and platelets play a significant role in common diseases, since they are involved in maintaining vascular integrity, responding to endothelial damage, as well as in activation of inflammatory and immune responses[33]. These critical roles have led to the study and analysis of these cells in different pathological process as Acute Coronary Syndrome (ACS) and other cardiovascular diseases.

## 3.1. Circulating Monocytes

Blood monocytes play an important role in a variety of homeostatic processes including host defense, inflammatory processes, and tumor surveillance [34,35,36]. Monocytes are activated during acute coronary syndromes (ACSs), and may reflect the pathophysiological processes occurring during this disorder. In fact, it has been established a clear relationship between the inflammatory activity in the plaque with infiltration of monocytes-macrophages and the ACS occurrence[37, 38].

Activated monocytes promote the synthesis of proinflammatory molecules, such as IL-6 and TNF-α.[39].The anti-inflammatory cytokine IL-10 is also upregulated in response to TNF-α in ACS, suggesting a control mechanism for inflammation[40]. In addition, nowadays it is accepted that macrophages (derived from circulating monocytes) degrade the extracellular matrix of the fibrotic capsule by secreting proteolytic enzymes that promote matrix weakness and facilitates its breaking by hemodynamic forces[41, 42, 43].

The monocyte differentiation into macrophages is an important process secondary to local inflammation and is the subject of several proteomic studies. Two dimensional gels and reference map of monocytes have been published[44]. Dupont et al. elaborated 2-DE reference maps of the human macrophages proteome and secretome in order to elucidate the macrophage dysfunction involved in inflammatory, immunological, and infectious diseases[45]. Seong et al. analyzed the effect of inflammation and oxidative stress on the proteomic profile of monocytes. They identified 28 proteins with altered expression pattern, involved in energy metabolism, translation and protein folding [46]

Barderas et al. analyzed the differential proteome of circulating human monocytes from patients suffering acute coronary syndrome, with no elevation-ST (NSTEACS), and stable patients. They found 18 proteins altered in admission compare with stable patients. Surprisingly 6 months after of the acute event, the proteomic profile of monocytes from ACS patients seems to resemble the monocytes profile of stable patients [47].

Most recently, this group also studied the effect of a statin (atorvastatin (ATV)) at different doses, in the protein profile of circulating human monocytes after an acute coronary syndrome. They have assessed the effects of intensive therapy with ATV after a NSTEACS on the protein expression of circulating monocytes, by combining 2-DE and MS[48]. They showed that high-dose ATV (80mg/dL) for two months as compared to standard therapy modifies the expression of 27 spots by circulating monocytes corresponding to 20 different proteins. Among the most striking results, they found normalization by intensive ATV of the expression of proteins that modulate inflammation and thrombosis such as PDI, Annexins I and II, and prohibitin, and of proteins which have other vascular protective effects, as HSP-70.The molecular mechanism by which ATV induces and/or up regulates the production of proteins that were previously inhibited in ACS monocytes is at present unknown. Therefore, ATV acts on arteries but also on circulating monocytes, a key cell involved in the formation and complication of atherome plaques.

## 3.2 Platelets

Platelets, also known as thrombocytes, are the smallest circulating blood particles. They are cytoplasmic fragments derived from megakaryocytes located in bone marrow and play critical roles in primary and secondary homeostasis (blood coagulation)[49]. Platelets play a significant role in common diseases, especially in atherotrombosis and coronary artery diseases. They are implicated in the maintenance of the vascular endothelium by sensing and responding to endothelium damage, in wound healing and in activation of inflammatory and immune responses [50] They contain proteins as well as mRNA. The remaining mRNA makes them able to keep on synthesizing some proteins and they possess the capability to modify the proteins post-translationally[51, 52]. These post-transcriptional pathways are potential targets for molecular intervention in atherotrombosis [53]

Although the underlying cellular and molecular mechanisms of ACS disease progression are complex, the adhesion of platelets and T-lymphocytes to the damaged arterial wall is characterized as an early event in vessel injury [54] Activated platelets deposit at sites of unstable plaque rupture [55] precipitating or exacerbating coronary vascular obstruction. It is well recognized that inflammatory and thrombotic mechanisms combine to obstruct or occlude the vascular lumen and activated platelets potentiate thrombus formation and ultimately promote restenosis[56,57].

Different proteomic studies have been developed to explore the proteome of platelets. Marcus et al. identified 186 proteins using 2-DE with broad pH range (pI 3-10)[58]. In a more complete study by 2-DE with different ranges of pH, O'Neill et al. identified 123 different gene products corresponding to proteins with very different functions as signal transduction, cytoskeleton, synthesis and processing of proteins, proteins associate with vesicles movement and proteins implicated in coagulation[59]. Other study published using narrower pI range (pI 4-5 and pI 5-11) identified 311 gene products, many of them resulting in proteins involved in signal transduction [60, 28]

Although they are anucleate, protein expression in platelets is quite dynamic, depending on their state of activation. It is therefore essential to study the proteome of activated as well as of inactivated platelets. Garcia et al. [61] detected 62 proteins differentially expressed in activated and inactivated platelets. Thirty-four of these were found in the pI 4-7 analytical range, with 18 being up-regulated and 16 down-regulated. In the pI 6-11 range, 8 proteins were up-regulated and 20 down-regulated. Forty-one of the 62 differentially expressed proteins were successfully identified by LC-MS/MS and mainly belonged to the cytoskeleton, signaling and processing proteins. In a different study, 41 proteins which were differentially phosphorylated after stimulation with TRAP (Thrombin Receptor-Activating Peptide) were identified. These included a novel protein, the adapter of downstream of tyrosine kinase 2 (Dok-2), which may play a role in thrombus formation [62] Zahedi et al. by means of/ through chromatography coupled with nano-LC-MS/MS identified 278 phosphorylated proteins in resting platelets [63] Quiescent platelets display minimal translational activity. Platelet activity leads to a rapid translation of the preexisting RNA with the release of platelet-secreted proteins, cytokines, and exosomes. Coppinger et al., by using thrombin stimulated platelets, identified several secreted proteins, as secretogranin III, cyclophilin A, and calumenin, previously identified in atherosclerotic lesions but absent in normal vasculature [64] Treatment with antihypertensive drugs can also modify the platelet protein profile of hypertensive patients [65]

## 3.3. Proteomics on Vascular Progenitors

In last time, research focused in stem, progenitor and precursor cells have raised notably the interest in vascular repair. Recent evidences suggest that in addition to hematopoietic precursor cells, endothelial precursor cells (EPC) and smooth muscle precursor cells (SMPC) are present in bone marrow and circulate in peripheral blood[66]. EPC are probably the most widely studied adult progenitor cell type, and are attracting considerable attention in cardiovascular research [68,67]but several issues regarding their characterization and activity remain unclear. Asahara et al., in 1997, detected and isolated circulating blood cells with endothelial cells potential (endothelial precursor cells); thereafter, this field have increased scientific attention. Since these cells derived from bone marrow, it have been suggested that the EPCs are stem cells and therefore may have therapeutic value in neovascularization or re-vascularization of ischemic tissue.

### *Endothelial Progenitor Cells (EPC)*

Recent research has shown that a good endothelial function is essential in many pathophysiological conditions, including infections, neoplasia, inflammation and cardiovascular disease. In fact, it is known that circulating endothelial cells (CEC) and endothelial progenitor cells (EPC) are markers of endothelial function. The increase in CEC, mature and presumably apoptotic or necrotic cells, reflects severe endothelial injury and is thought to potentially reflect different pathophysiological states. In parallel, it is thought that EPCs may be involved in repair processes / endothelial regeneration.

The EPCs have been known for years, initially thought to come from losses from the lumen of the endothelium. Noishiki suggested the bone marrow as the possible origin of these cells[67, 35], an idea that was confirmed and extended by others [69,70,71,72,73] Asahara et al. [68, 36]showed that angioblasts (endothelial cell progenitors) gave rise to what apparently seemed like adult endothelial cells which could be isolated from peripheral blood. Although there is currently some controversy in the definition of both cells types, the main criteria to define the endothelial cells (EC) is the presence / absence of certain cell surface glycoproteins by flow cytometry or immunobeads coupled to specific antibodies. In addition, multiple culture methods from peripheral blood mononuclear cells have been described obtaining EPCs, colony-forming unit (CFU) [74] EPCs are commonly identified by cell surface antigen expression of CD133, CD34, and the vascular endothelial growth factor receptor-2 (VEGFR-2 / KDR) [75]. CD34 and VEGFR-2, however, are also expressed in hematopoietic stem cells [76]/ To increase the phenotype controversy, it has been recently detected resident cells in the vasculature with potential progenitor capabilities.

In contrast to data obtained with CECs, it has been documented that the number of circulating EPCs decreased in patients with risk factors such as smoking, high cholesterol, diabetes and hypertension, most of which have been identified as prognostic markers of poor outcome after cerebral infarction [77] reported a decrease in the number of EPCs in subjects who had coronary artery disease compared with healthy individuals. They also noted that the number of EPCs showed an inverse correlation with risk factors. Eizawa et al. [78] reported a decrease of EPCs in haemodialysis patients and in patients with stable coronary disease [79]In addition, low levels of circulating EPCs have also been found in patients with unstable angina [77] cerebrovascular disease [80, 81]and aortic valve stenosis[82].

These and other studies have generated various reviews and comments which suggest that the EPCs are stem cells and therefore may have therapeutic value. EPCs have been associated with regeneration and neovascularisation of ischemic tissues [69, 83]It has been documented that mobilization of these cells enhances the repair of damaged arteries[84]. Transplantation of these progenitor cells after myocardial infarction is known to improve ventricular function [85, 86 ].

All these data suggest that EPCs are involved in these processes of endothelial repair / regeneration and their balance on the CECs may also be important in the evolution of certain pathologies [86, 87]Notably, after a decade of research, there is still no specific marker for their unambiguous identification, and small clinical trials using EPC as cell-based therapy following myocardial infarction produced controversial results [88]. Some articles have focused in the characterization of CD34+ cells, but this enrichment fraction represents a very heterogeneous group of different cell types. Recently, Pula et al. have published a proteomic characterization of endothelial progenitor cells in culture [89] This study use proteomic tools to analyze the secretome of EPCs and CFUs cultures. Among the angiogenic factors revealed by proteomics was thymidine phosphorylase (TP), also known as platelet derived endothelial cell growth factor (PD-ECGF). This growth factor and deoxyribose phosphatise (dRP), the product of its enzymatic activity, were shown to be essential for EPC survival and paracrine effects on endothelial cell migration and angiogenesis. It is possible that proteomics can help us to identify a more concrete phenotype, which is a necessity to improve our knowledge in this field and in the further therapeutic applications.

## 4. Tissue Proteomics

Although proteomic studies in ACS are frequently directed in the search for biomarkers in plasma, a tissue-based approach constitutes a valuable alternative, not only for basic research purposes, but also on a biomarkers discovery phase. Vascular tissue is in continuous contact with blood so that proteins present in the tissue are very frequently released to this fluid. The plasma proteome constitutes the most complex sample of the human body, in terms of dynamic range and number of protein species [90] Thus, plasma proteomic analysis constitutes a tough approach where complex depletion and/or prefractionation strategies are mandatory. In addition, such prefractionation methods are frequently unable to reach concentrations of proteins in the dynamic range of tissue leakage proteins. For these reasons, tissue-proteomic analysis is a complementary approach to plasma in the study of ACS Figure 3 shows different proteomic approaches used to study atherosclerosis and includes some representative proteins recently identified with each approach. However, the main disadvantage of tissue proteomic analysis for biomarker discovery is that altered levels of a protein in the vascular tissue is not always related with such variations in blood, and vascular biopsy analysis for diagnosis is not an option.

Aimed to ACS study, ideal tissue sources for analysis are coronary arteries and heart. As coronary artery specimens, especially from biopsy origin, are of small size and difficult to obtain, other arteries affected by atherosclerosis can be alternatively used in the search for atherosclerotic biomarkers, such as aorta, carotid or iliac/femoral arteries. Human samples for tissue proteomics in ACS may come from biopsy or necropsy origin. Artery biopsies can be obtained from bypass, heart transplant or arteriotomy surgery. In this case, control specimens for a differential abundance analysis should be a different artery type with low atherosclerosis affection collected from these patients (i.e. mammary or radial artery) since coronary, aorta, carotid and iliac/femoral arteries cannot be collected from healthy subjects. On the other hand, aortic aneurysm is most frequently produced by an atherosclerotic affection of this artery. Hence, recent findings in the atherosclerotic proteome profile have been achieved from the study of aortic aneurysms by 2-DE [91, 92]and from the analysis of intraluminal thrombus by SELDI-TOF[93]. Although small myocardium biopsies obtained also from bypass surgery have been used for proteomic analysis[94], better results may be obtained from transplant surgery hearts as more material can be collected. Human infarcted myocardium may be obtained from necropsy origin for proteomic analysis, but most frequently animal models where an obstruction of the coronary artery is forced are used[95]. Consequences of an ischemic/reperfusion event in heart tissue and cardioprotection derived from them have indeed been studied using *in vivo [96, 97]*or *ex vivo [98,99,100]*animal models. Additionally coronary effluent from these perfused hearts can be analyzed in the search for biomarkers of AMI released to the blood [100,101] These proceedings allow to easily obtain enough tissue material and to have a very precise control of the experimental conditions. Accordingly, human infarcted heart biopsies are rarely used.

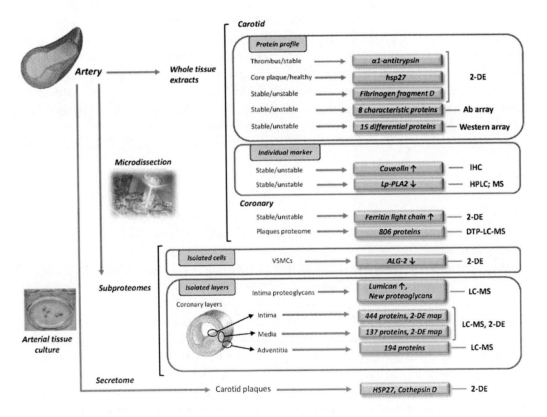

Figure 3. Overview of the different proteomic strategies and techniques used to study vascular proteomes in health and diseases.

Concerning necropsy material, samples from every desired source can be obtained, with the adequate legal consents. Every type of artery and the entire heart are available and unaffected tissue can be collected from subjects dying from non-cardiac events and without atherosclerosis affection. In addition, adjacent tissue healthier than the affected portions can be obtained, in some cases, to use as a control. The critical point while working with necropsy tissue is that the collection has to be done as soon as possible after death to avoid protein degradation. The convenience of using tissue specimens from autopsies for proteomic analysis has been assessed with brain material [102], and more recently on vascular tissue for the analysis of a subset of proteins using tissue microarrays (TMA) [103]An adequate election of control samples is very important in order to obtain protein alterations related to the concrete process under study: atherosclerosis development, plaque instability, ischemic damage, etc.

For a proteomic study, it is relevant to take into account that vascular tissue has a substantial complexity derived from the presence of myofilament proteins, which allow and control muscle contraction and constitute the most abundant proteins in this material [101]. These proteins include actin, myosin, tropomyosin, actin, desmin, etc, present in both artery and heart tissue, and troponins, which are particularly expressed in the heart. Its high abundance limits the ability to analyze lower abundant proteins in tissue extracts, and their difficulty to be solubilized affects protein separation, especially by 2-DE, and MS analysis. Prefractionation methods can be an option to reduce vascular tissue complexity and special mention deserves an approach named "*In sequence* myofilament protein extraction" to remove major abundant myofilament proteins based on its solubility at acidic pH levels [104].

Atherotrombotic arteries present additional difficulties to myofilament proteins presence for solubilization. Lipid core formation and calcification provide a high content in lipids and calcium, which affects solubilization and protein separation. Moreover, blood contamination coming from lumen and adventitial vascularization is difficult to avoid and distinguish from intraplaque hemorrhage contribution, as highlighted by Leppeda *et al.*, who identified the most abundant spots present in 2-DE gels of carotid plaque extracts resulting on a 70% of plasma-derived proteins [105]. Several washes of the specimens in buffer and an efficient removal of the adventitia are mandatory to obtain protein extracts with low plasma contamination. An observation of the proportion of albumin with respect to actin (major abundant proteins from plasma and arterial tissue, respectively) facilitates the evaluation of a proper extraction.

As detailed above, vascular tissue proteome's complexity is unquestionable. Thus, sub fractionation of vascular tissue to study its subproteomes simplifies the proteomic analysis and allows characterizing the specific role of a protein in the studied subproteome, somehow reducing possible contradictory behaviors in other regions of the tissue or cell organelles. An elegant way to specifically isolate cells/tissue areas and, therefore, focus on particular subproteomes is by microdissection. Firstly developed in 1996[106], it allows automated selection of regions of interest while minimizing surrounding tissue and plasma contamination. Studies performed by our group with intima and media layer from human coronary and aorta arteries isolated by laser microdissection (LMD) and analyzed by LC-MS/MS confirmed that plasma contamination can be avoided with this approach, since major abundant plasma proteins were not identified in these extracts except for albumin and hemoglobin, that were identified based on substantially less number of peptides than top rank identifications corresponding to actin variants [107] Manual microdissection constitutes an alternative to LMD when no laser devices are available and has been applied in certain studies to isolate concrete layers from atherotrombotic arteries for WB or LC-MS/MS analysis [108]. An improved variant of the LCM, the laser cutting microdissection, employs an ultraviolet laser to excise selected cells or tissue regions by cutting around the delimited area [109] This methodology permits to isolate regions of interest in a non-contact manner, but is not as faster as LCM when cell by cell microdissection is applied. Nevertheless, tissue heating produced by LCM affects tissue integrity and may be critical for proteomic analysis due to protein degradation effects.

LMD is only one of the possibilities that can be performed for sub fractionation. If a specific cell proteome is to be analyzed by proteomics, the analysis of cells directly isolated from tissue without a following culture process would reduce experimental variability, but low protein recovery is expected. In this sense, explants cultures from vascular tissue are frequently used as a greater cell yield is obtained. An interesting approach to isolate surface proteins from endothelial cells (ECs) of apo E- deficient mice was applied by Wu *et al.* recently [110] Perfusion of the blood vessels with an active biotin reagent was used to bind all accessible proteins. This methodology allowed the enrichment of ECs surface protein fraction for its analysis by LC-MS/MS. In a different approach, the study of the phosphoproteome of the heart mitochondrial has become a very popular field; since cardioprotection derived by ischemic pre- and post-conditioning has been associated to the phosphorylation state of several proteins in this organelle. Mitochondria can be isolated with high purity by differential centrifugation in a sucrose gradient and different approaches can be applied to study phosphorylation, such as pro Q Diamond staining (Molecular Probes, Invitrogen) [111] or anti-phospho antibodies [112, 113] applied to 2-DE or Blue Native gels. In a double-fractionation approach, proteoglycans from manually microdissected intimas of atherosclerotic and mammary arteries have been specifically extracted by ion exchange chromatography [108].

It is important to note that subfractionation of vascular tissue for proteomic analysis often implies scarce protein yield, especially while performing LMD. Results published by De Souza *et al.*, who invested 70 hours to collect enough material for a classical 2-DE analysis of microdissected myocytes and blood vessels from human hearts [114], illustrate this fact. This study is pioneer in the proteomic analysis of LMD-isolated vascular tissue. To overcome these limitations, a DIGE variant named saturation labeling DIGE, which allows running 5 μg of total protein amount in one gel with fine results, was recently developed. Thus, 2-DE analysis of microdissected tissue, as well as other scarce subproteomes, has been facilitated by this methodology. To our knowledge, only our group has applied this methodology for a 2-DE analysis of arterial tissue [102], despite of its emerging importance. This study has also complemented the protein catalogue of the coronary artery by LC-MS/MS analysis of intima and media from the preatherosclerotic artery [115]. The protein catalogue of atherosclerotic coronary artery was previously detailed in extent by Bagnato *et al.*, who analyzed whole artery and laser-microdissected intima, media and adventitia proteomes by LC-MS/MS [116]

In general, two different approaches are mainly used: descriptive and comparative in terms of proteins abundance. Differential protein abundance studies with atherosclerotic arteries have been mainly applied to compare preatherosclerotic and atherosclerotic samples, [117, 118] as well as to find out proteins related with plaque instability[105,119, 120] . Unstable plaques have been associated with increased risk of rupture and, consequently, of thrombosis. Biomarkers of instability could therefore be used to evaluate ACS risk. Besides, proteins varied in atherosclerotic arteries with respect to preatherosclerotic are potential ACS risk markers and therapeutic targets. *In vitro* studies performed with activated platelets compared to normal ones tend to mimic *in vivo* situation and are aimed to thrombosis biomarkers discovery[61,121, 60,122]. On the other hand, proteomic analysis of i.e. the thrombus should be done in a descriptive manner, as comparison with healthy tissue is not possible. To date, the proteome from *in vivo*-formed human thrombus has not been described, but a proteomic approach to do so has been described [123]. In general, descriptive approaches using LC-MS/MS have been pivotal to a better characterization of vascular tissue. In particular, the development of the catalog of human [124]and murine [125] cardiac proteins and their proteotypic peptides has opened the way to quantify these proteins by a recent methodology of LC-MS/MS named single reaction monitoring (SRM) or multiple reaction monitoring (MRM). Other methodologies for proteomic analysis of vascular tissues such as protein arrays, TMA or MS Imaging have been rarely used until today. Protein array technology has been improved in the latest years, with a substantial increase of commercial prearrayed platforms in diverse clinical fields. Its application in ACS proteomics is still to take off unless important results have been found when applying it to analyze plaque instability [119]. The utility of TMAs for vascular tissue analysis has been recently proved in a great cohort of human vessels [103], what suggests its use in the analysis of proteins already related with ACS or validation of proteins found varied in a discovery phase.

## Secretome

The term secretome was firstly introduced in 2000 in a genome-based global survey of secreted proteins of *Bacillus Subtilis* [126]. Since then, the sub-set of proteins released by a cell/tissue under certain conditions in a specific time frame is being increasingly investigated. Traditionally, biomarkers research has been focused on plasma or serum, as they are easily accessible sources and so, targets discovered in science can be directly transferred into clinical practice. Indeed, serum and plasma comprises a full set of proteins, such as cytokines, chemokines, hormones, growth factors, antibodies, etc., which are secreted from the cells of different organs and play pivotal biological roles. However, the very large dynamic range of protein concentrations in such body fluids makes their study very challenging, where high abundance proteins obscure detection of low abundance secreted molecules. One of the main advantages of studying the secretome is that it can be considered a sub-proteome of the serum/plasma and, in consequence, of reduced complexity; but, what it is more important is that it implies a more direct approximation to the key proteins that are influencing body's metabolism and mediating immune responses. Most studies are focused on the secretome obtained from in vitro cell cultures, particularly in the cancer field, assuming that such cells' behavior well simulates the in vivo condition [127] A further step in approximation to the physiological situation involves the use of tissue explants instead of cell lines (ex vivo approach), which provide with information from secretory molecules coming from all tissue components and as result of cross-talk between them. The difficulties that imply the study of the in vivo secretome have been partially overcome by implanting capillary ultrafiltration probes into tumor masses induced in mice, this being one of the few proteomics studies which best approach the real in vivo situation [128, 129]. One key point to take into account when designing the analytical strategy is that, two potential "contaminants" are present and should be minimized in the secretome sample, independently of the starting material (cells or tissue): a) intracellular proteins, released through cell damage, and b) serum. One can assume that it is very challenging to totally avoid the presence of intracellular proteins, as cell lysis always takes place during cell/tissue culture. However, it was shown that optimum culture conditions may favor secreted proteins enrichment [130] Related to serum presence as an undesirable external source of proteins, it is common to perform stringent washes of the cells to reduce BSA interference prior to final culture in serum-free media [131] However, lack of serum in culture conditions may slow down cell proliferation and even increase cell death. An alternative to serum deprivation in culture media has been recently applied to breast cancer cell lines grown in presence of FBS, based on "equalization" of proteins concentrations in the final sample [132] by means of Proteominer beads (BioRad), the protein dynamic range of the samples is reduced and detection of secreted proteins in presence of serum major ones is enhanced. When tissue explants are being cultured instead of cell lines, extensive washes of tissue pieces should be performed and tissue leakage should be removed by short incubation periods prior to final secretome obtention; in fact, the number of washes (replacement with fresh media) during tissue culture, as well as their distribution in time, may strongly influence the protein dynamic range and so the quality of the final sample for secretome analyses [103] In any case, validation of the true origin of the detected proteins as coming from the tissue itself can be approached by metabolic labeling: proteins incorporating the label are indeed synthesized by the cell/tissue under investigation and do not come from an external source [133, 134].

From the technical point of view, several proteomics platforms have been used, mainly gel-based and gel-free MS-based technologies. In a first approximation, comprehensive lists of proteins secreted by a certain cell line/tissue/organism were obtained in order to better understand disease mechanisms, commonly by means of 2DE separation combined with MALDI-MS(/MS) identification or by previous fractionation by SDS-PAGE and multi-dimensional LC which is further coupled to MS(/MS) [135, 136, 137]Classification of identified proteins as secreted ones is usually done by computational methods: classically secreted proteins (via the ER-Golgi pathway) can be predicted as containing a signal peptide by SignalP or being classified as extracellular via Gene Ontology analysis; non-classically secreted proteins, which do not contain N-terminal signal peptide, can be predicted by SecretomeP and more recently by SecretP [138]. Biological networks among the identified proteins can also be generated through i.e. Ingenuity Pathways (IPA), resulting in those biological functions and diseases that are most significant to the genes in the network [139].

In a further step, two conditions are to be compared (i.e. healthy/disease, drug treated/non-treated, reaction to presence/absence of stimuli). The stable isotope labeling with amino acids in cell culture (SILAC) approach allowed quantitative comparison; ensuring 100% incorporation of labeled amino acids into cells, a quantitative measurement of proteins abundance in the different conditions can be calculated[140] The 100% incorporation status is not so straightforward to set in tissue experiments, for which a novel approach has been recently proposed based on partial incorporation of light and heavy label in the two conditions whose ratios are lately compared (CILAIR) [141]Other strategies to perform relative quantitation are based on spectral counting [142]. This consists of an estimation of protein abundance based on the total number of MS/MS spectra assigned to it [143, 144, 145] However, absolute quantitation by MS should be performed by other strategies such as Single Reaction Monitoring (SRM) [146].

In the atherosclerosis field, few studies have been performed so far despite of the enormous value of the secretome as direct source of potential biomarkers. 2DE maps of the proteome and secretome of human macrophages and arterial smooth muscle cells have been established after 24h of cell culture in serum free media [145,45] In a pioneering work, secretomes of human arterial sections were evaluated by comparing radial artery segments (control) with carotid sections affected by atherosclerotic plaque of variable severity (non-complicated and ruptured plaques with thrombus). In general, tissue secretomes were comparatively analyzed by 2-DE [148] and 42, 154 and 202 proteins spots were detected for control artery segments, atherosclerotic lesion and plaque complicated with thrombus, respectively. This observation points to a greater metabolic activity of the diseased tissue compared to healthy arteries. In particular, HSP27 secretion was diminished in atherosclerosis, and correlates well with plaque complication; plasma levels pointed to the same direction [149]In a similar approach, 217 proteins spots showed higher expression levels in the secretome of the atherosclerotic plaques than in controls, and 43 proteins spots decreased or remained unchanged. From MS identification data, 34 out of 83 proteins identified in total were higher in atherome plaque secretome, whereas 31 proteins showed lower levels compared with the controls[150] Drugs effect on protein secretion was also investigated. Atorvastatin treatment influenced secretome patterns of carotid atherosclerotic sections in comparison with fibrous regions adjacent to plaques as controls: 66% of the proteins found to be differentially released reverted to control values after atorvastatin administration. In particular, cathepsin D not only reached control values after treatment, but was also found to have decreased in plaques obtained from patients who received atorvastatin treatment prior to carotid endarterectomy [151] However, atorvastatin alone was not able to increase the reduced levels of β-galactoside soluble lectin secreted by atherosclerotic lesions compared to the controls, in contrast to combined treatment with atorvastatin and amlodipine and similar effects are observed for retinol-binding protein, protein disulfide isomerase (PDI) and thioredoxin peroxidase B2 [150]. In a different study, arterial wall remodeling in hypertension was investigated in rats by comparison of aorta secretomes following treatment with a hypertensive drug (L-NAME). Ubiquitin, SM22α, thymosin β4 and C-terminal fragment of filamin A were found to be differentially secreted by SELDI-TOF-MS [152]. These are clear examples of relevant clinical information that can be obtained from secretome research. In this sense, one of the emerging fields in cardiovascular therapies is the use of stem cells as an alternative to transplantation, which is currently the unique effective therapy to replace damaged myocardium. Transplanted exogenous stem cells can influence neovascularization, myocardial protection, cardiac remodeling and contractility. Interestingly, it seems to be that these effects are possible not only based on the cells newly formed at the site of injury, but also through proteins secretion which induce changes in neighboring cells or in the originating cells itself

## 5. METABOLOMICS

In ACS, metabolites changes are expected as a response of the body to the disease process or to drug therapy. In general, there are about 3,000 endogenous metabolites, apart from diet compounds, xenobiotics and microbial metabolites in a broad range of concentrations. Their presence in human body is extremely influenced by different factors (age, gender, diet, drug therapy effects, and body metabolism) which may result in a confounding masking effect when varied levels are to be established as consequence of certain pathology. Besides, high interindividual variability is expected. Metabolites are cleared from the circulation into urine, so this is an ideal sample source. However, some metabolites have a rapid clearance rate and, in this sense, they may have difficult detention. As metabolites are small molecular products of enzyme reactions in various metabolic pathways, their final concentrations in biological fluids are at the end determined by protein activities. Besides, it is important to define the metabolite molecules to be analyzed or which of them are expected to be influenced, this means the original metabolite molecule or its biotransformations in i.e. the first phase of metabolism (oxidation and reduction) and in the second phase (conjugation). Metabolomics is an emerging field where a characteristic metabolite profile able to i.e. provide diagnosis, evaluate prognosis or distinguish cardiovascular disease severity, is demanded. Robust analytical techniques and bioinformatics tools are needed and, in this sense, nuclear magnetic resonance (NMR), GC-MS and LC-MS are the common platforms of choice [156] When plasma samples from atherosclerotic patients were compared to healthy individuals by combined GC-MS and $^1$H NMR, 24 metabolites related to insulin resistance were found significantly varied [157] Drug treatment effects on plaque progression in mice aorta resulted in differential urine metabolomic profiles obtained by NMR [158] The combination of liquid chromatography with a triple-quadrupole mass spectrometer for single reaction monitoring (SRM) experiments is a much more sensitive approach which has been applied in the search for biomarkers of myocardial ischemia [159]and early detection of myocardial injury by identifying changes in circulating metabolites in the following 10 minutes [160] In another study, 12 and 8 metabolites were found varied in plasma and urine, respectively, from atherosclerotic rats versus controls [161]

## ABBREVIATIONS

| |
|---|
| MMP: metaloproteasas |
| ECM: Extracellular Matrix |
| CVD: Cardiovascular Diseases |
| MS: Mass Spectrometry |
| MRM: Multiple Reaction Monitoring |
| SELDI-TOF: Surface Enhanced Laser Desorption Ionization-Time of Flight |
| HUPO: Human Proteome Organization |
| DVT: Deep Venous Thromboembolism |
| AMI: Acute Myocardial Infarction |
| ACS: Acute Coronary Syndrome |
| PAD: Peripheral Artery Disease |
| T2DM: Type 2 Diabetes Mellitus |
| LC-MS/MS: Liquid Chromatography tandem MS |
| CE: Capillary Electrophoresis |
| CAD: Coronary Artery Disease |
| PBMC: Peripheral Blood Mononuclear Cells |
| 2-DE: Two Dimensional Electrophoresis |

**(Continued)**

| |
|---|
| ATV: Atorvastatin |
| EPC: Endothelial Precursor Cell |
| SMPC: Smooth Muscle Precursor Cell |
| EC: Endothelial cell |
| CFU: Colony Forming Unit |
| CEC: Circulating Endothelial Cell |
| TMA: Tissue Microarray |
| LMD: Laser Microdissection |
| WB: Western Blotting |
| IHC: Immunohistochemistry |
| SRM: Single Reaction Monitoring |
| CILAIR: Comparison of Isotope Labeled Amino acids Incorporation rates |

## PROTEINS ABBREVIATIONS

| |
|---|
| TnI: Troponin I |
| Lpa: Lipoprotein Lipase a |
| SAA: Serum amyloid |
| TWEAK: Tumor necrosis-like weak induced of apoptosis |
| TTR: Transthyretin |
| APO H: Apolipoprotein H ($\beta_2$-glycoprotein) |
| TRAIL: TNF-related apoptosis induced ligand |
| YKL-40: YKL-Protein |
| CRP: Protein C-Reactive |
| MYO: Myoglobin |
| MPO: Myeloperoxidase |
| TNF: Tumor Necrosis Factor |
| PDI: Protein Disulfide Isomerase |
| HSP: Heat Shock Protein |
| TP: Thymidine Phosphorylase |

## REFERENCES

[1] Alvarez-Llamas G, de la Cuesta F, Barderas MG, Darde V, Padial LR, Vivanco F. Recent advances in aterosclerosis-based proteomics: new biomarkers and a future perspective. *Expert Rev. Proteomics* 2008; 5:679-691.

[2] Wheelock CE, Wheelock AM, Kawashima S, Diez D, Kanehisa M, van Erk M, Kleemann R, Haeggström JZ, Goto S. Systems biology approaches and pathway tools for investigating cardiovascular disease. *Mol. BioSyst.* 2009; 5:588-602.

[3] Ramsey SA, Gold ES, Aderem A. A systems biology approach to understanding atherosclerosis. *EMBO Mol. Med.* 2010; 2:79-89.

[4] Jain KK. *Technologies for discovery of biomarkers in The handbook of Biomarkers.* Springer 2010.

[5] Lusis AJ, Weiss JN. Cardiovascular networks: systems-based approaches to cardiovascular disease. *Circulation* 2010; 121:157-170.

[6] Anderson NL. The clinical plasma proteome: a survey of clinical assays for proteins in plasma and serum. *Clin Chem* 2010, 56(2):177-185.

[7] Hortin GL, Carr SA, Anderson NL. Advances in protein analysis for the clinical laboratory, *Clin Chem 2010, 56(2), 149-151.*

[8] Keshishian H, Addona T, Burgess M, Mani DR, Shi X, Kuhn E, Sabatine M, Gerszten RE, Carr S. Quantification of cardiovascular biomarkers in patient plasma by targeted mass spectrometry and stable isotope dilution. *Mol Cell Proteomics*, 2009; 8: 2339-2349.

[9] US Food and Drug Administration. FDA clears a test for ovarian cancer:*http://www.fda.gov/NewsEvents/Newsroom/PressAnnouncements/ucm182057.htm.*

[10] Anderson, N. L. and Anderson, N. G. The human plasma proteome: history, character, and diagnostic prospects. *Mol. Cell. Proteomics* 2002 ; 1 : 845–867.

[11] Berhane BT, Zong C, Liem DA, Huang A, Le S, Edmondson RD, Jones RC, Qiao X, Whitelegge JP, Ping P, Vondriska TM. Cardiovascular-related proteins identified in human plasma by the HUPO Plasma Proteome Project Pilot Phase. *Proteomics* 2005; 5: 3520-3530.

[12] Berhane BT, Zong C, Liem DA, Huang A, Le S, Edmondson RD, Jones RC, Qiao X, Whitelegge JP, Ping P, Vondriska TM. Cardiovascular-related proteins identified in human plasma by the HUPO Plasma Proteome Project Pilot Phase. *Proteomics* 2005; 5: 3520-3530.

[13] Huang P, Lo L, Chen Y, Lin R, Shiea J, Liu C. Serum free hemoglobin as a novel potential biomarker for acute ischemic stroke. *J Neurol* 2009, 256: 625-631.

[14] Zhang G, Zhou B, Zheng Y, Feng K, Rao L, Zhang J, Xin J, Zhang B, Zhang L. Time course proteomic profile of rat acute myocardial infarction by SELDI-TOF MS analysis. *Int J Cardiol* 2009, 131: 225-233.

[15] Florian-Kujawski M, Chyna B, et al, Biomarker profiling of plasma from acute coronary syndrome patients. Application of ProteinChip array analysis *Int Angiol* 2004, 23:246-254.

[16] Zhang X, Guo T, Wang H, He W, Mei H, Hong M, Yu J, Hu Y, Song S. Potential biomarkers of acute cerebral infarction detected by SELDI-TOF-MS. *Am J Clin Pathol* 2008, 130:299-304.

[17] Hong M, Zhang X, Hu Y, Wang h, He W, Mei H, Yu J, Guo T, Song S. The potential biomarkers for thromboembolism detected by SELDI-TOF-MS. *Thrombosis Research.* 2009, 123, 556-564.

[18] Ganesh S K, Sharma Y, Dayhoff J, Fales H M, Van Eyk J, Kickler T S, Billings E M, Nabel E G. Detection of venous thromboembolism by proteomic serum biomarkers. *PLoS ONE* 2007; 2(6):e544.

[19] Howes J M, Keen J N, Findlay B C, Carter A M. The application of proteomics technology to thrombosis research: the identification of potential therapeutic targets in cardiovascular diseases. Diabetes *Vasc Dis Res* 2008; 5:205-212.

[20] Blanco-Colio L, Martin-Ventura J L, Muñoz-Garcia B, Orbe J, Paramo J A, Michel J B, Ortiz A, Meilhac O, Egido J. Identification of soluble tumour necrosis factor-like weak inducer of apoptosis (sTWEAK) as a possible biomarker of subclinical atherosclerosis. *Arterioscler Thromb Vas Biol* 2007; 27:916-922.

[21] Wilson AM, Kimura E, Harada RK, Nair N, Narasimhan B, Meng X, Zhang F, Beck KR, Olin JW, Fung ET, Cooke JP. β2-Microglobulin as a biomarker in peripheral arterial disease. *Circulation*. 2007 ; 116 : 1396-1403.

[22] Sundsten T, Zethelius B, Berne C, Bergsten P. Plasma proteome changes in subjects with type 2 diabetes mellitus with a low or high early insulin response. *Clin Science* 2008, 114:499-507.

[23] Liu R X, Chen H B, Tu K, Zhao S H, Li S J, Dai J, Li Q R, Nie S, Li Y X, Jia W P, Wu J R. Localized-statistical quantification of human serum proteome associated with type 2 diabetes. *PLoS ONE* 2008; 3: e3224.

[24] Abdul-Salam V, Ramrakha P, Krishnan U, Owen DR, Snalhoub J, Davies AH., et al. Identification and assessment of plasma lysozyme as a putative biomarker of atherosclerosis. *Arterioscler Thromb Vasc Biol*. 2010; 30: (in press).

[25] Derer W, Barnathan ES, Safak E, Argawal P, Heidecke H, Mockel M., et al. Vitronectin concentrations predict risk in patients undergoing coronary stenting. *Circ Cardiovasc Intervent.* 2009, 2:14-19.

[26] Secchiero P, Corallini F, ceconi C, Parrinello G, Volpato S, Ferrari R, Zauli G. Potential prognostic significance of decreased Serum levels of TRAIL after acute myocardial infarction. *PLoS ONE* 2008; 4(2):e4442.

[27] Broedi UC, Lebherz C, Lerhke M, Stark R, Greif M, Becker A, Von Ziegler F, Tittus J. et al. Low adiponectin levels are an independent predictor of mixed and non-calcified coronary atherosclerotic plaques. *PLoS ONE* 2009; 4(3):e4733.

[28] Rathcke C N, Vestergaard H. YKL-40 an emerging biomarker in cardiovascular disease and diabetes. *Cardiovasc. Diabet.* 2009, 8.61-67.

[29] Coon J, Zurbig P, Dakna M, Dominiczak A, Decramer et al. CE-MS analysis of the human urinary proteome for biomarker discovery and disease diagnostics. *Proteomics Clin Appl* 2008; 2:964-973.

[30] Zimmerli LU, Schiffer E, Zürbig P, Good DM, Kellmann M, Mouls L, Pitt AR, Coon JJ, Schmieder RE, Peter KH, Mischak H, Kolch W, Delles C, Dominiczak AF. Urinary proteomic biomarkers in coronary artery disease. *Mol. Cell. Proteomics* 2008; 7: 290-298.

[31] Von zur Muhlen C, Schiffer E, Zuerbig P, Kellmann M, Brasse M, Meert N, Vanholder RC, Dominiczak AF, Chen YC, Mischak H, Bode C, Peter K. Evaluation of urine proteome pattern analysis for its potential to reflect coronary artery atherosclerosis in symptomatic patients. *J. Proteome Res* 2009; 8, 335-345.

[32] Floriano P N, Christodoulides N, Miller CS, Ebersole J., et al. Use of saliva-based nano biochip tests for acute myocardial infarction at the point of care: a feasibility study. *Clinical Chemistry* 2009, 55 (8), 1530-1538.

[33] Macaulay IC, Carr P, Gusnanto A, Ouwehand WH, Fitzgerald D, Watkins NA. Platelet genomics and proteomics in human health and disease. *J Clin Invest*. 2005, 115, 3370-3377.

[34] Fedorko ME, Hirsch JG: Structure of monocytes and macrophages. *Semin Hematol* 1970, 7(2):109-124.

[35] Johnston RBJ: Current concepts: immunology. Monocytes and macrophages. *N Engl J Med* 1988, 318(12):747-752.

[36] Taylor PR, Gordon S: Monocyte heterogeneity and innate immunity. *Immunity* 2003, 19(1):2-4.

[37] van der Wal AC, Becker AE, van der Loos CM, Das PK. Site of intimal rupture or erosion of thrombosed coronary atherosclerotic plaques is characterized by an inflammatory process irrespective of the dominant plaque morphology. *Circulation* 1994 ;89:36-44.

[38] Moreno PR, Falk E, Palacios IF, Newell JB, Fuster V, Fallon JT. Macrophage infiltration in acute coronary syndromes. Implications for plaque rupture. *Circulation* 1994; 90:775-8.

[39] Liuzzo, G., Vallejo, A. N., Kopecky, S. L., Frye, R. L. et al., Molecular fingerprint of interferon-gamma signaling in unstable angina. *Circulation* 2001, *103*, 1509–1514.

[40] Riese U, Brenner S, Do¨cke WD, Pro¨sch S, Reinke P, Oppert M, Volk HD, Platzer C. Catecholamines induce IL-10 release in patients suffering from acute myocardial infarction by transactivating its promoter in monocytic but not in T-cells. *Mol Cell Biochem*. 2000; 212:45–50.

[41] Falk E, Shah PK, Fuster V. Coronary plaque disruption. *Circulation* 1995;92:657-71.

[42] Matrisian LM. The matrix-degrading metalloproteinases. *Bioessays* 1992;14:455-63.

[43] Bauriedel G, Hutter R, Welsch U, Bach R, Sievert H, Luderitz B. Role of smooth muscle cell death in advanced coronary primary lesions: implications for plaque instability. *Cardiovasc Res* 1999; 41:480-8.

[44] Ming Jin, Philip T Diaz, Tran Bourgeois, Charis Eng, Clay B Marsh, and Haifeng M Wu. Two-dimensional gel proteome reference map of blood monocytes. *Proteome Sci.* 2006; 4: 16.

[45] Dupont A., Tokarski C., Dekeyzer O., Guihot A. L., Amouyel P., RolandoC., Pinet_F. Two-dimensional maps and databases of the human macrophage proteome and secretome. *Proteomics* 2004, 4, 1761-1778.

[46] Seong J.K., Kim D.K., Choi K.H.,Oh S.H., Kim K.S., Lee S.S., Um H.D. Proteomic analysis of the cellular proteins induced by adaptive concentrations of hydrogen peroxide in human U937 cells. *Exp. Mol. Med* 2002, 34, 374-378.

[47] Barderas MG, Tunon J, Darde VM, et al: Circulating human monocytes in the acute coronary syndrome express a characteristic proteomic profile. *J Proteome Research* 2007, 6:876-886).

[48] María G. Barderas, José Tuñón, Verónica M. Dardé, Fernando De la Cuesta, José J. Jiménez-Nácher, Nieves Tarín, Lorenzo López-Bescós, Jesús Egido and Fernando Vivanco. Atorvastatin modifies the protein profile of circulating human monocytes after an acute coronary syndrome. *Proteomics* 2009, *9,* 1982–1993.

[49] Stenberg PE, Hill RL. Platelets and megakaryocytes. In: Lee G, Foerster J, Lukens J, eds. *Wintrobe's Clinical Hematology.* Philadelphia, PA: Lippincott Williams & Wilkins; 1999:615-660.

[50] Macaulay IC, Carr P, Gusnanto A, Ouwehand WH, Fitzgerald D, Watkins NA. Platelet genomics and proteomics in human health and disease. *J Clin Invest*. 2005, 115, 3370-3377.

[51] Kieffer N, Guichard J, Farcet JP, Vainchenker W, Breton-Gorius J. Biosynthesis of major platelet proteins in human blood platelets. Eur J Biochem. 1987, 164:189-195.

[52] Weyrich AS, Dixon DA, Pabla R, et al. *Signal-dependent translation of a regulatory protein, Bcl-3, in activated human platelets.* Proc Natl Acad Sci U S A. 1998;95:5556-5561).

[53] Davi G, Patrono C. Platelet activation and atherotrhombosis. *N Engl J Med.* 2007, 357:2482-2494.

[54] Fuster V, Badimon L, Badimon JJ, et al. The pathogenesis of coronary artery disease and the acute coronary syndromes. *N Engl J Med.* 1992;326:242–250.

[55] FitzGerald DJ, Roy L, Catella F, et al. Platelet activation in unstable coronary disease. *N Engl J Med.* 1986;315:983–989.

[56] Chesebro JH, Rauch U, Fuster V, et al. Pathogenesis of thrombosis in coronary artery disease. *Haemostasis.* 1997;27(suppl 1):12–18.

[57] Massberg S, Schulz C, Gawaz M. Role of platelets in the pathophysiology of acute coronary syndrome. *Semin Vasc Med.* 2003 May;3(2):147-62.

[58] Marcus KG, Immler D, Sternberger J, Meyer HE. Identification of platelet proteins separated by two-dimensional gel electrophoresis and analyzed by matrix assisted laser desorption/ionization-time of flight-mass spectrometry and detection of tyrosine-phosphorylated proteins. *Electrophoresis* 2000, 21, 2622-2636.

[59] O'Neill EE, Brock CJ, von Kriegsheim AF, Pearce AC, Dwek RA, Watson SP, Hebestreit HF. Towards complete analysis of the platelet proteome. *Proteomics* 2002,2,288-305.

[60] Garcia A, Prabhakar S, Brock CJ, Pearce AC, Dwek RA, Watson SP, Hebestreit HF et al. Extensive analysis of the human platelet proteome by two-dimensional gel electrophoresis and mass spectrometry. *Proteomics* 2004, 4, 656-668.

[61] Angel Garcia, Sripadi Prabhakar, Sascha Hughan, Tom W. Anderson, Chris J. Brock, Andrew C. Pearce, Raymond A. Dwek,Steve P. Watson, Holger F. Hebestreit, and Nicole Zitzmann. Differential proteome analysis of TRAP-activated platelets *Blood*, 15 March 2004,vol 103, n° 6, 2088-2095.

[62] Garcia A. Proteomics analysis of signaling cascades in human platelets. *Blood Cells Mol Dis* 2006; 36:152-156.

[63] Zahedi RP, Lewandrowski U, Wiesner J et al. Phosphoproteomics of resting human platelets. *J Proteom Res* 2008, 7:526-534.

[64] Coppinger JA, Gagney G, Toomey S, et al. Characterization of the proteins releases from activated platelets leads to localization of novel platelet proteins in human atherosclerotic lesions. *Blood* 2004,; 103:2096-2104.

[65] Sacristan D, Marques M, Zamorano J et al. Modifications by Olmesartan medoxomil treatment of the platelet profile of moderate hypertensive patients. *Proteomics Clin Appl* 2008; 2:1300-1312.

[66] Simper D, Stalboerger PG, Panneta CJ et al. Smooth muscle progenitor cells in human cells. *Circulation* 2002, 106:1119-1204.

[67] Asahara T, Masuda H, Takahashi T, Kalka C, Pastore C, Silver M, Kearne M, Magner M, Isner JM. Bone marrow origin of endothelial progenitor cells responsible for postnatal vasculogenesis in physiological and pathological neovascularization. *Circ Res.* 1999;85:221–228.

[68] Asahara T, Murohara T, Sullivan A, Silver M, van der Zee R, Li T, Witzenbichler B, Schatteman G, Isner JM. Isolation of putative progenitor endothelial cells for angiogenesis. *Science.* 1997;275:964–967.

[69] Noishiki Y, Tomizawa Y, Yamane Y, Matsumoto A. Autocrine angiogenic vascular protesis with bone marrow transplantation. *Nat Med* 1996; 2:90-3.

[70] Reyes M, Dudek A, Jahagirdar B, et al. Origin of endothelial progenitors in human postnatal bone marrow. *J Clin Invest* 2002; 109:337-46.

[71] Shi Q, Rafii S, Wu MH, et al. Evidence for circulating bone marrow derived endothelial cells. *Blood* 1998; 92:362-7.

[72] Ikpeazu C, Davidson MK, Halteman D, Browning PJ, Brandt SJ. Donor origin of circulating endothelial progenitors alters allogenic bone marrow transplantation. *Biol Blood Marrow Transpl* 2000; 6:301-8.

[73] Rookmaaker MB, Tolboom H, Goldschmeding R et al. Bone marrow derived cells contribute to endothelial repair alters thrombotic micrioangiopathy. *Blood* 2002; 99:1095 letters.

[74] Reinisch A, Hohmann NA, Obenauf AC, Kashofer K, Rohde E, Schallmoser K, Flicker K, Lanzer G, Linkesch W, Speicher MR and Strunk D. Humanized large-scale expanded endothelial colony forming cells function in vitro and in vivo. *Blood* 2009 113: 6716-6725.

[75] Urbich C, Dimmeler S. Endothelial progenitor cells: characterization and role in vascular biology. *Circ Res.* 2004;95:343–353.)

[76] Hristov M, Erl W, Weber PC. Endothelial progenitor cells: mobilization, differentiation, and homing. *Arterioscler Thromb Vasc Biol.* 2003;23: 1185–1189.).

[77] Vasa M, Fichtlscherer S, Aicher A et al. Number and migratory activity of circulating endothelial progenitor cells inversely correlate with risk factors for coronary artery disease. *Circ Res* 2001; 89:E1-7.

[78] Eizawa T, Murakami Y, Matsui K et al. Circulating endothelial progenitor cells are reduced in haemodialysis patients. *Curr Med res Opin* 2003; 19:627-33.

[79] Eizawa T, Ikeda U, Murakami Y, et al. Decrease in circulating endothelial progenitors cells in patients with stable coronary artery disease. *Heart* 2004:90:685-6.

[80] Asahara T, Masuda H, Takahashi T, Kalka C, Pastore C, Silver M, Kearne M, Magner M, Isner JM. Bone marrow origin of endothelial progenitor cells responsible for postnatal vasculogenesis in physiological and pathological neovascularisation. *Circ Res.* 1999; 85:221–228.

[81] Cesari F, Nencini P, Nesi M, Caporale R, Giusti B, Abbate R, Gori AM and Inzitari D. Bone marrow-derived progenitor cells in the early phase of ischemic stroke: relation with stroke severity and discharge outcome. *J Cer Blood Flow & Met.* 2009; 29: 1983-1990.

[82] Matsumoto Y, Adams V, Walther C, Kleinecke C, Brugger P, Linke A, Walther T, Mohr FW and Schuler G. Reduced number and function of endothelial progenitor cells in patients with aortic valve stenosis: a novel concept for valvular endothelial cell repair. *Eur Heart J.* 2009 30: 346-355.

[83] Hu Y, Davison F, Zhang Z, Xu Q. Endothelial replacement and angiogenesis in arteriosclerotic lesions of allograft are contributed by circulating progenitor cells. *Circulation.* 2003; 108:3122–3127.

[84] Goldstein LB, Bertels C, Davis JN. Interrater reliability of the NIH Stroke Scale. *Arch Neurol.* 1989; 46:660–662.

[85] Muir KW, Weir CJ, Murray GD, Povey C, Lees KR. Comparison of neurological scales and scoring systems for acute stroke prognosis. *Stroke.* 1996; 27:1817–1820.

[86] Lambiase PD, Edwards RJ, Anthopoulos P, Rahman S, Meng YG, Bucknall CA, Redwood SR, Pearson JD, Marber MS. Circulating humoral factors and endothelial progenitor cells in patients with differing coronary collateral support. *Circulation.* 2004; 109:2986 –2992.

[87] Rustemeyer P, Wittkowski W, Greve B, Stehling M. Flow-cytometric identification, enumeration, purification, and expansion of CD133_ and VEGF-R2_ endothelial progenitor cells from peripheral blood. *J Immunoass Immunoch.* 2007; 28:13–23.

[88] Hristov M, Zernecke A, Schober A, Weber C. Adult progenitor cells in vascular remodelling during atherosclerosis *Biol Chem* 2008, 389:837-844.

[89] Giordano Pula,* Ursula Mayr,* Colin Evans, Marianna Prokopi, Dina S. Vara, Xiaoke Yin, Zoe Astroulakis, Qingzhong Xiao, Jonathan Hill, Qingbo Xu, Manuel Mayr. Proteomics Identifies Thymidine Phosphorylase As a Key Regulator of the Angiogenic Potential of Colony-Forming Units and Endothelial Progenitor Cell Cultures. *Circ. Res.* 2009;104;32-40.

[90] Polkinghorne VR, Standeven KF, Schroeder V, Carter AM. Role of proteomic technologies in understanding risk of arterial thrombosis. *Expert Rev Proteomics* 2009; 6(5):539-50.

[91] PilopC, Aregger F, Gorman RC, Brunisholz R, Gerrits B, Schaffner T et al. Proteomic analysis of patients with Marfan syndrome reveals increased activity of Calpain 2 in aortic aneurysms. *Circulation* 2009; 120:983-91.

[92] Urbonavicius S, Lindholr JS, Vorum H, Urbonaviciene G, Henneberg EW, Honoré B. Proteomic identification of differentially expressed proteins in aortic wall of patients with ruptured and nonruptured abdominal aortic aneurysms. *J Vasc Surg* 2009;49:455-63

[93] Dejouvencel T, Féron D, Rossignol P, Sapoval M, Kauffman C, Piot JM et al. Hemorphin 7 reflects hemoglobin proteolysis in abdominal aortic aneurysm. *Arterioscler Thromb Vasc Biol* 2010; 30:269-75.

[94] McDonough JL, Neverova I, Van Eyk JE. Proteomic analysis of human biopsy samples by single two-dimensional electrophoresis: Coomassie, silver, mass spectrometry, and Western blotting. *Proteomics* 2002; 2(8):978-87.

[95] Scobioala S, Klocke R, Kuhlmann M, Tian W, Hasib L, Milting H et al. Up-regulation of nestin in the infarcted myocardium potentially indicates differentiation of resident cardiac stem cells into various lineages including cardiomyocytes. *FASEB J* 2008; 22(4):1021-31.

[96] Liu B, Tewari AK, Zhang L, Green-Church KB, Zweier JL, Chen YR et al. Proteomic analysis of protein tyrosine nitration after ischemia reperfusion injury: mitochondria as the major target. *Biochim Biophys Acta* 2009; 1794(3):476-85.

[97] Nicolaou P, Rodriguez P, Ren X, Zhou X, Qian J, Sadayappan S et al. Inducible expression of active protein phosphatase-1 inhibitor-1 enhances basal cardiac function and protects against ischemia/reperfusion injury. *Circ Res* 2009; 104(8):1012-20.

[98] Chen CH, Budas GR, Churchill EN, Disatnik MH, Hurley TD, Mochly-Rosen D. Activation of aldehyde dehydrogenase-2 reduces ischemic damage to the heart. *Science* 2008; 321(5895):1493-5.

[99] Feng J, Zhu M, Schaub MC, Gehrig P, Roschitzki B, Lucchinetti E et al. Phosphoproteome analysis of isoflurane-protected heart mitochondria: phosphorylation

of adenine nucleotide translocator-1 on Tyr194 regulates mitochondrial function. *Cardiovasc Res* 2008; 80(1):20-9.

[100] Fert-Bober J, Basran RS, Sawicka J, Sawicki G. Effect of duration of ischemia on myocardial proteome in ischemia/reperfusion injury. *Proteomics* 2008; 8(12):2543-55

[101] Jacquet S, Yin X, Sicard P, Clark J, Kanaganayagam GS, Mayr M et al. Identification of cardiac myosin-binding protein C as a candidate biomarker of myocardial infarction by proteomics analysis. *Mol Cell Proteomics* 2009; 8(12):2687-99.

[102] Hynd MR, Lewohl JM, Scott HL, Dodd PR. Biochemical and molecular studies using human autopsy brain tissue. *J Neurochem* 2003; 85(3):543-62.

[103] Halushka MK, Cornish TC, Lu J, Selvin S, Selvin E. Creation, validation and quantitative analysis of protein expression in vascular tissue microarrays. *Cardiovascular Pathology In press*. 2010.

[104] Kane LA, Neverova I, Van Eyk JE. Subfractionation of heart tissue: the "in sequence" myofilament protein extraction of myocardial tissue. *Methods Mol Biol* 2007; 357:87-90.

[105] Lepedda AJ, Cigliano A, Cherchi GM, Spirito R, Maggioni M, Carta F et al. A proteomic approach to differentiate histologically classified stable and unstable plaques from human carotid arteries. *Atherosclerosis* 2009; 203(1):112-8.

[106] Emmert-Buck MR, Bonner RF, Smith PD, Chuaqui RF, Zhuang Z, Goldstein SR et al. Laser capture microdissection. *Science* 1996; 274(5289):998-1001.

[107] De la Cuesta F, Alvarez-Llamas G., Maroto A.S., Donado A., Juarez-Tosina R., Rodriguez-Padial L et al. An optimum method designed for 2-D DIGE analysis of human arterial intima and media layers isolated by laser microdissection. *Proteomics Clin.Appl.* 3, 1-11. 2009.

[108] Talusan P, Bedri S, Yang S, Kattapuram T, Silva N, Roughley PJ et al. Analysis of intimal proteoglycans in atherosclerosis-prone and atherosclerosis-resistant human arteries by mass spectrometry. *Mol Cell Proteomics* 2005; 4(9):1350-7.

[109] Kondo T, Hirohashi S. Application of highly sensitive fluorescent dyes (CyDye DIGE Fluor saturation dyes) to laser microdissection and two-dimensional difference gel electrophoresis (2D-DIGE) for cancer proteomics. *Nat Protoc* 2006; 1(6):2940-56.

[110] Wu J, Liu W, Sousa E, Qiu Y, Pittman DD, Maganti V et al. Proteomic identification of endothelial proteins isolated in situ from atherosclerotic aorta via systemic perfusion. *J Proteome Res* 2007; 6(12):4728-36.

[111] Nicolaou P, Rodriguez P, Ren X, Zhou X, Qian J, Sadayappan S et al. Inducible expression of active protein phosphatase-1 inhibitor-1 enhances basal cardiac function and protects against ischemia/reperfusion injury. *Circ Res* 2009; 104(8):1012-20.

[112] Chen CH, Budas GR, Churchill EN, Disatnik MH, Hurley TD, Mochly-Rosen D. Activation of aldehyde dehydrogenase-2 reduces ischemic damage to the heart. *Science* 2008; 321(5895):1493-5.

[113] Feng J, Zhu M, Schaub MC, Gehrig P, Roschitzki B, Lucchinetti E et al. Phosphoproteome analysis of isoflurane-protected heart mitochondria: phosphorylation of adenine nucleotide translocator-1 on Tyr194 regulates mitochondrial function. *Cardiovasc Res* 2008; 80(1):20-9.

[114] De Souza AI, McGregor E, Dunn MJ, Rose ML. Preparation of human heart for laser microdissection and proteomics. *Proteomics* 2004; 4(3):578-86.

[115] De la Cuesta F, Alvarez-Llamas G., Maroto A.S., Donado A., Juarez-Tosina R., Rodriguez-Padial L et al. An optimum method designed for 2-D DIGE analysis of human arterial intima and media layers isolated by laser microdissection. *Proteomics Clin.Appl.* 3, 1-11. 2009.

[116] Bagnato C, Thumar J, Mayya V, Hwang SI, Zebroski H, Claffey KP et al. Proteomics analysis of human coronary atherosclerotic plaque: a feasibility study of direct tissue proteomics by liquid chromatography and tandem mass spectrometry. *Mol Cell Proteomics* 2007; 6(6):1088-102.

[117] Sung HJ, Ryang YS, Jang SW, Lee CW, Han KH, Ko J. Proteomic analysis of differential protein expression in atherosclerosis. *Biomarkers* 2006; 11(3):279-90.

[118] You SA, Archacki SR, Angheloiu G, Moravec CS, Rao S, Kinter M et al. Proteomic approach to coronary atherosclerosis shows ferritin light chain as a significant marker: evidence consistent with iron hypothesis in atherosclerosis. *Physiol Genomics* 2003; 13(1):25-30.

[119] Slevin M, Elasbali AB, Miguel TM, Krupinski J, Badimon L, Gaffney J. Identification of differential protein expression associated with development of unstable human carotid plaques. *Am J Pathol* 2006; 168(3):1004-21.

[120] Donners MM, Verluyten MJ, Bouwman FG, Mariman EC, Devreese B, Vanrobaeys F et al. Proteomic analysis of differential protein expression in human atherosclerotic plaque progression. *J Pathol* 2005; 206(1):39-45.

[121] Garcia A, Senis YA, Antrobus R, Hughes CE, Dwek RA, Watson SP et al. A global proteomics approach identifies novel phosphorylated signaling proteins in GPVI-activated platelets: involvement of G6f, a novel platelet Grb2-binding membrane adapter. *Proteomics* 2006; 6(19):5332-43.

[122] Maguire PB, Wynne KJ, Harney DF, O'Donoghue NM, Stephens G, Fitzgerald DJ. Identification of the phosphotyrosine proteome from thrombin activated platelets. *Proteomics* 2002; 2(6):642-8.

[123] Howes JM, Keen JN, Findlay JB, Carter AM. The application of proteomics technology to thrombosis research: the identification of potential therapeutic targets in cardiovascular disease. *Diab Vasc Dis Res* 2008; 5(3):205-12.

[124] Kline KG, Frewen B, Bristow MR, Maccoss MJ, Wu CC. High quality catalog of proteotypic peptides from human heart. *J Proteome Res* 2008; 7(11):5055-61.

[125] Bousette N, Kislinger T, Fong V, Isserlin R, Hewel JA, Emil A et al. Large-scale characterization and analysis of the murine cardiac proteome. *J Proteome Res* 2009; 8(4):1887-901.

[126] Tjalsma H, Bolhuis A, Jongbloed JD, Bron S, van Dijl JM. Signal peptide-dependent protein transport in Bacillus subtilis: a genome-based survey of the secretome. *Microbiol Mol Biol Rev* 2000; 64(3):515-47.

[127] Hathout Y. Approaches to the study of the cell secretome. *Expert Rev Proteomics* 2007; 4(2):239-48.

[128] Huang CM, Ananthaswamy HN, Barnes S, Ma Y, Kawai M, Elmets CA. Mass spectrometric proteomics profiles of in vivo tumor secretomes: capillary ultrafiltration sampling of regressive tumor masses. *Proteomics* 2006; 6(22):6107-16.

[129] Xue H, Lu B, Lai M. The cancer secretome: a reservoir of biomarkers. *J Transl Med* 2008; 6:52.

[130] Mbeunkui F, Fodstad O, Pannell LK. Secretory protein enrichment and analysis: an optimized approach applied on cancer cell lines using 2D LC-MS/MS. *J Proteome Res* 2006; 5(4):899-906.

[131] Pellitteri-Hahn MC, Warren MC, Didier DN, Winkler EL, Mirza SP, Greene AS et al. Improved mass spectrometric proteomic profiling of the secretome of rat vascular endothelial cells. *J Proteome Res* 2006; 5(10):2861-4.

[132] Colzani M, Waridel P, Laurent J, Faes E, Ruegg C, Quadroni M. Metabolic labeling and protein linearization technology allow the study of proteins secreted by cultured cells in serum-containing media. *J Proteome Res* 2009; 8(10):4779-88.

[133] Alvarez-Llamas G, Szalowska E, de Vries MP, Weening D, Landman K, Hoek A et al. Characterization of the human visceral adipose tissue secretome. *Mol Cell Proteomics* 2007; 6(4):589-600.

[134] Zwickl H, Traxler E, Staettner S, Parzefall W, Grasl-Kraupp B, Karner J et al. A novel technique to specifically analyze the secretome of cells and tissues. *Electrophoresis* 2005; 26(14):2779-85.

[135] Chevallet M, Diemer H, Van DA, Villiers C, Rabilloud T. Toward a better analysis of secreted proteins: the example of the myeloid cells secretome. *Proteomics* 2007; 7(11):1757-70.

[136] Chan XC, McDermott JC, Siu KW. Identification of secreted proteins during skeletal muscle development. *J Proteome Res* 2007; 6(2):698-710.

[137] Strande V, Canelle L, Tastet C, Burlet-Schiltz O, Monsarrat B, Hondermarck H. The proteome of the human breast cancer cell line MDA-MB-231: Analysis by LTQ-Orbitrap mass spectrometry. *Proteomics Clin.Appl.* 3, 41-50. 2009.

[138] Yu L, Guo Y, Zhang Z, Li Y, Li M, Li G et al. SecretP: A new method for predicting mammalian secreted proteins. *Peptides* 2010; In press.

[139] Lawlor K, Nazarian A, Lacomis L, Tempst P, Villanueva J. Pathway-based biomarker search by high-throughput proteomics profiling of secretomes. *J Proteome Res* 2009; 8(3):1489-503.

[140] Gronborg M, Kristiansen T, Iwahori A, Chang R, Reddy R, Sato N et al. Biomarker discovery from pancreatic cancer secretome using a differential proteomic approach. *Mol.CellProteomics* 5, 157-71. 2006.

[141] Roelofsen H, Dijkstra M, Weening D, de Vries MP, Hoek A, Vonk RJ. Comparison of isotope-labeled amino acid incorporation rates (CILAIR) provides a quantitative method to study tissue secretomes. *Mol Cell Proteomics* 2009; 8(2):316-24.

[142] Liu H, Sadygov RG, Yates JR, III. A model for random sampling and estimation of relative protein abundance in shotgun proteomics. *Anal Chem* 2004; 76(14):4193-201.

[143] Strande V, Canelle L, Tastet C, Burlet-Schiltz O, Monsarrat B, Hondermarck H. The proteome of the human breast cancer cell line MDA-MB-231: Analysis by LTQ-Orbitrap mass spectrometry. *Proteomics Clin.Appl.* 3, 41-50. 2009.

[144] Lawlor K, Nazarian A, Lacomis L, Tempst P, Villanueva J. Pathway-based biomarker search by high-throughput proteomics profiling of secretomes. *J Proteome Res* 2009; 8(3):1489-503.

[145] Yoon JH, Yea K, Kim J, Choi YS, Park S, Lee H et al. Comparative proteomic analysis of the insulin-induced L6 myotube secretome. *Proteomics* 2009; 9(1):51-60.

[146] Colzani M, Waridel P, Laurent J, Faes E, Ruegg C, Quadroni M. Metabolic labeling and protein linearization technology allow the study of proteins secreted by cultured cells in serum-containing media. *J Proteome Res* 2009; 8(10):4779-88.

[147] Dupont A, Corseaux D, Dekeyzer O, Drobecq H, Guihot AL, Susen S et al. The proteome and secretome of human arterial smooth muscle cells. *Proteomics* 2005; 5(2):585-96.

[148] Duran MC, Mas S, Martin-Ventura JL, Meilhac O, Michel JB, Gallego-Delgado J et al. Proteomic analysis of human vessels: application to atherosclerotic plaques. *Proteomics* 2003; 3(6):973-8.

[149] Martin-Ventura JL, Duran MC, Blanco-Colio LM, Meilhac O, Leclercq A, Michel JB et al. Identification by a differential proteomic approach of heat shock protein 27 as a potential marker of atherosclerosis. *Circulation* 2004; 110(15):2216-9.

[150] Martin-Ventura JL, Tunon J, Duran MC, Blanco-Colio LM, Vivanco F, Egido J. Vascular protection of dual therapy (atorvastatin-amlodipine) in hypertensive patients. *J Am Soc Nephrol* 2006; 17(12 Suppl 3):S189-S193.

[151] Duran MC, Martin-Ventura JL, Mohammed S, Barderas MG, Blanco-Colio LM, Mas S et al. Atorvastatin modulates the profile of proteins released by human atherosclerotic plaques. *Eur J Pharmacol* 2007; 562(1-2):119-29.

[152] Delbosc S, Haloui M, Louedec L, Dupuis M, Cubizolles M, Podust VN et al. Proteomic analysis permits the identification of new biomarkers of arterial wall remodeling in hypertension. *Mol Med* 2008; 14(7-8):383-94.

[153] Stastna M, Chimenti I, Marban E, Van Eyk JE. Identification and functionality of proteomes secreted by rat cardiac stem cells and neonatal cardiomyocytes. *Proteomics* 2010; 10(2):245-53.

[154] Stastna M, Abraham MR, Van Eyk JE. Cardiac stem/progenitor cells, secreted proteins, and proteomics. *FEBS Lett* 2009; 583(11):1800-7.

[155] Gnecchi M, Zhang Z, Ni A, Dzau VJ. Paracrine mechanisms in adult stem cell signaling and therapy. *Circ Res* 2008; 103(11):1204-19.

[156] Grainger DJ. Metabolic profiling in heart disease. *Heart Metab*. 2006; 32:22-25.

[157] Teul J, Ruperez FJ, Garcia A, Vaysse J, Balayssac S, Gilard V, Malet-Martino M, Martin-Ventura JL, Blanco-Colio LM, Tuñon J, Egido J, Barbas C. Improving metabolite knowledge in stable atherosclerotic patients by association and correlation of GC-MS and $^1$H NMR fingerprints. *J. Proteome Res*. 2009;8:5580-5589.

[158] Leo GC, Darrow AL. NMR-based metabolomics of urine for the atherosclerotic mouse model using apolipoprotein-E deficient mice. *Magn. Reson. Chem* 2009; DOI 10.1002/mrc.2470

[159] Sabatine MS, Liu E, Morrow DA, Heller E, McCarroll R, Wiegand R, Berriz GF, Roth FP, Gerszten RE. Metabolomic identification of novel biomarkers of myocardial ischemia. *Circulation* 2005;112:3868-3875.

[160] Lewis GD, Wei R, Liu E, Yang E, Shi X, Martinovic M, Farrell L, Asnani A, Cyrille M, Ramanathan A, Shaham O, Berriz G, Lowry PA, Palacios IF, Tasan M, Roth FP, Min J, Baumgartner C, Keshishian H, Addona T, Mootha VK, Rosenzweig A, Carr SA, Fifer MA, Sabatine MS, Gerszten RE. Metabolite profiling of blood from individuals undergoing planned myocardial infarction reveals early markers of myocardial injury. *J. Clin. Invest* 2008;118:3503-3512.

[161] Zhang F, Jia Z, Gao P, Kong H, Li X, Chen J, Yang Q, Yin P, Wang J, Lu X, Li F, Wu Y, Xu G. Metabonomics study of atherosclerosis rats by ultra fast liquid chromatography coupled with ion trap-time of flight mass spectrometry. *Talanta* 2009;79:836-844.

In: Ventricular Fibrillation and Acute Coronary Syndrome
Editor: Joyce E. Mandell

ISBN: 978-1-61728-969-9
© 2011 Nova Science Publishers, Inc.

*Chapter III*

# MAJOR BLEEDING IN ACUTE CORONARY SYNDROME: DEFINITIONS, MAGNITUDE OF THE PROBLEM, PREDICTORS, OUTCOMES, MANAGEMENT, AND PREVENTION

*Douraid K. Shakir and Jassim Al Suwaidi**
Department of Cardiology and Cardiovascular Surgery,
Hamad Medical Corporation (HMC), Doha, Qatar

## ABSTRACT

Acute coronary syndrome forms the vast majority of cases seen in daily cardiology clinical practice. It is usually managed using antiplatelet, antithrombotic, and anticoagulation agents, all of which are double-edged swords that also increase the risk of bleeding with an associated increase in morbidity and mortality. Predicting the occurrence of major bleeding and preventing it may help save lives, improve outcomes, and reduce costs. The definition of major bleeding in acute coronary syndrome poses a great challenge when using data from studies and registries around the world to explore the magnitude, predictors, and management of this problem. Different definitions have resulted in inconsistent prevalence and outcomes data. In this chapter, we explore these issues based on data extracted from a large number of clinical trials and registries, and suggest strategies to address this serious complication of acute coronary syndrome management.

## INTRODUCTION

Coronary heart disease (CHD) is the most common cause of death globally [1]. In the USA, CHD accounted for nearly one in every six deaths in 2006, representing 425,425

---

* Correspondence: Jassim Al Suwaidi, MB, ChB, FACC, FSCAI, FESC, Director of the Cardiac Catheterization Laboratory, Department of Cardiology and Cardiovascular Surgery, Hamad General Hospital (HMC), P.O Box 3050, Doha, Qatar, Tel: +974-4392464, Fax: +9744392454

deaths, and CHD is the number one cause of mortality for both men and women. In an estimate for 2010, nearly 785,000 Americans will have a new coronary artery event, around 470,000 will have a recurrent attack, and an additional 195,000 will suffer a silent myocardial infarction (MI). Every 25 seconds an American will suffer a coronary event and each minute one patient will die from it [2]. As a primary diagnosis for hospitalization, acute coronary events accounted for 733,000 of hospital discharges in 2006; while when reported as a secondary cause of discharge, the number rose to 1,365,000 [2]. In the United Kingdom, cardiovascular disease (CVD) accounts for 198,000 deaths each year, which translates to one in five deaths for men, and one in six deaths for women. In England, the prevalence of CHD was 6.5% in men and 4% in women, while 3.4 million people in the UK reported having experienced angina or a heart attack, and CVD was the second most commonly reported longstanding illness in Great Britain [3]. The death rates from CHD in Eastern and Central Europe have substantially increased, accounting for 4.35 million deaths each year.

Acute coronary syndrome (ACS) consists of unstable angina (UA) and myocardial infarction (both ST-segment elevation [STEMI] and non-ST-segment elevation [NSTEMI]). It represents the largest contributor to mortality in CHD and accounts for the vast majority of cases seen daily in cardiology clinical practice. ACS is triggered by atherosclerotic plaque rapture and exposure of the arterial media, which leads to platelet activation and aggregation, thrombin activation, and occlusive thrombus formation [4]. Embolization of microthrombi to distal vascular beds causes myocardial ischemia and its sequelae [5]. The primary goal in the management of ACS is to prevent thrombus formation or its expansion, and hence reduce the burden of ischemia. This is often achieved through the liberal use of antiplatelet, antithrombotic, and thrombolytic agents in various combinations and regimens. However, these agents represent double-edged swords; enhancing recovery but also increasing risk of bleeding along with an associated increase in mortality and morbidity [6]. Increasing awareness of the association between major bleeding and adverse outcomes in ACS has resulted in reports showing that approximately 5% of ACS cases have major bleeding in the 30 days following the primary event [7-11]. This complication thus needs to be seriously addressed to reverse its adverse effects on outcomes in ACS.

Predicting and preventing the occurrence of major bleeding are the first steps toward saving lives, improving outcomes, and reducing costs. Extensive data exploring the magnitude, predictors, and management of major bleeding in ACS are available from studies and registries around the world. However, the wide variation in the definitions of major bleeding in ACS seen across different studies complicates the use of these data in delineating predictors of major bleeding in ACS or estimating its incidence and impact on outcomes. In this chapter, we discuss these issues and derive conclusions based on data from a large number of major clinical trials and registries.

## DEFINITIONS OF MAJOR BLEEDING IN ACS

The definition of major bleeding is of great importance, since the incidence and magnitude of this complication are significantly altered by the different classifications and definitions currently in use. The wide variation in data derived using definitions based on laboratory criteria compared to those that emphasize clinical parameters has prompted recent recommendations to combine these two definitions. Two main definitions have been widely used to classify bleeding in ACS:

1. In the thrombolysis in myocardial infarction (TIMI) study group [12], "Hemorrhage was defined as "major" if there was a reduction of hemoglobin of 5 g/dl or more (or >15% in hematocrit) or any intracranial bleeding. Hemorrhage was classified as "minor" if there was an observed blood loss and a drop in hemoglobin of 3 to 5 g/dl (or in hematocrit from 10% to 15%) from study entry to the time of the lowest hemoglobin (hematocrit) and this was within 10 days; if there was spontaneous gross hematuria or hematemesis (>120 ml), even if the hemoglobin or hematocrit drop was less than 3 g or less than 10%, respectively; or if there was an unobserved loss 4 g/dl or more in hemoglobin or 12% or more in hematocrit. Blood loss attributable to revascularization or other surgical procedures was not classified as a TIMI hemorrhagic event."
2. In the global use of strategies to open occluded coronary arteries (GUSTO) trial [13], "Bleeding complications were classified as severe or life-threatening if they were intracerebral or if they resulted in substantial hemodynamic compromise requiring treatment. Moderate bleeding was defined by the need for transfusion. Minor bleeding referred to other bleeding, not requiring transfusion or causing hemodynamic compromise."

The TIMI definition relies primarily on laboratory values with a few clinical parameters, whereas the GUSTO definition was based exclusively on clinical indicators. Other less commonly used definitions of major bleeding in ACS are shown in Table 1. The PARAGON study (Platelet IIb/IIIa Antagonism for the Reduction of Acute coronary syndrome events in a Global Organization Network) defined bleeding as major or life threatening if there was any intracranial hemorrhage, bleeding requiring transfusion, or a decrease in hemoglobin of $\geq 5$ g/dl (or decrease in hematocrit $\geq 15\%$) [14]. In the ACUITY trial (acute catheterization and urgent intervention triage), Manoukian et al. [15] defined major bleeding as any intracranial or intraocular bleeding; access site bleeding requiring intervention; a 5-cm diameter hematoma; hemoglobin reduction of 4 g/dl without or 3 g/dl with an overt source; any reoperation for bleeding; or requirement for blood product transfusion. In a case-control study, Karjalainen et al defined major bleeding as a hemoglobin decrease of $\geq 4.0$ g/dl, transfusion of $\geq 2$ units of blood products, need for corrective surgery, or intracranial or retroperitoneal hemorrhage [16]. The OASIS-2 study (organization to assess strategies in acute ischemic syndrome) defined bleeding as life-threatening if it was fatal, intracranial, required surgical intervention or $\geq 4$ units of blood or plasma expanders; major if it required transfusion of 2 to 3 units or was judged to be disabling; and all other bleeds regarded as minor [17]. Other definitions of bleeding in ACS have emerged from studies such as the CRUSADE (Can rapid risk stratification of unstable angina patients suppress adverse outcome with early implementation [18]), ISTH (international society on thrombosis and hemostasis [19]), CURE trial (clopidogrel in unstable angina to prevent recurrent ischemic events [20]), STEEPLE (safety and efficacy of enoxaparin in percutaneous coronary intervention patients [21]), OASIS-6 [22], HORIZONS study [23], and the REPLACE-2 trial [24].

## Table 1. Definitions of major bleeding used in clinical trials.

| Study/ Registry | Degree of bleeding | Definition of bleeding |
|---|---|---|
| TIMI [12] | Major | Reduction of hemoglobin of 5 g/dl or more (or > 15% in hematocrit) or any intracranial bleeding |
| | Minor | Observed blood loss and a drop in hemoglobin of 3 to 5 g/dl (or in hematocrit from 10 to 15%) from study entry to the time of the lowest hemoglobin |
| | Minimal | Clinical overt hemorrhage with a < 3 g/dl decrease in the hemoglobin or < 9 % decrease in hematocrit. |
| GUSTO [13] | Severe or life-threatening | Intracranial bleeding with hemodynamic compromise requiring intervention |
| | Moderate | Bleeding requiring blood transfusion not associated with hemodynamic compromise. |
| | Mild | All other bleeding events. |
| Cure [100] | Life-threatening | Bleeding episode was fatal or led to a reduction in the hemoglobin level of at least 5 g/dl or to substantial hypotension requiring use of intravenous inotropic agents, necessitated a surgical intervention, was a symptomatic intracranial hemorrhage, or necessitated transfusion of 4 or more units of blood |
| | Minor | Bleeding episodes included other hemorrhages that led to the interruption of the study medication |
| PARAGON–B [101] | Major or life-threatening | Intracranial hemorrhage or bleeding with hemodynamic compromise requiring intervention |
| | Intermediate | Bleeding requires blood transfusion or a decrease in hemoglobin of > 5 g/dl or a decrease in hematocrit of > 15%. |
| Canadian ACS registry [45] | Major | Blood transfusion of > 2 units of packed red blood cells, or a decrease of > 10% in hematocrit or fatal hemorrhage. |
| PRISM-PLUS [102] | Major | Decrease in hemoglobin level by > 4g/dl, the need of > 2 units of blood for transfusion, the need for corrective surgery, intracranial, retroperitoneal hemorrhage, or any combination of these. |
| | Mild | All other bleeding complications. |
| GRACE registry [10] | Major | Life-threatening bleeding necessitates blood transfusion of ≥ 2 units of packed red blood cells, or bleeding that resulting in ≥ 10% decrease in hematocrit, death, hemorrhagic, or subdural hematoma. |
| ACUITY study [81] | Major | Intracranial or intraocular bleeding, hemorrhage at access site requiring intervention, hematoma ≥ 5 cm, hemoglobin fall ≥ 4 g/dl without overt bleeding site or ≥ 3g/dl with source, reoperation for bleeding, or transfusion of blood products. |
| OASIS-5 [66] | Major | Fatal, intracranial, retroperitoneal, intraocular leading to loss of vision, hemoglobin fall ≥ 3 g/dl adjusted for transfusion, or transfusion of 2 units of blood |
| | Minor | Any clinically significant bleeding not meeting major criteria leading to study drug interruption, surgery, or transfusion of one unit of blood. |
| Suggested Standardized definition [30] | Red ( essential for all studies) | Clinical bleeding events, date/time of the diagnosis Location- gastrointestinal, genitourinary, intracranial, vascular access site, and other related to a procedures yes/no<br>Laboratory parameters: record dates and times of values and most recent hemoglobin value before bleeding is recognized. Lowest hemoglobin value within 24 hours after onset of bleeding has been recognized, change in hemoglobin associated with clinical events.<br>Consequences of bleeding: death related to bleeding (yes/no), blood transfusion type, number of units, associated with overt bleeding (yes/no), hemoglobin value at the time of transfusion, date and times of administration, resulted in permanent disability (yes/no). |
| | Orange (recommended for all studies) | Bleeding resulted in discontinuation of therapy (yes/no), bleeding prompted dose alteration of therapy (yes/no). |
| | Green (optional for all studies) | Bleeding resulted in hemodynamic compromise (yes/no), bleeding resulted in increase length of stay (yes/no)(number of hospital days added, number of intensive care unit days added), hemoglobin decrease associated with procedures. |

Rao et al. [25] compared the two major definitions (TIMI and GUSTO). The median time from the primary event to the most severe TIMI bleeding was 1 day, compared to 2 days in GUSTO. There were 1151 patients who met the GUSTO criteria but did not meet TIMI criteria, while 765 patients met the TIMI criteria but did not meet the GUSTO bleeding criteria. Using the TIMI classification, 12.7% had minimal bleeding, 8.5% had minor bleeding and 8.2% had major bleeding while in GUSTO the classification 19.2% had mild bleeding, 11.4% had moderate bleeding, and only 1.2% had major bleeding. There was a graded increase in the short and intermediate-term adverse outcomes correlating with GUSTO classes but not with TIMI classes after adjusting for background risk factors. There were also stepwise increases in the 30-day and 6-month mortality and rates of MI with worsening GUSTO class, but no significant association with the TIMI classification. The authors concluded that, in predicting outcomes, assessment of major bleeding based on clinical criteria is more important than laboratory-based criteria [25]. The PURSUIT trial also used the two classifications in the assessment of major bleeding [26]. Using the TIMI classification, the incidence of major bleeding was 10.6% in the eptifibatide arm vs. 9.1% in the placebo group. In contrast, the GUSTO classification placed the incidence of severe bleeding at 1.5 and 0.9% respectively in the eptifibatide and placebo group. In the SYNERGY trial, the incidence of major bleeding was 7.6-9.1% using the TIMI scale, and 2.2-2.7% using the GUSTO scale [27]. The same finding was seen in the PRISM-PLUS study in which the two classifications also showed different incidences [28]. These figures illustrate the wide variation caused by different classifications used in these trials, and suggest that the laboratory-based definitions result in higher estimates of incidence while the clinically-based definitions may better predict outcomes. It is also interesting to note that there is a substantial group of patients who satisfy one definition and not the other.

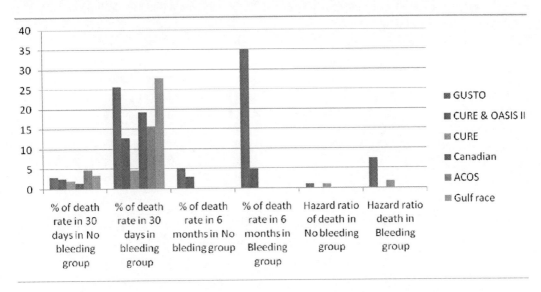

Figure 1. Comparison of 30-day and 6-month mortality among different studies

Seto et al. [29] found that centers also differ widely in their definitions and reporting of major bleeding depending on the size of the center. Small centers had less precise definitions for bleeding and less reporting compared to bigger centers that have more rigid definitions and higher reporting. This further elaborates for the need for a unified definition for major bleeding as well as stricter reporting. To provide consistency, the Academic Bleeding Consensus proposed a standardized reporting system for bleeding complications in clinical investigations of ACS [30]. They analyzed the existing evidence on bleeding in ACS and its impact on clinical outcomes. Criteria for the assessment of bleeding were then developed by an expert panel that suggested dividing bleeding-related events to be reported in the clinical trials into three categories (Table 1):

1. Red category includes clinical data on bleeding events, laboratory parameters, and the consequences of bleeding (essential for all studies).
2. Orange category includes everything in the red category plus whether bleeding resulted in discontinuation or alteration of therapy (recommended for all studies).
3. Green category includes the red and orange criteria plus whether bleeding resulted in hemodynamic instability, disability, increased length of stay or a decrease in hemoglobin (optional for all studies).

## MAGNITUDE OF THE PROBLEM

As discussed in the previous section, the incidence of major bleeding in ACS varies among different trials, ranging from 0.7 to 19.2% [17, 31]. The incidence was 3.9% in the GRACE study [10], 15% in TIMI-1 [32], and 4.1% in TIMI-2 [33]. The death rates in ACS complicated by major bleeding also varied widely, ranging from 0.1 to 38% in different trials [11, 31]. These huge discrepancies are primarily due to the different definitions used in the trials as evidenced by the trials that compared the TIMI and GUSTO definitions [25-28]. Another contributing factor is the difference in drug regimens used: monotherapy vs. dual or triple combinations, the doses used with or without loading doses, and the duration of use of antiplatelet, anticoagulant, or thrombolytic agents. The availability of interventional facilities at the site also plays a role in increasing bleeding complications. Patient characteristics including age, presence of comorbidities, renal function, Killip class at presentation, GRACE score, and the type of ACS event also play a role in the different rates of major bleeding in various clinical studies (Tables 2, 3, and 4).

## PREDICTORS OF MAJOR BLEEDING

A large number of trials have studied the predictors of major bleeding in an attempt to anticipate and prevent this complication in daily clinical practice (Table 4).

## Table 2. Major clinical trials identifying incidence and mortality rates for major bleeding in ACS

| Study | Study Type | No. of Pts. | Patient Type | Invasive Proc. (%) | Year | Follow-Up | Prevalence of Bleeding (%) | Mean age (y) | Mortality in Patients with Bleeding (%) |
|---|---|---|---|---|---|---|---|---|---|
| Prism-Plus[28] | RCT | 1915 | UA & NSTEMI | | 1994-1996 | 6 months | 3-4% With TIMI 1.4-0.8% | 63±11 | |
| Yusuf [20] | RCT | 12 562 | ACS | | 1998-2000 | 12 months | 3.7% | 64.2±11.3 | 0.2% |
| Oasis -2 [17] | RCT | 10 141 | ACS | | 1996-1998 | 7 days | 0.7-1.2% | 64 | 0.1% |
| GUSTO IIb [103] | RCT | 12 142 | MI & ACS | | 1994-1995 | Up to 1 year | All bleeding 9% in both arms | 63 | |
| PURSUIT Trial [26] | RCT | 10 948 | ACS | | 1995-1997 | 30 days | TIMI scale 9.1-10.9 GUSTO scale 9.9-14.8 | 64 | |
| PRISM Trial [104] | RCT | 3232 | ACS | | 1994-1996 | 3 days | Major bleeding 0.4% Intracranial bleeding 0.1% | | |
| SYNERGY Trial [27] | RCT | 10027 | NSTEMI | 46.5% | 2001-2003 | 30 days | TIMI 9.1% GUSTO 2.7% | 68 | |
| GRACE study [10] | GRACE | 24,045 | ACS | | 2003 | In-hospital | 3.9% (4.8%, STEMI; 4.7%, NSTEMI; 2.3%, unstable angina) | 71.1 | 18.6 (22.8 STEMI, 15.3 NSTEMI, 16.1 unstable angina) |
| Eikelboom et al. [38] | Registry + 2 RCT† (OASIS, OASIS-2, CURE) | 34,146 | NSTEMI-ACS | 28-38 | 2006 | 6 months | 2.3% | 67.9 | 5.3 (at 3 months) |
| Rao SV et al. [31] | 2 RCT (PURSUIT, PARAGON) | 15,454 | NSTE-ACS | 43-69.4 | 2006 | 6 months | TIMI (12.7%, 8.5%, 8.2%‡) GUSTO (19.2%, 11.4%, 1.2%‡) | 65≈ | 24.9% (TIMI severe) 59.5% (GUSTO severe, defined as death or MI) |
| Al Mallah et al. [105] (Gastrointestinal bleeding only) | Registry | 3045 | ACS | 40-44.9 | 2006 | In-hospital | 3% | 64.8-70.1 | 36% |
| Klein et al. [37] | ACOS registry | | | | 2007 | | 1.7% | 74.6 | |
| Manoukian et al. [9] | RCT (ACUITY) | 13,819 | Moderate to high risk ACS | 63-70 | 2007 | 30 days | 3%-5.7%* | | 7.3% |
| Mortensen et al. [36] | Registry (Danish) vs. RCT (CURE) | 195/ 6259 | NSTE-ACS | 81.5-35.4% | 2008 | 6 months | 17.6% | 68± 12.4 | NA |
| Yan AT et al. [11] | RCT (INTERACT) | 746 | High-risk NSTE-ACS | ≈60% | 2008 | 2.4 years | 4.6%, HR§ 3.48, P value 0.003 | 71 | 38% |
| Al Sallami H et al. [106] | Retrospective study | 446 | NSTE-ACS | 74-79 | 2008 | In-hospital | 10.5% | 71 | NA |
| Mehran R et al. [107] | ACUITY | 13,819 | Moderate to high risk NSTE-ACS | 100 | 2009 | 30 days | 4.7% | 63-70 | |
| Nikolsky E et al. [108] (Gastrointestinal bleeding only) | ACUITY | 13,819 | Moderate to high risk NSTE-ACS | PCI (56.3-60.1) | 2009 | 30 days | 1.3% | 63-70 | 9.6% |

## Table 2. (continued)

| Study | Study Type | No. of Pts. | Patient Type | Invasive Proc. (%) | Year | Follow-Up | Prevalence of Bleeding (%) | Mean age (y) | Mortality in Patients with Bleeding (%) |
|---|---|---|---|---|---|---|---|---|---|
| Budaj A et al. [42] | OASIS-5 | 20,078 | ACS | | | 180 days | 4.9% | 66.3-72.4 | 14.3% |
| Spencer et al. [35] | | 40,087 | AMI | 52% | 2007 | 180 days | 2.8% | 74 | 10% |
| Oldgren et al. [34] | Registry | 14,732 | AMI | | 2009 | | 1.4%-4 | | |
| Sorensen R et al. [109] | Registry | 40812 | AMI | 29.1% | 2000-2005 | 476.5 days | | | |
| Gulf RACE [40] | Registry | 8166 | ACS | 11.8 % | 2009 | In-hospital | 0.83% | 63 | 27.9 % |

Abbreviations: ACS, acute coronary syndrome; ACUITY, Acute Catheterization and Urgent Intervention Triage Strategy; AMI, acute myocardial infarction; CURE, Clopidogrel in Unstable angina to prevent Recurrent Events; GUSTO, Global Use of Strategies To Open occluded coronary arteries; GRACE, Global Registry of Acute Coronary Events; INTERACT, INTegrilin and Enoxaparin Randomized assessment of the Acute Coronary syndrome Treatment; NA, not available; OASIS, Organization to ASsess Ischemic Syndromes registries; PARAGON, Platelet IIb/IIIa Antagonism for the Reduction of Acute coronary events in a Global Organization Network; PCI, Percutaneous Coronary Intervention; PURSUIT, Platelet Glycoprotein IIb/IIIa inhibitor in Unstable angina: Receptor Suppression Using Integrilin Therapy; RBC, red blood cells; TIMI, Thrombolysis In Myocardial Infarction.
* Heparin plus Glycoprotein IIb/IIIa inhibitor inhibitors (GPI) vs. bivalirudin monotherapy.
† Combining data from OASIS, OASIS-2, and CURE. ‡ Severe bleeding. § HR Hazard ratio

## Age

Advanced age is one of the strongest predictors of major bleeding in ACS as established by numerous studies (Table 3). In the GRACE trial [10], the mean age among bleeders was 71.1 (range 61.5-79.5 years) compared to 66.2 years in non-bleeders (OR 1.28, $p < 0.001$), and older patients, particularly those $\geq 80$ years, were at higher risk. The same was reported in SWEDEHEART [34], by Spencer et al. [35] with mean age of 74 years (range 64-81, $p < 0.001$), the Real-Life study (mean age $68 \pm 12.4$ years) [36], and the German ACOS trial [37] with a mean age of 74.6 years (range 66-79 years). The INTERACT trial [11] also reported a mean age of 71 years for bleeders, while Eikelboom et al. [38] reported a mean age of $67.9 \pm 10.4$ years ($p < 0.0001$). Because most of the participants in the Gulf RACE study were young immigrant workers, they reported a younger age distribution of 53-72 years (mean 63 years) among bleeders compared to 47-65 years (mean 55 years) among non-bleeders. In all the studies, advanced age correlated with higher risk of major bleeding. Possible explanations for this include baseline changes in hemostasis with advance age, changes in sensitivity to drugs, and altered pharmacokinetics.

## Table 3. Predictors of major bleeding in major clinical trials

| Predictor | Non-bleeders | Bleeders | P value Ppp |
|---|---|---|---|
| Age in Years | | | |
| GRACE study [10] median age, years | 66.2 years | 71.1 years | <0.001 |
| Age ( per 10-year increase) | | OR 1.28 | <0.0001 |
| ACUITY trial [9] | | 67.6 years | <0.001 |
| Canadian ACSR [45](n) | 66 | 75 | <0.001 |
| Canadian ACSR [45] (per 10 years) OR | | 1.8 | <0.0001 |

## Table 3. (continued)

| Predictor | Non-bleeders | Bleeders | P value Ppp |
|---|---|---|---|
| **Age in Years** | | | |
| INTERACT trial [11] | 63 | 71 | 0.01 |
| ACOS [37] | | 74.6 years | |
| Al-Sallami H et al. [110] | 71 | 71 | NS |
| Eikelboom JW et al. [38] | 63.7±11.2 | 67.9±10.4 | <0.0001 |
| Rao et al. [31] | 63.8 | 70 | <0.001 |
| Gulf RACE [40] | 55(47-65) | 63(53-72) | <0.0001 |
| **Gender** | | | |
| GRACE study [10] | | | |
| Female sex% | | OR 1.43 | <0.0001 |
| ACUITY trial [9] | | | |
| Female sex% | | 7.6% | <0.001 |
| Canadian ACSR [45] | | | |
| Female sex % | 34.8 | 41.8 | 0.2 |
| INTERACT trial [12] | | | |
| Female % | 30.8 | 41.2 | 0.2 |
| ACOS [37] equal sex distribution | | | |
| Sorensen R et al. [109] male % | | 63% | HR 1.33 |
| Eikelboom JW et al. [32] | | | |
| Female% | 38.4% | 38.8% | 0.82 |
| Rao et al. [25] | | | |
| Female% | 33.1% | 37.5 | <0.001 |
| Gulf RACE [40] | | | |
| Male% | 76.5% | 75.7 | NS |
| Mortensen, J et al Real life study [36] female % | | 38.5% | |
| **History of bleeding** | | | |
| GRACE study [10] | | OR 2.83 | <0.0001 |
| GRACE study [35] % | 1.1 | 3.7 | <0.001 |
| Sorensen R et al. [109]% | 4% | 14.3% | HR 2.46 |
| Rao et al. [25]% | 4.5% | 10.4% | <0.001 |
| **Renal insufficiency** | | | |
| GRACE study [10]OR | | OR 1.48 | 0.0004 |
| ACUITY trial [9] Cr.cl ml/min | | 77 | <0.001 |
| Canadian ACSR [45] Cr.cl ml/min | 90 | 104 | 0.002 |
| Canadian ACSR [45] OR (per every 10 units increase) | | 1.02 | 0.026 |
| INTERACT trial [12] Cr µmol/L | 86 | 97 | 0.02 |
| ACOS [37]% | | 9.9% | 0.0001 |
| Sorensen R et al. [109] (%) | 1.1% | 2.5% | HR 1.35 |
| Budaj A et al. [42] Cr µmol/L | | 102 | <0.001 |
| Al-Sallami H et al. [110] mean Cr.cl ml/min | 60 | 54 | |
| Eikelboom JW et al. [32] Cr µmol/L | 94.3±33.7 | 104.2±43.1 | <0.0001 |
| Rao et al. [25] % | 0.7% | 2% | <0.001 |
| Gulf RACE [40] Cr µmol/L | 0.97 | 1.17 | 0.0003 |
| **STEMI** | | | |
| GRACE study [10]% | | 4.8% | <0.001 |
| ACUITY trial [9] n(%) | | 290 (6%) | <0.001 |
| Canadian ACSR [45] (%) | 18.4 | 36.7 | <0.0001 |
| Canadian ACSR [45] OR | | 1.52 | 0.10 |
| INTERACT trial [12] % | 22.4 | 24.2 | 0.8 |
| ACOS [37]% | | 50.4% | NS |
| Gulf RACE [40] % | 39% | 60.3% | 0.002 |
| **Killip class IV** | | | |
| GRACE study [10]% | | 13.1% | <0.001 |
| Canadian ACSR [45]% | 15.4 | 28.9 | 0.01 |
| Canadian ACSR [45] OR | | 1.61 | 0.08 |
| INTERACT trial [12] % | 0.8 | 3 | 0.01 |
| Budaj A et al. [42]% | | 7.6% | <0.001 |
| Rao et al. [25]% | 1.3% | 3.9% | <0.001 |
| Gulf RACE [40] % | 8.8% | 2.1% | <0.0001 |
| **Grace score** | | | |
| Gulf RACE [40]% | 32% | 58% | 0.0004 |

## Table 3. (continued)

| Predictor | Non-bleeders | Bleeders | P value Ppp |
|---|---|---|---|
| **Weight BMI kg/m$^2$** | | | |
| GRACE study [10] | 26.9 | 26.2 | <0.001 |
| Al-Sallami H et al. [110] | 27.5 | 26.6 | |
| Rao et al. [25] median Weight Kg | 77 | 76 | <0.001 |
| **Anemia** | | | |
| ACUITY trial [9] Mean (SD) | | 13.3 (2) | <0.001 |
| INTERACT trial [12] mean Hb g/L | 142 | 131 | 0.001 |
| GRACE study [10]% | 96.4% | 3.6% | <0.05 |
| REPLACE -2 [24] | 2.8% | 4.9% | 0.0001 |
| **Cardiac Markers** | | | |
| ACUITY trial [9] n (%) | | 414 (5.5) | <0.001 |
| INTERACT trial [12] CK-MB ng/dl | 84.8 | 73.5 | 0.08 |
| Gulf RACE [40] TnT ng/dl | 0.77 | 2.6 | 0.0027 |
| **Diabetes Mellitus** | | | |
| GRACE study [10]% | 3.7% | 4.4% | 0.03 |
| Canadian ACSR [45] DM% | 25.8 | 36.4 | 0.04 |
| INTERACT trial [12]% | 22.6 | 23.4 | 0.90 |
| ACOS [37]% | | 34.8% | NS |
| Sorensen R et al. [109]% | 4.4% | 6.6% | HR 1.03 |
| Eikelboom JW et al. [32]% | 21.6% | 25% | 0.02 |
| Rao et al. [25] % | 20% | 29% | <0.001 |
| Gulf RACE [40] % | 40.4% | 42.6% | 0.71 |
| **Arterial pressure** | | | |
| GRACE study [10]OR | | OR 1.11 | 0.0016 |
| Canadian ACSR [45]OR | | 1.72 | 0.05 |
| INTERACT trial [12] mean sys BP mm Hg | 134 | 133 | 0.83 |
| INTERACT trial [12] mean dia BP mm Hg | 77 | 77 | 0.87 |
| ACOS [37]% | | 75.2% | |
| Budaj A et al. [42] mean sys BP mm Hg | | 138.8 | 0.17 |
| Budaj A et al. [42] mean dia BP mm Hg | | 77.7 | 0.002 |
| Al-Sallami H et al. [110] mean BP mm Hg | 89.3 | 86.3 | |
| Rao et al. [25]% | 51% | 60.3% | <0.001 |
| Gulf RACE [40]% | 49.4% | 57.4% | 0.23 |
| **Thrombolytic therapy** | | | |
| GRACE study [10] OR | | OR 1.43 | 0.0017 |
| Eikelboom JW et al. [32]% | 1.1% | 2% | 0.009 |
| Gulf RACE [40] % | 58% | 54% | 0.61 |
| **Heparin** | | | |
| GRACE study [10]% | 95.4% | 4.6% | <0.001 |
| ACOS [37]% | | 71.6% | |
| Budaj A et al. [42]% | | 35.8% | <0.001 |
| Eikelboom JW et al. [32]% | 51% | 56.8% | 0.001 |
| Gulf RACE [40]% | 58% | 54% | 0.61 |
| **LMWH** | | | |
| GRACE study [10] OR | | OR 0.7 | <0.0001 |
| INTERACT trial [12] % | 51.5 | 38.2 | 0.13 |
| ACOS [37]% | | 34.8% | |
| Eikelboom JW et al. [32]% | 20.4% | 28% | <0.0001 |
| Gulf RACE [40]% | 47% | 41% | 0.44 |
| **Aspirin** | | | |
| GRACE study [10] % | 96.3% | 3.7% | <0.001 |
| ACOS [37] % | | 81% | |
| Budaj A et al. [42] % | | 94% | 0.17 |
| Al-Sallami H et al. [110] % | 62% | 72% | |
| Gulf RACE [40] % | 98% | 92% | 0.011 |
| **Clopidogrel** | | | |
| Gulf RACE [40] % | 53% | 61% | 0.25 |
| INTERACT trial [12] % | 15.3 | 26.5 | 0.08 |
| ACOS [37] % | | 64.5% | |
| Budaj A et al. [42] % | | 66% | <0.001 |
| Al-Sallami H et al. [110]% | | | |

| | | | |
|---|---|---|---|
| Al-Sallami H et al. [110]% | 64% | 60% | |
| GPIIa/IIIb | | | |
| GRACE study [10] OR | | OR 1.93 | <0.0001 |
| ACOS [37] % | | 45.4% | |
| Al-Sallami H et al. [110] % | 19% | 17% | |
| Eikelboom JW et al. [32] % | 1.6% | 3.7% | < 0.0001 |
| Gulf RACE [40] % | 11% | 15% | 0.3 |
| Coronary intervention | | | |
| GRACE study [10] | | OR 1.63 | <0.0001 |
| ACUITY trial [9] n (%) | | 460 (5.9) | <0.001 |
| Canadian ACSR [45] (%) | 18.2 | 21.5 | 0.44 |
| INTERACT trial [12] % | 28.8 | 26.5 | 0.77 |
| Sorensen R et al. [109] % | 37.3% | 29.1 | HR 0.88 |
| Al-Sallami H et al. [110] % | 74% | 79% | |
| Eikelboom JW et al. [32] % | 10.4% | 11.2% | 0.46 |
| Rao et al. [25] % | 15.8% | 16.6% | <0.001 |
| Gulf RACE [40] % | 11.7% | 11.8% | NS |
| Diuretics | | | |
| GRACE study [10] OR | | 1.69 | <0.0001 |
| Sorensen R et al. [109] % | 37.5% | 57.5% | HR 1.49 |
| Inotropic agents | | | |
| GRACE study [10] OR | | 2.05 | <0001 |
| Sorensen R et al. [109] % | 0.8% | 1.2% | HR 0.94 |
| Vasodilators | | | |
| GRACE study [10] OR | | 1.35 | 0.0068 |
| Right heart catheterization | | | |
| GRACE study [10] OR | | 2.48 | <0.0001 |

OR= Odd ratio, HR= hazard ratio

## Gender

Gender was inconsistently found to be a predictor of major bleeding in different trials (Table 3). In the GRACE trial, females had a higher bleeding tendency (5 vs. 3.3%, OR 1.43, $p < 0.0001$) compared to males [10]. A similar female predominance was reported by Spencer et al. [35] and in the SWEDEHEART trial [34]. In contrast, the ACUITY trial [39] reported more major bleeding in males with $p < 0.0001$ as did Ferguson et al., who reported a male predominance with $p < 0.001$ [27]. In the Real-Life study, Mortensen et al. also reported a higher proportion of males among bleeders at 61.5% [36]. Other studies such as the German ACOS trial [37] and Eikelboom et al. [38] reported equal gender distribution for major bleeding in ACS events. These differences could be explained by differences in socio-economic status and demographics of the populations studied. In the Gulf RACE trial, for example, young male expatriate workers constituted more than half of the study participants [40], which represents a great demographical difference from the populations in other studies.

## History of Bleeding

Prior history of bleeding was also identified as a risk for major bleeding in patients with ACS (Table 3). This was reported in GRACE trial [10], in which the incidence of major bleeding in those who had a bleeding history was 11.5% compared to 3.8% in those with no previous history ($p < 0.0001$). Spencer et al. [35] also reported an increased risk of bleeding in patients with ACS from 1.1% in non-bleeders to 3.7% in previous bleeders. Increased awareness and reporting history of bleeding in ACS trials may draw more attention to this important risk factor.

**Table 4. Major bleeding and hospital outcomes**

| Hospital outcome | Mortality | One year mortality | Congestive heart failure | Re-infarction | Mechanical ventilation | Stroke | Recurrent ischemia | Median hospital stay (days) | Cardiogenic shock | Others |
|---|---|---|---|---|---|---|---|---|---|---|
| Gulf RACE [40] | 23% P value <0.0001 | | 48% P value <0.0001 | 8% P value <0.0001 | 32% P value <0.0001 | 8% P value <0.0001 | | 8 days P value <0.0001 | 29% P value <0.0001 | |
| Meta-analysis Rao et al. [25] | 25.7%, HR 10.6 | 35.1%, HR 7.5 | | 32.7% 1-month | | | | | | |
| Meta-analysis OASIS-1, OASIS-2, CURE Eikelboom et al. [32] | 12.8-4.6% in 1-6 months | | | 10.6-1.6% in 1-6 months | | 2.6-0.8% in 1-6 months | | | | |
| GRACE study [10] | 20.9% OR 1.64, HR 1.9 | | | | | | | | | |
| ACUITY trial [107] | 7.3% HR 7.55 for early mort. | HR 3.5 P <0.001 | | 14.6% | | | | | | Stent thrombosis is 3.4% |
| Canadian ACSR [45] | OR 9.82 <0.0001 | P OR 3.92 P < 0.0001 | | | | | | | | |
| INTERACT trial [12] | HR 3.48 P value 0.003 | | | | | | | | | |
| ACOS [37] Budaj A et al. [42] | 15.6% 21% | | 21% | | | 1.7% 3% P value <0.0001 | 8.3% P value <0.0001 | 15 | 20% | |
| Kinnaird et al. [43] | 7.5% HR 5.3 | | | | | | Higher rate | Longer stay | | |
| REPLACE-2 [24] | 13% | 16.7% | | | | | | | | |
| OASIS-5 [66] | 13.2% | | | | | | 3.5% | 11.9% | | |

OR= Odd ratio, HR= hazard ratio

## Renal Impairment

Renal impairment is another strong predictor of major bleeding in ACS patients. The GRACE trial [10] reported an increase in major bleeding from 3.8% in patients with normal renal function to 11.5% in patients with renal impairment (p < 0.001), and Spencer et al. [35] reported a similar increase from 7.7 to 14% respectively. As for the level of renal impairment, Fox et al. [41] reported higher incidence of major bleeding in patients receiving enoxaparin over fondaparinux for non-ST-segment elevation ACS among patients with renal dysfunction especially in those with GFR less than 58 ml/min/1.7m$^2$, and Budaj et al. [42] reported significant increase in major bleeding in those with GFR less than 63.6 ml/min (p <0.001).

Other studies, including the INTERACT trial [11], ACUITY trial [9, 39], the German ACOS trial [37], Eikelboom et al. [38], Gulf RACE study [40], and Mortensen et al. [36] also report the association between major bleeding in ACS and renal impairment (Table 3). Renal impairment is reported as an independent risk factor for major bleeding with an odds ratio of 1.48-1.53 in different trials [10, 43, 44]. The increased incidence of bleeding may be related to the hematological abnormalities that are associated with impaired renal function. These include decreased activity of platelet factor III, abnormal platelet adhesiveness and aggregation, and impaired prothrombin consumption. Each of these factors can contribute to increased risk of bleeding, prolonged bleeding, or spontaneous GI bleeding. Impaired renal excretion of drugs such as low molecular weight heparins and the resulting prolonged half-life also increase the risk of bleeding.

Table 5. Bleeding sites in ACS major bleeding

| Study/Registry | Cerebral | Gastrointestinal | Respiratory | Urogenital | Puncture site | Post OP | retroperitoneal | others |
|---|---|---|---|---|---|---|---|---|
| Sorensen R et al. [109] | 35(30.4%) | 34(29.6%) | 1(0.9%) | 2(1.7%) | 39(33.9%) | --- | --- | --- |
| OASIS-2 [17] | --- | 38(0.3%) | 3(0.02%) | 11(0.1 %) | 6(0.05%) | 15(0.1%) | 6(0.05 %) | 14(0.1 %) |
| Gulf RACE [40] | 10.3% | 50% | 3 % | 26.5% | --- | --- | --- | 9.4% |
| Yusuf S et al. [20] | --- | 83(1.3 %) | | 4(0.1 %) | 36(0.6 %) | 56(0.9 %) | 8(0.1 %) | |

## Type of ACS

Among the different constituents of ACS, most clinical trials reported that STEMI is a strong predictor of major bleeding since it is usually treated more aggressively. Thrombolytic therapy is often combined with antiplatelet agents, and more invasive interventions, leading to a higher incidence of major bleeding. The GRACE trial [10] reported a significantly higher incidence of major bleeding in STEMI and NSTEMI compared to UA (4.8 and 4.7% vs. 2.3% respectively, p < 0.001). Spencer et al. [35] reported that 58% of bleeders had STEMI vs. 42% for NSTEMI (p <0.001), while the ACUITY trial [9, 39] reported 45% (p < 0.0001), and the INTERACT trial [11] reported 44.8% (p = 0.03). Other trials including the German ACOS trial [37] and the Gulf RACE study [40] also reported significantly higher incidence of major bleeding in STEMI (Table 3). The consistently higher rates of major bleeding in STEMI are due to the more intensive use of medications such as fibrinolytics and platelet GP IIb/IIIa inhibitors, combined with higher use of invasive procedures in STEMI.

## Killip Class

The patient's cardiopulmonary status at the time of the ACS event plays a big role in predicting major bleeding as evidenced by the fact that Killip class III or IV correlates with increased major bleeding events. This was seen in the GRACE trial [10], in which 13.1% of patients with major bleeding were classified as advanced Killip class with p < 0.001. The Canadian ACS registry [45] also reported more patients with major bleeding had advanced

Killip class (28.9 vs. 15.4%, OR 1.61, p = 0.01). The INTERACT trial [11], Budaj et al. [42], and Rao et al. [32] also support a role for advanced Killip class in increased risk of major bleeding (Table 3). Patients with advanced Killip class receive more intensive therapy and invasive procedures which leads to more major bleeding events.

The same applies for increased GRACE score, which was associated with an increase major bleeding events in Gulf RACE study [40].

## Diabetes Mellitus

Diabetes mellitus (DM) is studied intensively as it is a growing problem globally. Its complications include impaired renal function with nephropathy and proteinuria, which drastically affects the coagulation system and endothelial functions. Comorbidities ranging from increased body weight to hypertension and atherosclerosis also lead to increased incidence of major bleeding in ACS. A large number of studies reported the association between DM and major bleeding (Table 3), but there are discrepancies in whether its presence significantly affects outcomes in ACS patients. No study has shown DM to be an independent risk factor for major bleeding in ACS through a multi-variate analysis; thus, its effects must be investigated further. There are many other factors that increase bleeding tendency in DM. DM is associated with the development of celiac disease and malabsorption, which affects the clotting factor synthesis [46]; and some oral hypoglycemic agents such as glibenclamide, have been reported to increase bleeding tendency [47]. Wolfram syndrome, a congenital abnormality that is linked to DM has increased bleeding tendency [48]. Immunosuppression therapy in renal transplantation suppresses bone marrow activity and thus platelet production. Finally, there are many reports indicating some changes in hemostatic and fibrinolytic activities in DM [49, 50].

## Choice of Antiplatelet, Antithrombotic, and Fibrinolytic Agents

All the medications used in the management of ACS inhibit thrombosis and platelet function, and thus increase the risk of bleeding. Many trials have studied the impact of different agents on major bleeding (Table 3). Although the protocols used, doses, duration of use, and varying combinations of these drugs all play a role in precipitating major bleeding, their impact and significance is unclear due to discrepancies among different clinical trials (Table 3). This is discussed further later in this chapter.

## Invasive Procedures

Coronary interventions and right heart catheterizations increase major bleeding as reported in many clinical trials (Table 3). Medications used in the procedures including heparins and GP IIb/IIIa inhibitors, the use of higher loading doses of antiplatelet agents, and the puncture site wound from the procedure itself, all contribute to increased incidence of major bleeding.

## Blood Transfusion

Major bleeding leads to hypoxemia secondary to hypoperfusion, hypotension, and anemia. The liberal use of blood transfusions to avoid morbidity and mortality, however, was associated with adverse outcomes in many studies of ACS with major bleeding [51-54], and the adverse effects increased with the number of units transfused [52, 55]. Decreased tissue oxygenation [56-58] due to decreased nitric oxide in stored blood, as well as vasoconstriction and increase in platelet aggregation have been reported [59, 60]. ACS mortality at 30 days was increased 3- to 4-fold in the transfused group compared to those without transfusion [53]. Rao et al. [53] and Yang et al. [54] reported increased mortality, and myocardial infarctions. The mechanism by which transfusion adversely affects outcomes in major bleeding in ACS is mainly attributed to prolonged storage, which leads to functional and structural changes in red blood cells. Decreased levels of 2,3-bisphosphoglycerate, nitric oxide, and adenosine triphosphate, as well as reduced deformability of red blood cells, all lead to decrease in oxygen delivering capacity to tissues, vasoconstriction, tissue ischemia, and inflammation [60-64]. Blood transfusion also increases infection rates, stimulates immune reactions, results in total volume increases, and increases blood viscosity.

## Anemia

Many trials demonstrate that hemoglobin level at the time of an ACS event may be a factor in precipitating major bleeding [9-11]. Higher incidence of bleeding complications was reported in those with low or high hemoglobin, while hemoglobin levels between 14-16 g/dl were associated with lower bleeding in a J-shaped relationship [65]. Anemia is also an independent risk factor for major adverse cardiovascular events in both STEMI and NSTEMI; with increased mortality and heart failure at hemoglobin levels below 14 g/dl in STEMI, while in NSTEMI, the same is seen with hemoglobin below 11 g/dl [65]. Drop in hemoglobin on day 9 increases the risk of death, MI, and stroke, yet blood transfusion are also potentially dangerous [66]. Aronson et al. [67] reported that 50% of admitted ACS patients had a drop in hemoglobin of > 1.3 g/dl due to oozing from procedure site or occult loss. The discharge hemoglobin level was a major predictor of increased death and heart failure rates. Anemia can increase the inflammatory response and affect myocardial remodeling through higher oxygen consumption, increased diastolic wall stress, accelerated myocardial cell loss, and neuro-hormonal activation [67]. In a review of anemia in ACS, Voeltz et al. [68] noticed that around 40% of ACS patients developed some degree of anemia, which was a major risk factor for bleeding, transfusion, cardiovascular events, mortality, prolonged hospital stay, and increased cost.

## HOSPITAL OUTCOMES AND MAJOR BLEEDING

Outcomes for patients hospitalized with ACS are greatly affected by the occurrence of major bleeding. The mortality of ACS at 1, 3, and 6 months, and at 1 year increases with increasing incidence of major bleeding, ranging from 0.1-38%, OR 1.64-3.92 (Tables 2 and

4). Both major and minor bleeding are associated with increased mortality and morbidity in ACS, with a graded worsening of outcomes in those with more serious bleeding [38, 43]. A multivariate analysis of the ACUTY trial [69] at 1 year found that major bleeding was a stronger predictor of mortality compared to peri-procedural MI (hazards ratio 2.89 vs. 2.47). Both congestive heart failure and re-infarction rates are increased in ACS patients with major bleeding (21-48% and 8-50%, respectively, all the increases were statistically significant, Table 4). The rates of the cardiogenic shock were also significantly increased by major bleeding (20-29% with significant p-values). These complications may be due to anemia, hypotension, overuse of inotropic agents, and the associated tachycardia. Rates of mechanical ventilation are also higher in major bleeding (32%), and incidence of stroke also increases from 0.8-8% with significant impact on outcomes. This is mostly due to use of drugs at higher doses or in combinations. Increase in the length of hospital stay (8 to 15 days) due to complications of major bleeding has effects ranging from increased rates of hospital-acquired infections to increased costs and overuse of hospital resources.

## Mechanisms by Which Major Bleeding Affects Outcomes

Many mechanisms have been suggested to explain how major bleeding affects outcomes in ACS. Anemia as a consequence of bleeding, results in a decrease in oxygen delivery to vital organs, including the already vulnerable myocardium, thereby exacerbating ischemia. Hypotension from loss of a large amount of blood (especially from non-compressible areas) also compounds hypoxemia and hypo-perfusion of the vital organs including the myocardium. Both hypotension and bleeding lead to activation of the sympathetic nervous system, release of noradrenalin, endothelin, vasopressin, and exaggeration of inflammatory response, all of which result in increased platelet activation, adhesion, and increased thrombosis. Thus discontinuation or dose adjustment of antiplatelet, anticoagulant, and fibrinolytic agents to minimize bleeding will promote continuation of thrombotic events thus increasing ischemia and its sequelae. In addition to these direct mechanisms, other drawbacks of major bleeding are the increase in the length of hospital stay, which is associated with increased risk of hospital-acquired infections and adverse effects of blood transfusions as discussed above.

## Prevention and Management

The main goal in the management of major bleeding in ACS is to minimize its adverse effects on total body hemodynamic integrity and oxygenation, and preventive measures should form the corner stone of any management strategy. Most reviews suggest that appropriate antithrombotic or antiplatelet agent selection with proper dose adjustment in the context of careful selection and matching of patients with procedures and protocols may help to reduce the incidence of major bleeding.

Dosing and combination of antithrombotic therapies plays a significant role in the incidence of major bleeding. In his review of the CURE trial [70], Peters et al. found a dose-dependent increase in major bleeding without an increase in efficacy as the dose of aspirin was increased. The same review found that post-CABG bleeding was only reduced when clopidogrel was stopped 5 days prior to the procedure. Triple therapy with aspirin, clopidogrel and unfractionated heparin (UFH) led to increased incidence of major bleeding (GRACE investigators, [71]). The ISAR-REACT 2 randomized trial [72] used quadruple therapy with aspirin, clopidogrel, UFH and abciximab, a platelet glycoprotein IIb/IIIa inhibitor (GPI). At 30 days, the mortality, MI rates, and urgent target vessel revascularization were significantly lower in the abciximab arm compared to placebo, with no significant difference in major bleeding as measured by blood transfusion requirements. The TARGET trial [73] used the same quadruple strategy and found no significant differences in major bleeding between abciximab and another GPI, tirofiban. The CRUSADE trial [18] however, reported that excessive dosing of UFH, low molecular weight heparin (LMWH) or GPIs, led to increased major bleeding and mortality in those who received the GPI, and increased length of hospital stay in those on high doses of LMWH or GPI. In a meta-analysis of UFH use in PCI, higher doses and higher active clotting times (ACT, a measure of UFH effect) were associated with increased incidence of minor and major bleeding, with linear increase as ACT increased [74]. Weight-indexed dosing of UFH was independently associated with higher bleeding rates for each 10 units/kg (OR 1.04, $p = 0.001$). The SYNERGY trial [27] studied the effect of LMWH on major bleeding and found no difference between LMWH and UFH in all causes of mortality at 30 days, and higher rates of major bleeding. Dose adjustment for UFH in the GUSTO IIb trial led to a decreased rate of bleeding [75] as was the case for LMWH in patients with renal impairment [76, 77], suggesting that appropriate dosing, timing, and careful combination of agents can impact the incidence of major bleeding.

Glycoprotein IIb/IIIa inhibitors are superior to UFH in reducing the adverse effects of ongoing ischemia. Aguirre et al. [78] compared abciximab used as an infusion or bolus doses to placebo on a base of UFH and aspirin. There were more major bleeds in the infusion group than the bolus arm, with the lowest incidence in the placebo group ($p < 0.001$). The need for blood transfusions was also significantly increased in the abciximab group [78]. These complications can be avoided if lower doses of UFH are used, as in the EPILOG study (Evaluation in PTCA to Improve Long Term Outcome with Abciximab GP IIb/IIIa Blockade) [79]. Minor bleeding was lower in GPI group, also depending on the dose and protocol used for UFH.

Newer agents may also help in decreasing the incidence of major bleeding. Use of the direct thrombin inhibitor, bivalirudin is associated lower risk of bleeding in ACS than UFH or GPI, with non-inferior outcomes for ischemia. In the REPLACE-2 trial, bivalirudin and GPI was compared to UFH and GPI in a PCI protocol, with significant reduction in major bleeding and lower one-year mortality in patients who received bivalirudin and GPI [9, 24, 80-82]. A multivariate analysis of the ACUTY trial [69] at one year found that the incidence of major bleeding in PCI patients was lower in bivalirudin monotherapy compared to UFH and GPI. In a review by same group [81] looking at non-CABG bleeding, there was a 47% reduction in bleeding and superiority in the net clinical outcomes in the bivalirudin group compared to UFH and GPI. PROTECT-TIMI 30 [83] showed better coronary flow reserve, lower minor and major bleeding complications and lower transfusion requirements in the bivalirudin group. OASIS-2 investigators [17] compared lepirudin (a recombinant hirudin) to UFH in the management of NSTEMI. The lepirudin group had significantly lower cardiovascular mortality, re-infarction rates, and refractory angina, but there was a significant increase in major bleeding that required blood transfusion in the lepirudin group. Fondaparinux sodium is a synthetic pentasaccharide that inhibits activated factor X. This agent was evaluated in OASIS-5 [41, 66] in patients with UA or NSTEMI and showed significantly decreased incidence of major bleeding, with better short-term outcomes as measured by MI, recurrent ischemia, and mortality. Interestingly, this was more prominent in patients with renal impairment. However, there were more catheter thromboses that led to use UFH during PCI procedures. Fondaparinux use in STEMI was studied in OASIS-6 [22] and it significantly reduced risk of death, re-infarction at 30 days, with lower major bleeding (HR 0.83).

New antiplatelet agents are now also emerging. Prasugrel is a thienopyridine pro-drug that requires conversion to an active metabolite before binding to the platelet P2Y12 receptor. It inhibits adenosine diphosphate more rapidly and consistently than clopidogrel. In TRITON-TIMI 38 [84], a randomized, double-blind trial for patients scheduled for PCI, prasugrel 60 mg loading dose was compared to clopidogrel 300 mg, with maintenance doses of 10 mg prasugrel and 75 mg clopidogrel with up to 15 months follow up. The prasugrel group had significantly lower rates of MI, urgent target vessel revascularization and stent thrombosis, but there was an increase in major bleeding events (HR 1.32, $p = 0.03$). There was also a significant increase in life-threatening bleeding, including both fatal and nonfatal bleeding. Ticagrelor is a reversible and direct acting oral P2Y12 receptor antagonist that provides greater and more consistent platelet inhibition than clopidogrel. The PLATO trial [85], a double-blind study compared ticagrelor (180 mg loading dose followed by 90 mg twice daily) and clopidogrel (300-600 mg loading and 75 mg maintenance dose) in the management of ACS with 12 months follow up. Cardiovascular death, MI and stroke were significantly lower in ticagrelor arm (HR 0.84, $p = 0.0025$), with no difference in major bleeding. Cangrelor, an adenosine triphosphate analogue, is an intravenous antiplatelet agent that reversibly binds to and inhibits P2Y12 ADP receptor. In the CHAMPION PLATFORM trial [86], a randomized, double-blind, placebo-controlled trial, in the setting of PCI, the rate of stent thrombosis and mortality from any cause were both significantly decreased in cangrelor group. There was an increase in major bleeding due to groin hematomas in the cangrelor group.

Procedural protocols in different institutions also affect the rates of major bleeding. Higher risk of bleeding with femoral punctures vs. the radial approach [87, 88], has prompted certain centers to increase use of the radial approach to more than 98% of PCI cases. Bigger puncture sites also lead to more site bleeding [89]. Use of arterial puncture closing devices did not decrease the risk of puncture site bleeding but was associated with increased hematoma size and pseudo-aneurysm formation [90]. Longer procedure times significantly increase the risk of developing a major bleed [78], as does the use of devices such as intra-aortic balloon counter pulsation [43]. From this discussion, radial puncture with smaller size sheath, shorter procedures, and avoiding intra-aortic balloons or closure devices may decrease the risk of major bleeding [91].

Major bleeding from gastrointestinal sites can be minimized through the use of proton pump inhibitors (PPIs) as Chan et al. [92] demonstrated using a combination of aspirin and esomeprazole in patients with history of gastrointestinal bleeding. The same finding was reported by Ng et al. [93]. There are many reports suggesting the inhibitory effect of PPIs on clopidogrel. Gilard et al. [94] found that omeprazole significantly decreased clopidogrel's inhibitory effect on platelet P2Y12 as assessed by the VASP phosphorylation test. Pantoprazole may be superior to omeprazole in patients receiving clopidogrel to avoid any potential negative interaction with CYP2C19 [95]. In their report dated November 17, 2009 [96], the Food and Drug Administration suggested that some PPIs and cimetidine should be avoided for the time being until further reports become available. New antiplatelet agents such as prasugrel may be the agents of choice as they require less dose adjustment with PPIs [97]. In contrast, a meta-analysis of 13 studies showed no significant association between PPI use and overall mortality (RR 1.09, 95% CI 0.94 -1.26, p = 0.23). Clinicians should thus weigh the potential harm from ulcers and hemorrhage with the risk of ACS before stopping clopidogrel [98].

In many trials, hemodynamic stability in major bleeding is achieved using blood transfusion, but this increases the risk of morbidity and mortality [53, 54]. The increase in worse outcomes is directly related to the number of units transfused, thus aggressive blood transfusion is not recommended in ACS, even with low hemoglobin levels [61]. Although erythropoietin increases the RBC mass when used in renal failure, is does not help in the acute setting of ACS and it was associated with increased cardiovascular events [99]. It thus has no role in the management of anemia associated with ACS.

## CONCLUSION

Major bleeding represents a serious complication that adversely affects outcomes in the treatment of ACS. Increasing awareness of the factors that contribute to major bleeding in ACS can help reduce the incidence of this complication and prevent its sequelae. Based on evidence from a large number of clinical trials, we conclude that appropriate selection of antithrombotic or antiplatelet agent, combined with proper dose adjustment and regimen selection, and careful patient selection may help to reduce the incidence of major bleeding in ACS and the adverse outcomes associated with it.

## REFERENCES

[1] Murray Cj, Lopez Ad. Mortality By Cause For Eight Regions Of The World: Global Burden Of Disease Study. *Lancet1997* May 3;349(9061):1269-76.

[2] Lloyd-Jones D, Adams Rj, Brown Tm, Carnethon M, Dai S, De Simone G, Et Al. Heart Disease And Stroke Statistics--2010 Update. A Report From The American Heart Association. *Circulation2009* Dec 17.

[3] British Heart Foundation Statistics Website. *British Heart Foundation*; 2008 [Updated 4th Decemeber 2009; Cited 2010].

[4] Fuster V, Badimon L, Badimon Jj, Chesebro Jh. The Pathogenesis Of Coronary Artery Disease And The Acute Coronary Syndromes (1). *N Engl J Med*1992 Jan 23;326(4):242-50.

[5] Roe Mt, Ohman Em, Maas Ac, Christenson Rh, Mahaffey Kw, Granger Cb, Et Al. Shifting The Open-Artery Hypothesis Downstream: The Quest For Optimal Reperfusion. *J Am Coll Cardiol*2001 Jan;37(1):9-18.

[6] Collaborative Meta-Analysis Of Randomised Trials Of Antiplatelet Therapy For Prevention Of Death, Myocardial Infarction, And Stroke In High Risk Patients. *Bmj2002* Jan 12;324(7329):71-86.

[7] Cannon Cp, Battler A, Brindis Rg, Cox Jl, Ellis Sg, Every Nr, Et Al. American College Of Cardiology Key Data Elements And Definitions For Measuring The Clinical Management And Outcomes Of Patients With Acute Coronary Syndromes. A Report Of The American College Of Cardiology Task Force On Clinical Data Standards (Acute Coronary Syndromes Writing Committee). *J Am Coll* Cardiol2001 Dec;38(7):2114-30.

[8] Holmes Dr, Jr., Kereiakes Dj, Kleiman Ns, Moliterno Dj, Patti G, Grines Cl. Combining Antiplatelet And Anticoagulant Therapies. *J Am Coll Cardiol* 2009 Jul 7;54(2):95-109.

[9] Manoukian Sv, Feit F, Mehran R, Voeltz Md, Ebrahimi R, Hamon M, Et Al. Impact Of Major Bleeding On 30-Day Mortality And Clinical Outcomes In Patients With Acute Coronary Syndromes: An Analysis From The Acuity Trial. *J Am Coll Cardiol* 2007 Mar 27;49(12):1362-8.

[10] Moscucci M, Fox Ka, Cannon Cp, Klein W, Lopez-Sendon J, Montalescot G, Et Al. Predictors Of Major Bleeding In Acute Coronary Syndromes: The Global Registry Of Acute Coronary Events (Grace). *Eur Heart J*2003 Oct;24(20):1815-23.

[11] Yan At, Yan Rt, Huynh T, Deyoung P, Weeks A, Fitchett Dh, Et Al. Bleeding And Outcome In Acute Coronary Syndrome: Insights From Continuous Electrocardiogram Monitoring In The Integrilin And Enoxaparin Randomized Assessment Of Acute Coronary Syndrome Treatment (Interact) Trial. *Am Heart J*2008 Oct;156(4):769-75.

[12] Chesebro Jh, Knatterud G, Roberts R, Borer J, Cohen Ls, Dalen J, Et Al. Thrombolysis In Myocardial Infarction (Timi) Trial, Phase I: A Comparison Between Intravenous Tissue Plasminogen Activator And Intravenous Streptokinase. Clinical Findings Through Hospital Discharge. *Circulation1987* Jul;76(1):142-54.

[13] An International Randomized Trial Comparing Four Thrombolytic Strategies For Acute Myocardial Infarction. The Gusto Investigators. *N Engl J Med*1993 Sep 2;329(10):673-82.

[14] International, Randomized, Controlled Trial Of Lamifiban (A Platelet Glycoprotein Iib/Iiia Inhibitor), Heparin, Or Both In Unstable Angina. The Paragon Investigators. Platelet Iib/Iiia Antagonism For The Reduction Of Acute Coronary Syndrome Events In A Global Organization Network. *Circulation*1998 Jun 23;97(24):2386-95.

[15] Manoukian Sv, Feit F, Mehran R, Voeltz Md, Ebrahimi R, Hamon M, Et Al. Impact Of Major Bleeding On 30-Day Mortality And Clinical Outcomes In Patients With Acute Coronary Syndromes: An Analysis From The Acuity Trial. *Journal Of The American College Of Cardiology*2007;49(12):1362-8.

[16] Karjalainen Pp, Porela P, Ylitalo A, Vikman S, Nyman K, Vaittinen Ma, Et Al. Safety And Efficacy Of Combined Antiplatelet-Warfarin Therapy After Coronary Stenting. *Eur Heart J*2007 Mar;28(6):726-32.

[17] Effects Of Recombinant Hirudin (Lepirudin) Compared With Heparin On Death, Myocardial Infarction, Refractory Angina, And Revascularisation Procedures In Patients With Acute Myocardial Ischaemia Without St Elevation: A Randomised Trial. Organisation To Assess Strategies For Ischemic Syndromes (Oasis-2) Investigators. *Lancet1999* Feb 6;353(9151):429-38.

[18] Alexander Kp, Chen Ay, Roe Mt, Newby Lk, Gibson Cm, Allen-Lapointe Nm, Et Al. Excess Dosing Of Antiplatelet And Antithrombin Agents In The Treatment Of Non-St-Segment Elevation Acute Coronary Syndromes. *Jama2005* Dec 28;294(24):3108-16.

[19] Schulman S, Kearon C. Definition Of Major Bleeding In Clinical Investigations Of Antihemostatic Medicinal Products In Non-Surgical Patients. *J Thromb Haemost*2005 Apr;3(4):692-4.

[20] Yusuf S, Zhao F, Mehta Sr, Chrolavicius S, Tognoni G, Fox Kk. Effects Of Clopidogrel In Addition To Aspirin In Patients With Acute Coronary Syndromes Without St-Segment Elevation. *N Engl J Med*2001 Aug 16;345(7):494-502.

[21] Montalescot G, White Hd, Gallo R, Cohen M, Steg Pg, Aylward Pe, Et Al. Enoxaparin Versus Unfractionated Heparin In Elective Percutaneous Coronary Intervention. *N Engl J Med*2006 Sep 7;355(10):1006-17.

[22] Yusuf S, Mehta Sr, Chrolavicius S, Afzal R, Pogue J, Granger Cb, Et Al. Effects Of Fondaparinux On Mortality And Reinfarction In Patients With Acute St-Segment Elevation Myocardial Infarction: The Oasis-6 Randomized Trial. *Jama*2006 Apr 5;295(13):1519-30.

[23] Stone Gw, Witzenbichler B, Guagliumi G, Peruga Jz, Brodie Br, Dudek D, Et Al. Bivalirudin During Primary Pci In Acute Myocardial Infarction. *N Engl J Med*2008 May 22;358(21):2218-30.

[24] Lincoff Am, Bittl Ja, Harrington Ra, Feit F, Kleiman Ns, Jackman Jd, Et Al. Bivalirudin And Provisional Glycoprotein Iib/Iiia Blockade Compared With Heparin And Planned Glycoprotein Iib/Iiia Blockade During Percutaneous Coronary Intervention: Replace-2 Randomized Trial. *Jama*2003 Feb 19;289(7):853-63.

[25] Rao Sv, O'grady K, Pieper Ks, Granger Cb, Newby Lk, Mahaffey Kw, Et Al. A Comparison Of The Clinical Impact Of Bleeding Measured By Two Different Classifications Among Patients With Acute Coronary Syndromes. *J Am Coll Cardiol*2006 Feb 21;47(4):809-16.

[26] Inhibition Of Platelet Glycoprotein Iib/Iiia With Eptifibatide In Patients With Acute Coronary Syndromes. The Pursuit Trial Investigators. Platelet Glycoprotein Iib/Iiia In Unstable Angina: Receptor Suppression Using Integrilin Therapy. N Engl J Med1998 Aug 13;339(7):436-43.

[27] Ferguson Jj, Califf Rm, Antman Em, Cohen M, Grines Cl, Goodman S, Et Al. Enoxaparin Vs Unfractionated Heparin In High-Risk Patients With Non-St-Segment Elevation Acute Coronary Syndromes Managed With An Intended Early Invasive Strategy: Primary Results Of The Synergy Randomized Trial. *Jama*2004 Jul 7;292(1):45-54.

[28] Inhibition Of The Platelet Glycoprotein Iib/Iiia Receptor With Tirofiban In Unstable Angina And Non-Q-Wave Myocardial Infarction. Platelet Receptor Inhibition In Ischemic Syndrome Management In Patients Limited By Unstable Signs And Symptoms (Prism-Plus) Study Investigators. *N Engl J Med*1998 May 21;338(21):1488-97.

[29] Seto A, Bernotas A, Crowther M, Wittkowsky Ak. Definition Of Major Bleeding Used By Us Anticoagulation Clinics. *Thromb Res*2009 Jun;124(2):239-40.

[30] Rao Sv, Eikelboom J, Steg Pg, Lincoff Am, Weintraub Ws, Bassand Jp, Et Al. Standardized Reporting Of Bleeding Complications For Clinical Investigations In Acute Coronary Syndromes: A Proposal From The Academic Bleeding Consensus (Abc) Multidisciplinary Working Group. *Am Heart J*2009 Dec;158(6):881-6 E1.

[31] Rao Sv, O'grady K, Pieper Ks, Granger Cb, Newby Lk, Van De Werf F, Et Al. Impact Of Bleeding Severity On Clinical Outcomes Among Patients With Acute Coronary Syndromes. *Am J Cardiol* 2005 Nov 1;96(9):1200-6.

[32] Rao Ak, Pratt C, Berke A, Jaffe A, Ockene I, Schreiber Tl, Et Al. Thrombolysis In Myocardial Infarction (Timi) Trial--Phase I: Hemorrhagic Manifestations And Changes In Plasma Fibrinogen And The Fibrinolytic System In Patients Treated With Recombinant Tissue Plasminogen Activator And Streptokinase. *J Am Coll Cardiol* 1988 Jan;11(1):1-11.

[33] Bovill Eg, Terrin Ml, Stump Dc, Berke Ad, Frederick M, Collen D, Et Al. Hemorrhagic Events During Therapy With Recombinant Tissue-Type Plasminogen Activator, Heparin, And Aspirin For Acute Myocardial Infarction. Results Of The Thrombolysis In Myocardial Infarction (Timi), Phase Ii Trial. *Ann Intern Med* 1991 Aug 15;115(4):256-65.

[34] Oldgren J, Wernroth L, Stenestrand U. Fibrinolytic Therapy And Bleeding Complications: Risk Predictors From Swedeheart. *J Am Coll Cardiol* 2009 March 10, 2009;53(10_Suppl_A):A323.

[35] Spencer Fa, Moscucci M, Granger Cb, Gore Jm, Goldberg Rj, Steg Pg, Et Al. Does Comorbidity Account For The Excess Mortality In Patients With Major Bleeding In Acute Myocardial Infarction? *Circulation* 2007 Dec 11;116(24):2793-801.

[36] Mortensen J, Thygesen Ss, Johnsen Sp, Vinther Pm, Kristensen Sd, Refsgaard J. Incidence Of Bleeding In 'Real-Life' Acute Coronary Syndrome Patients Treated With Antithrombotic Therapy. *Cardiology* 2008;111(1):41-6.

[37] Klein B, Wienbergen H, Heer T, Gitt Ak, Junger C, Senges J, Et Al. Impact Of Bleeding Complications With The Need For Blood Transfusion In Patients With Acute Coronary Syndrome. *Results Of The German Acos Registry*. Esc 9/20072007.

[38] Eikelboom Jw, Mehta Sr, Anand Ss, Xie C, Fox Ka, Yusuf S. Adverse Impact Of Bleeding On Prognosis In Patients With Acute Coronary Syndromes. *Circulation* 2006 Aug 22;114(8):774-82.

[39] Mehran R, Nikolsky E, Lansky Aj, Kirtane Aj, Kim Yh, Feit F, Et Al. Impact Of Chronic Kidney Disease On Early (30-Day) And Late (1-Year) Outcomes Of Patients With Acute Coronary Syndromes Treated With Alternative Antithrombotic Treatment Strategies: An Acuity (Acute Catheterization And Urgent Intervention Triage Strategy) Substudy. *Jacc Cardiovasc Interv* 2009 Aug;2(8):748-57.

[40] Shakir D, Zubaid M, Al-Mallah M, Mahmeed Wa, Alsheikh-Ali Aa, Rajivir Singh, Et Al. Bleeding Complications With Acute Coronary Syndrome In Six Middle Eastern Countries. *Circulation* 2010;Abstract, Wcc (June).

[41] Fox Ka, Bassand Jp, Mehta Sr, Wallentin L, Theroux P, Piegas Ls, Et Al. Influence Of Renal Function On The Efficacy And Safety Of Fondaparinux Relative To Enoxaparin In Non St-Segment Elevation Acute Coronary Syndromes. *Ann Intern Med* 2007 Sep 4;147(5):304-10.

[42] Budaj A, Eikelboom Jw, Mehta Sr, Afzal R, Chrolavicius S, Bassand Jp, Et Al. Improving Clinical Outcomes By Reducing Bleeding In Patients With Non-St-Elevation Acute Coronary Syndromes. *Eur Heart J* 2009 Mar;30(6):655-61.

[43] Kinnaird Td, Stabile E, Mintz Gs, Lee Cw, Canos Da, Gevorkian N, Et Al. Incidence, Predictors, And Prognostic Implications Of Bleeding And Blood Transfusion Following Percutaneous Coronary Interventions. *Am J Cardiol* 2003 Oct 15;92(8):930-5.

[44] Manoukian Sv, Voeltz Md, Eikelboom J. Bleeding Complications In Acute Coronary Syndromes And Percutaneous Coronary Intervention: Predictors, Prognostic Significance, And Paradigms For Reducing Risk. *Clin Cardiol*2007 Oct;30(10 Suppl 2):Ii24-34.

[45] Segev A, Strauss Bh, Tan M, Constance C, Langer A, Goodman Sg. Predictors And 1-Year Outcome Of Major Bleeding In Patients With Non-St-Elevation Acute Coronary Syndromes: Insights From The Canadian Acute Coronary Syndrome Registries. *Am Heart J*2005 Oct;150(4):690-4.

[46] Walsh Ch, Cooper Bt, Wright Ad, Malins Jm, Cooke Wt. Diabetes Mellitus And Coeliac Disease: A Clinical Study. *Qjm1978* January 1, 1978;47(1):89-100.

[47] Israeli A, Matzner Y, Or R, Raz I. Glibenclamide Causing Thrombocytopenia And Bleeding Tendency: Case Reports And A Review Of The Literature. *Klin Wochenschr*1988 Mar 1;66(5):223-4.

[48] Al-Sheyyab M, Jarrah N, Younis E, Shennak Mm, Hadidi A, Awidi A, Et Al. Bleeding Tendency In Wolfram Syndrome: A Newly Identified Feature With Phenotype Genotype Correlation. *Eur J Pediatr*2001 Apr;160(4):243-6.

[49] Aronson D, Weinrauch La, D'elia Ja, Tofler Gh, Burger Aj. Circadian Patterns Of Heart Rate Variability, Fibrinolytic Activity, And Hemostatic Factors In Type I Diabetes Mellitus With Cardiac Autonomic Neuropathy. *Am J Cardiol*1999 Aug 15;84(4):449-53.

[50] Weniger J, Panzram G. [Circadian Behavior Of Hemostaseologic Parameters In Diabetic Patients And Metabolically Healthy Individuals]. *Z Gesamte Inn Med*1985 Aug 15;40(16):489-92.

[51] Hebert Pc, Wells G, Blajchman Ma, Marshall J, Martin C, Pagliarello G, Et Al. A Multicenter, Randomized, Controlled Clinical Trial Of Transfusion Requirements In Critical Care. Transfusion Requirements In Critical Care Investigators, Canadian Critical Care Trials Group. *N Engl J Med*1999 Feb 11;340(6):409-17.

[52] Murphy Gj, Reeves Bc, Rogers Ca, Rizvi Si, Culliford L, Angelini Gd. Increased Mortality, Postoperative Morbidity, And Cost After Red Blood Cell Transfusion In Patients Having Cardiac Surgery. *Circulation*2007 Nov 27;116(22):2544-52.

[53] Rao Sv, Jollis Jg, Harrington Ra, Granger Cb, Newby Lk, Armstrong Pw, Et Al. Relationship Of Blood Transfusion And Clinical Outcomes In Patients With Acute Coronary Syndromes. *Jama*2004 Oct 6;292(13):1555-62.

[54] Yang X, Alexander Kp, Chen Ay, Roe Mt, Brindis Rg, Rao Sv, Et Al. The Implications Of Blood Transfusions For Patients With Non-St-Segment Elevation Acute Coronary Syndromes: Results From The Crusade National Quality Improvement Initiative. *J Am Coll Cardiol*2005 Oct 18;46(8):1490-5.

[55] Perrotta Pl, Snyder El. Non-Infectious Complications Of Transfusion Therapy. *Blood Rev*2001 Jun;15(2):69-83.

[56] Casutt M, Seifert B, Pasch T, Schmid Er, Turina Mi, Spahn Dr. Factors Influencing The Individual Effects Of Blood Transfusions On Oxygen Delivery And Oxygen Consumption. *Crit Care Med*1999 Oct;27(10):2194-200.

[57] Dietrich Ka, Conrad Sa, Hebert Ca, Levy Gl, Romero Md. Cardiovascular And Metabolic Response To Red Blood Cell Transfusion In Critically Ill Volume-Resuscitated Nonsurgical Patients. *Crit Care Med*1990 Sep;18(9):940-4.

[58] Fortune Jb, Feustel Pj, Saifi J, Stratton Hh, Newell Jc, Shah Dm. Influence Of Hematocrit On Cardiopulmonary Function After Acute Hemorrhage. *J Trauma*1987 Mar;27(3):243-9.

[59] Mcmahon Tj, Moon Re, Luschinger Bp, Carraway Ms, Stone Ae, Stolp Bw, Et Al. Nitric Oxide In The Human Respiratory Cycle. *Nat Med*2002 Jul;8(7):711-7.

[60] Stamler Js, Jia L, Eu Jp, Mcmahon Tj, Demchenko It, Bonaventura J, Et Al. Blood Flow Regulation By S-Nitrosohemoglobin In The Physiological Oxygen Gradient. *Science1997* Jun 27;276(5321):2034-7.

[61] Welch Hg, Meehan Kr, Goodnough Lt. Prudent Strategies For Elective Red Blood Cell Transfusion. *Ann Intern Med1*992 Mar 1;116(5):393-402.

[62] Basran S, Frumento Rj, Cohen A, Lee S, Du Y, Nishanian E, Et Al. The Association Between Duration Of Storage Of Transfused Red Blood Cells And Morbidity And Mortality After Reoperative Cardiac Surgery. *Anesth Analg*2006 Jul;103(1):15-20, Table Of Contents.

[63] Marik Pe, Sibbald Wj. Effect Of Stored-Blood Transfusion On Oxygen Delivery In Patients With Sepsis. *Jama1993* Jun 16;269(23):3024-9.

[64] Wallis Jp. Nitric Oxide And Blood: A Review. *Transfus Med*2005 Feb;15(1):1-11.

[65] Sabatine Ms, Morrow Da, Giugliano Rp, Burton Pb, Murphy Sa, Mccabe Ch, Et Al. Association Of Hemoglobin Levels With Clinical Outcomes In Acute Coronary Syndromes. *Circulation2005* Apr 26;111(16):2042-9.

[66] Yusuf S, Mehta Sr, Chrolavicius S, Afzal R, Pogue J, Granger Cb, Et Al. Comparison Of Fondaparinux And Enoxaparin In Acute Coronary Syndromes. *N Engl J Med*2006 Apr 6;354(14):1464-76.

[67] Aronson D, Suleiman M, Agmon Y, Suleiman A, Blich M, Kapeliovich M, Et Al. Changes In Haemoglobin Levels During Hospital Course And Long-Term Outcome After Acute Myocardial Infarction. *Eur Heart J*2007 Jun;28(11):1289-96.

[68] Md V, F F, Gw S, Sv M. Anemia And Outcomes In Acute Coronary Syndrome. *Acute Coron Synd*2005;7:47-55.

[69] Gw S. A Prospective, Randomized Trial Of Bivalirudin In Acute Coronary Syndromes: Final One-Year Results From The Acuity Trial. Presented At: 56th Annual Session Of The American College Of Cardiology. 2007 [Cited 2010]; Available From: *Http:// Www.Cardiosource.Com/Annualmtg /Acc07/Lectures.Asp?Sessiontitle = Latebreaking%20clinical%20 Trials %20follow-Up&Sessionid = 22&Date=3/26/2007.*

[70] Peters Rj, Mehta Sr, Fox Ka, Zhao F, Lewis Bs, Kopecky Sl, Et Al. Effects Of Aspirin Dose When Used Alone Or In Combination With Clopidogrel In Patients With Acute Coronary Syndromes: Observations From The Clopidogrel In Unstable Angina To Prevent Recurrent Events (Cure) Study. *Circulation2003* Oct 7;108(14):1682-7.

[71] Lim Mj, Eagle Ka, Gore Jm, Anderson Fa, Jr., Dabbous Oh, Mehta Rh, Et Al. Treating Patients With Acute Coronary Syndromes With Aggressive Antiplatelet Therapy (From The Global Registry Of Acute Coronary Events). *Am J Cardiol*2005 Oct 1;96(7):917-21.

[72] Kastrati A, Mehilli J, Neumann Fj, Dotzer F, Ten Berg J, Bollwein H, Et Al. Abciximab In Patients With Acute Coronary Syndromes Undergoing Percutaneous Coronary Intervention After Clopidogrel Pretreatment: The Isar-React 2 Randomized Trial. *Jama2006* Apr 5;295(13):1531-8.

[73] Topol Ej, Moliterno Dj, Herrmann Hc, Powers Er, Grines Cl, Cohen Dj, Et Al. Comparison Of Two Platelet Glycoprotein Iib/Iiia Inhibitors, Tirofiban And Abciximab, For The Prevention Of Ischemic Events With Percutaneous Coronary Revascularization. *N Engl J Med*2001 Jun 21;344(25):1888-94.

[74] Brener Sj, Moliterno Dj, Lincoff Am, Steinhubl Sr, Wolski Ke, Topol Ej. Relationship Between Activated Clotting Time And Ischemic Or Hemorrhagic Complications: Analysis Of 4 Recent Randomized Clinical Trials Of Percutaneous Coronary Intervention. *Circulation2004* Aug 24;110(8):994-8.

[75] Gilchrist Ic, Berkowitz Sd, Thompson Td, Califf Rm, Granger Cb. Heparin Dosing And Outcome In Acute Coronary Syndromes: The Gusto-Iib Experience. Global Use Of Strategies To Open Occluded Coronary Arteries. *Am Heart J*2002 Jul;144(1):73-80.

[76] Antman Em, Morrow Da, Mccabe Ch, Murphy Sa, Ruda M, Sadowski Z, Et Al. Enoxaparin Versus Unfractionated Heparin With Fibrinolysis For St-Elevation Myocardial Infarction. N Engl J Med2006 Apr 6;354(14):1477-88.

[77] Lim W, Dentali F, Eikelboom Jw, Crowther Ma. Meta-Analysis: Low-Molecular-Weight Heparin And Bleeding In Patients With Severe Renal Insufficiency. *Ann Intern Med*2006 May 2;144(9):673-84.

[78] Aguirre Fv, Topol Ej, Ferguson Jj, Anderson K, Blankenship Jc, Heuser Rr, Et Al. Bleeding Complications With The Chimeric Antibody To Platelet Glycoprotein Iib/Iiia Integrin In Patients Undergoing Percutaneous Coronary Intervention. Epic Investigators. *Circulation1995* Jun 15;91(12):2882-90.

[79] Platelet Glycoprotein Iib/Iiia Receptor Blockade And Low-Dose Heparin During Percutaneous Coronary Revascularization. The Epilog Investigators. *N Engl J Med1*997 Jun 12;336(24):1689-96.

[80] Lincoff Am, Kleiman Ns, Kereiakes Dj, Feit F, Bittl Ja, Jackman Jd, Et Al. Long-Term Efficacy Of Bivalirudin And Provisional Glycoprotein Iib/Iiia Blockade Vs Heparin And Planned Glycoprotein Iib/Iiia Blockade During Percutaneous Coronary Revascularization: Replace-2 Randomized Trial. *Jama2004* Aug 11;292(6):696-703.

[81] Stone Gw, Mclaurin Bt, Cox Da, Bertrand Me, Lincoff Am, Moses Jw, Et Al. Bivalirudin For Patients With Acute Coronary Syndromes. *N Engl J Med*2006 Nov 23;355(21):2203-16.

[82] Stone Gw, White Hd, Ohman Em, Bertrand Me, Lincoff Am, Mclaurin Bt, Et Al. Bivalirudin In Patients With Acute Coronary Syndromes Undergoing Percutaneous Coronary Intervention: A Subgroup Analysis From The Acute Catheterization And Urgent Intervention Triage Strategy (Acuity) Trial. *Lancet2007* Mar 17;369(9565):907-19.

[83] Gibson Cm, Morrow Da, Murphy Sa, Palabrica Tm, Jennings Lk, Stone Ph, Et Al. A Randomized Trial To Evaluate The Relative Protection Against Post-Percutaneous Coronary Intervention Microvascular Dysfunction, Ischemia, And Inflammation Among Antiplatelet And Antithrombotic Agents: The Protect-Timi-30 Trial. *J Am Coll Cardiol*2006 Jun 20;47(12):2364-73.

[84] Wiviott Sd, Braunwald E, Mccabe Ch, Montalescot G, Ruzyllo W, Gottlieb S, Et Al. Prasugrel Versus Clopidogrel In Patients With Acute Coronary Syndromes. *N Engl J Med*2007 Nov 15;357(20):2001-15.

[85] Cannon Cp, Harrington Ra, James S, Ardissino D, Becker Rc, Emanuelsson H, Et Al. Comparison Of Ticagrelor With Clopidogrel In Patients With A Planned Invasive

Strategy For Acute Coronary Syndromes (Plato): A Randomised Double-Blind Study. *Lancet2010* Jan 23;375(9711):283-93.

[86] Bhatt Dl, Lincoff Am, Gibson Cm, Stone Gw, Mcnulty S, Montalescot G, Et Al. Intravenous Platelet Blockade With Cangrelor During Pci. *N Engl J Med*2009 Dec 10;361(24):2330-41.

[87] Louvard Y, Benamer H, Garot P, Hildick-Smith D, Loubeyre C, Rigattieri S, Et Al. Comparison Of Transradial And Transfemoral Approaches For Coronary Angiography And Angioplasty In Octogenarians (The Octoplus Study). *Am J Cardiol*2004 Nov 1;94(9):1177-80.

[88] Cantor Wj, Mahaffey Kw, Huang Z, Das P, Gulba Dc, Glezer S, Et Al. Bleeding Complications In Patients With Acute Coronary Syndrome Undergoing Early Invasive Management Can Be Reduced With Radial Access, Smaller Sheath Sizes, And Timely Sheath Removal. *Catheter Cardiovasc Interv*2007 Jan;69(1):73-83.

[89] Blankenship Jc, Hellkamp As, Aguirre Fv, Demko Sl, Topol Ej, Califf Rm. Vascular Access Site Complications After Percutaneous Coronary Intervention With Abciximab In The Evaluation Of C7e3 For The Prevention Of Ischemic Complications (Epic) Trial. *Am J Cardiol*1998 Jan 1;81(1):36-40.

[90] Koreny M, Riedmuller E, Nikfardjam M, Siostrzonek P, Mullner M. Arterial Puncture Closing Devices Compared With Standard Manual Compression After Cardiac Catheterization: Systematic Review And Meta-Analysis. *Jama*2004 Jan 21;291(3):350-7.

[91] Hamon M, Sabatier R, Zhao Q, Niculescu R, Valette B, Grollier G. Mini-Invasive Strategy In Acute Coronary Syndromes: Direct Coronary Stenting Using 5 Fr Guiding Catheters And Transradial Approach. *Catheter Cardiovasc Interv*2002 Mar;55(3):340-3.

[92] Chan Fk, Ching Jy, Hung Lc, Wong Vw, Leung Vk, Kung Nn, Et Al. Clopidogrel Versus Aspirin And Esomeprazole To Prevent Recurrent Ulcer Bleeding. *N Engl J Med*2005 Jan 20;352(3):238-44.

[93] Ng Fh, Wong Sy, Lam Kf, Chang Cm, Lau Yk, Chu Wm, Et Al. Gastrointestinal Bleeding In Patients Receiving A Combination Of Aspirin, Clopidogrel, And Enoxaparin In Acute Coronary Syndrome. *Am J Gastroenterol*2008 Apr;103(4):865-71.

[94] Gilard M, Arnaud B, Cornily Jc, Le Gal G, Lacut K, Le Calvez G, Et Al. Influence Of Omeprazole On The Antiplatelet Action Of Clopidogrel Associated With Aspirin: The Randomized, Double-Blind Ocla (Omeprazole Clopidogrel Aspirin) Study. *J Am Coll Cardiol*2008 Jan 22;51(3):256-60.

[95] Cuisset T, Frere C, Quilici J, Poyet R, Gaborit B, Bali L, Et Al. Comparison Of Omeprazole And Pantoprazole Influence On A High 150-Mg Clopidogrel Maintenance Dose The Paca (Proton Pump Inhibitors And Clopidogrel Association) Prospective Randomized Study. *J Am Coll Cardiol*2009 Sep 22;54(13):1149-53.

[96] Fda. Information For Healthcare Professionals: Update To The Labeling Of Clopidogrel Bisulfate (Marketed As Plavix) To Alert Healthcare Professionals About A Drug Interaction With Omeprazole (Marketed As Prilosec And Prilosec Otc) 2009; Available From:
*Http://Www.Fda.Gov/Drugs/Drugsafety/Postmarketdrugsafetyinformationforpatientsandproviders/Drugsafetyinformationforheathcareprofessionals/Ucm190787.Htm.*

[97] Small Ds, Farid Na, Payne Cd, Weerakkody Gj, Li Yg, Brandt Jt, Et Al. Effects Of The Proton Pump Inhibitor Lansoprazole On The Pharmacokinetics And Pharmacodynamics Of Prasugrel And Clopidogrel. *J Clin Pharmacol*2008 Apr;48(4):475-84.

[98] Kwok Cs, Loke Yk. Meta-Analysis: Effects Of Proton Pump Inhibitors On Cardiovascular Events And Mortality In Patients Receiving Clopidogrel. *Aliment Pharmacol* Ther2010 Jan 22.

[99] Besarab A, Bolton Wk, Browne Jk, Egrie Jc, Nissenson Ar, Okamoto Dm, Et Al. The Effects Of Normal As Compared With Low Hematocrit Values In Patients With Cardiac Disease Who Are Receiving Hemodialysis And Epoetin. *N Engl J Med*1998 Aug 27;339(9):584-90.

[100] Fox Ka, Mehta Sr, Peters R, Zhao F, Lakkis N, Gersh Bj, Et Al. Benefits And Risks Of The Combination Of Clopidogrel And Aspirin In Patients Undergoing Surgical Revascularization For Non-St-Elevation Acute Coronary Syndrome: The Clopidogrel In Unstable Angina To Prevent Recurrent Ischemic Events (Cure) Trial. *Circulation2004* Sep 7;110(10):1202-8.

[101] Randomized, Placebo-Controlled Trial Of Titrated Intravenous Lamifiban For Acute Coronary Syndromes. *Circulation2002* Jan 22;105(3):316-21.

[102] Huynh T, Piazza N, Dibattiste Pm, Snapinn Sm, Wan Y, Pharand C, Et Al. Analysis Of Bleeding Complications Associated With Glycoprotein Iib/Iiia Receptors Blockade In Patients With High-Risk Acute Coronary Syndromes: Insights From The Prism-Plus Study. *Int J Cardiol*2005 Apr 8;100(1):73-8.

[103] Armstrong Pw, Fu Y, Chang Wc, Topol Ej, Granger Cb, Betriu A, Et Al. Acute Coronary Syndromes In The Gusto-Iib Trial: Prognostic Insights And Impact Of Recurrent Ischemia. The Gusto-Iib Investigators. *Circulation1998* Nov 3;98(18):1860-8.

[104] A Comparison Of Aspirin Plus Tirofiban With Aspirin Plus Heparin For Unstable Angina. Platelet Receptor Inhibition In Ischemic Syndrome Management (Prism) Study Investigators. *N Engl J Med*1998 May 21;338(21):1498-505.

[105] Al-Mallah M, Bazari Rn, Jankowski M, Hudson Mp. Predictors And Outcomes Associated With Gastrointestinal Bleeding In Patients With Acute Coronary Syndromes. *J Thromb Thrombolysis*2007 Feb;23(1):51-5.

[106] Al-Sallami H, Ferguson R, Wilkins G, Gray A, Medlicott Nj. Bleeding Events In Patients Receiving Enoxaparin For The Management Of Non-St-Elevation Acute Coronary Syndrome (Nsteacs) At Dunedin Public Hospital, New Zealand. *N Z Med J*2008 Nov 14;121(1285):87-95.

[107] Mehran R, Pocock Sj, Stone Gw, Clayton Tc, Dangas Gd, Feit F, Et Al. Associations Of Major Bleeding And Myocardial Infarction With The Incidence And Timing Of Mortality In Patients Presenting With Non-St-Elevation Acute Coronary Syndromes: A Risk Model From The Acuity Trial. *Eur Heart J*2009 Jun;30(12):1457-66.

[108] Nikolsky E, Stone Gw, Kirtane Aj, Dangas Gd, Lansky Aj, Mclaurin B, Et Al. Gastrointestinal Bleeding In Patients With Acute Coronary Syndromes: Incidence, Predictors, And Clinical Implications: Analysis From The Acuity (Acute Catheterization And Urgent Intervention Triage Strategy) T*rial*. *J Am Coll Cardiol*2009 Sep 29;54(14):1293-302.

[109] Sorensen R, Hansen Ml, Abildstrom Sz, Hvelplund A, Andersson C, Jorgensen C, Et Al. Risk Of Bleeding In Patients With Acute Myocardial Infarction Treated With Different Combinations Of Aspirin, Clopidogrel, And Vitamin K Antagonists In Denmark: A Retrospective Analysis Of Nationwide Registry Data. *Lancet2009* Dec 12;374(9706):1967-74.

[110] Al-Sallami H, Ferguson R, Wilkins G, Gray A, Medlicott Nj. Bleeding Events In Patients Receiving Enoxaparine For The Management Of Non- St-Elevation Acute Coronary Syndrome (Nsteacs) At Dunedin Public Hospital, New Zealand. *Journal Of The New Zealand Medical Association*2008;121:87-95.

In: Ventricular Fibrillation and Acute Coronary Syndrome  ISBN: 978-1-61728-969-9
Editor: Joyce E. Mandell  © 2011 Nova Science Publishers, Inc.

*Chapter IV*

# NOVEL ANTIPLATELETS IN ACUTE CORONARY SYNDROMES

### *Burak Pamukcu*[*a] *and Huseyin Oflaz*[b]

[a]University Department of Medicine, Centre for Cardiovascular Sciences,
City Hospital, Birmingham, England UK.
[b]Istanbul University, Istanbul Faculty of Medicine,
Department of Cardiology, Capa, Istanbul, Turkey

## ABSTRACT

Atherosclerotic coronary artery disease and acute coronary syndromes are the major cause of death in developed countries and their prevalance are increasing in the developing world. Damaged endothelium, impaired coronary flow and finally almost always rupture in a vulnerable atherosclerotic plaque results with thrombus formation and total luminal occlusion at the atherosclerotic lesion site. Atherothrombosis, the latest phase of the atherosclerotic process, is one of the most studied stages that recent studies provided important evidence for its prevention. In 1980s, aspirin became the first line antiaggregant agent in patients with acute coronary syndromes. However, researchers aimed to discover optimal antiplatelet agents with improved efficacy and reasonable safety profile. Developments in the percutaneous coronary interventions (PCI) and especially the stent technology established requirement for newer antiplatelet agents, which was the beginning of 'age of thienopyridines'. Ticlopidine was the first line thienopyridine, however, serious side effects (neutropenia and severe allergic reactions) limited its clinical use. Then, the ADP $P_2Y_{12}$ receptor antagonist 'clopidogrel' became the most commonly used antiplatelet agent after PCI. Subsequently, new generation and more potent ADP receptor antagonists, prasugrel and ticagrelor were developed. The spectrum of antithrombotics is enlarging by the development of vonWillebrand (eg, ARC1779), thrombin (PAR-1 antagonists, eg, SCH530348) and thromboxane receptor antagonists (eg, terutroban). Novel antiplatelet agents aim to reduce atherothrombosis more efficiently than recent ones but without increasing major or life threatenning

---

* Correspondance: Burak Pamukcu, MD, University Department of Medicine, Centre for Cardiovascular Sciences, City Hospital, Birmingham B18 7QH England UK. E-mail: bpamukcu@gmail.com

bleeding. In this chapter we aim to focus on recent developments and future therapeutic antithrombotic perspectives in patients with acute coronary syndromes.

## INTRODUCTION

Atherothrombotic vascular disease is the leading cause of morbidity and mortality in developed countries (1). Atherothrombosis is a later phase of the atherosclerotic vascular disease that platelets have pivotal contribution in thrombus formation at the site of injured endothelium (2). This process generally affects coronary, cerebral and peripheral arteries (3). Many cytokines are released at the lesion site by both leukocytes and platelets that mediate inflammatory and thrombotic processes in patients with acute coronary syndromes (ACS) (4). Frequently, serum levels of inflammatory markers are increased at presentation (4). Platelets, play pivotal roles (eg, triggering the inflammatory cascade, thrombosis) as cells that contain significant amounts of inflammatory mediators (eg, CD40, thrombospondin, phospholipase A2) (5). In addition, more than 35 platelet-associated messenger ribonucleic acid (RNA) mediators involved in arterial injury and inflammation have been determined (6).

Platelet adhesion to the exposed subendothelial matrix at the atherosclerotic lesion site is the initial step in thrombus formation (7). Endothelial injury allows platelets to adhere subendothelial collagen and von Willebrand factor (vWF) via interactions with platelet surface receptors. Typically, rupture of an atherosclerotic plaque exposes collagen and vWF that binds to the platelets by glycoprotein-Ib-IX (GP-Ib-IX) receptor (8). Contact with subendothelial collagen activates platelets via GP VI (9) which is followed by the generation and release of thromboxane A2 (TxA2) and adenosine diphosphate (ADP). ADP binds to the platelet P2Y12 receptor and increases response to agonists (eg, thrombin) (10). TxA2, ADP and thrombin, generated by the coagulation cascade, stimulate and recruit additional platelets at the lesion site (7). Activation of the glycoprotein GP IIb/IIIa ($\alpha$IIb$\beta$3) receptors allow platelets to extend fibrinogen bridges between platelets and establish a platelet rich clot (11).

Most of the platelet activation and aggregation steps summarized above consists potential targets for the antithrombotic therapy in patients with ACS. More powerful blockade of platelets but without increasing bleeding is the goal of optimal antiplatelet therapy to be achieved. Novel potent, fast, long, short, reversible and irreversible acting agents are under development. These agents with different pharmacokinetics and pharmacodynamics include; ADP receptor antagonists, inhibitors of thromboxane synthesis, direct thrombin inhibitors, thromboxane receptor antagonists, vWF receptor antagonists and glycoprotein inhibitors. In this chapter we aim to overview current literature concerning classic and novel antiplatelet agents and to discuss newer strategies to prevent atherothrombosis in patients with acute coronary syndromes.

## ASPIRIN (ACETYLSALICYLIC ACID, ASA)

Aspirin was used as a powerful and reliable analgesic and anti-inflammatory drug since the end of 19th century. Aspirin's protective effect against myocardial infarction was first discovered in the 1950s (12). Twenty years later researchers discovered that aspirin was acting by the inhibition of prostaglandin synthesis (13). Aspirin achieved to provide a 51% decrease in myocardial infarction (MI) prevalence in one year follow-up in patients with unstable angina (14, 15). Aspirin's antiplatelet effect has been proven by subsequent studies and two important meta-analyses emphasized its importance in both primary and secondary prevention of MI and stroke (16-19).

'Physician's Health Study' established the efficiency of aspirin in primary prevention of MI and ischemic cerebrovascular disease (16). In "The Antithrombotic Trialists' Collaboration" meta-analysis of 145 randomized studies in patients with coronary artery disease (prior MI, unstable angina pectoris) and cerebrovascular disease, 75 to 300 mg daily aspirin therapy reduced the risk of non-fatal MI by 35% (p<0.00001) and the risk of vascular events by 18% (p<0.00001) (17). The antithrombotic effects of aspirin in patients with acute MI were confirmed by the second and third "International Study of Infarct Survival" (ISIS) trials (18, 19).

Under the light of these studies, in the last two decades, aspirin became the essential antiplatelet drug in management of patients with atherosclerotic cardiovascular disease. Lower doses of aspirin (80-300 mg/day) were shown to inhibit platelets as well as higher doses in patients with ACS (20, 21).

Aspirin's position in antiplatelet therapy was investigated after recurrent vascular events under regular aspirin therapy. However, none of the studies has suggested stopping aspirin but higher doses of aspirin and or additional therapies may have value in case of aspirin resistance (22, 23).

## THIENOPYRIDINES

### Ticlopidine

Ticlopidine is a first line thienopyridine that inhibits ADP receptors irreversibly. Ticlopidine's antiplatelet activity occurs due to its active metabolites in 24 to 48 hours after oral administration (24). Ticlopidine provided 46% reduction of cardiovascular death and MI in a cohort of 662 patients with unstable angina pectoris (p=0.009) (25). Ticlopidine was supposed to be a good option for antiplatelet therapy especially after percutaneous coronary interventions (PCI), however, clinical experiences and subsequent clinical studies established its limiting side effects such as severe neutropenia which is seen in about 1% of patients, necessitating close monitoring of blood counts during the first few weeks or months of treatment and its delayed antiplatelet action (26). Furthermore, liver dysfunction and allergic reactions (eg, rash) may occur after ticlopidine therapy (27).

### Clopidogrel

The second line thienopyridine, ADP receptor antagonist clopidogrel became the most commonly used drug in the last decade after stenting. Clinical trials investigated clopidogrel's efficacy and safety in patients both with ACS and stable coronary artery disease.

The CAPRIE trial (Clopidogrel versus Aspirin in Patients at Risk of Ischemic Events) aimed to directly compare clopidogrel and aspirin in a broad range of patients with atherosclerotic disease for the secondary prevention of ischemic events (28). Patients in the clopidogrel arm of the CAPRIE trial did not receive aspirin. The study concluded that clopidogrel reduced the primary outcome of vascular death, MI or ischemic stroke by 8.7% (95% confidence interval [CI], 0.3% to 16.5%) compared to aspirin arm at a mean follow-up of 1.9 years (28).

The 'Clopidogrel in Unstable angina to prevent Recurrent Events' (CURE) trial showed the benefits of combined aspirin and clopidogrel therapy in the reduction of major cardiovascular events (29). A reduction of 20% (p<0.00009) in cardiovascular death, MI and stroke was determined with combination therapy in a broad range of patients with ACS (29). A substudy of CURE trial, 'PCI CURE' aimed to investigate the impact of pretreatment with clopidogrel plus aspirin before angioplasty compared with placebo and benefits of long-term therapy after PCI against placebo. Clopidogrel pretreatment achieved a substantial risk reduction (31% RRR, 12.6% versus 8.8%; relative risk (RR), 0.69; 95% CI, 0.54 to 0.87; p<0.002) in patients undergoing PCI in PCI-CURE trial independently from timing of PCI. Addiotinally, efficacy and safety benefits of combined aspirin and clopidogrel therapy persisted for up to one year (30).

The 'Clopidogrel for Reduction of Events During Observation' (CREDO) trial aimed to evaluate the benefit of 12-month treatment with clopidogrel after PCI. CREDO investigated also potential benefits of preprocedural clopidogrel loading in addition to aspirin therapy. The results established that clopidogrel therapy was associated with a 26.9% relative reduction in the combined risk of death, MI or stroke at the end of one year follow-up (95% CI, 3.9%-44.4%; p=0.02; absolute risk reduction, 3%) but a loading dose of clopidogrel given at least 3 hours before the procedure did not reduce events at 28 days (31).

The 'ClOpidogrel and Metoprolol in Myocardial Infarction Trial' (Commit-CCS2) investigated the role of clopidogrel in 45,852 patients with suspected acute MI (93% STEMI). Clopidogrel therapy provided a significant reduction (9%) in death, reinfarction or stroke (9.2% in clopidogrel group versus 10.1% in placebo; p=0.002). Considering all kind of bleeding no additional risk was determined with clopidogrel therapy. As conclusion Commit-CCS2 trial established that adding clopidogrel 75 mg daily to aspirin and other standard treatments safely reduced inpatients' mortality and major vascular events rates (32).

The 'Clopidogrel as Adjunctive Reperfusion Therapy' (CLARITY) study investigated the efficacy and safety of clopidogrel in patients with STEMI who received fibrinolytic therapy. The investigators determined that clopidogrel therapy reduced primary efficacy end point (composite of occluded infarct-related artery defined by a Thrombolysis in Myocardial Infarction (TIMI) flow grade of 0 or 1 on angiography or death or recurrent MI before angiography) by 36% (95% CI, 24 to 47%; p<0.001) (21.7% vs15% in the placebo and clopidogrel groups respectively). Bleeding rates were similar between the placebo and clopidogrel groups. The investigators conclude that additional clopidogrel therapy improved the patency rate of infarct related artery in patients receiving aspirin and standard fibrinolytic therapy (33).

Another clinical trial performed with clopidogrel, the PCI-CLARITY study, aimed to determine if clopidogrel pretreatment before PCI is superior to clopidogrel treatment initiated at the time of PCI in preventing major adverse cardiovascular events in patients with STEMI. The results demonstrated that pretreatment with clopidogrel significantly reduced the incidence of cardiovascular death, MI or stroke following PCI (3.6% versus 6.2%; p=0.008). As conclusion PCI-CLARITY established that clopidogrel pretreatment significantly reduces the incidence of cardiovascular death or ischemic complications both before and after PCI and it does not increase bleeding significantly (34).

These evidence consolidated clopidogrels position in current antiplatelet regimens. It became a pivotal drug in patients with ACS undergoing PCI. However, antiplatelet responsiveness problem appeared also for clopidogrel as well as aspirin. Current efforts for generating novel, more efficient and safe ADP receptor antagonists added new options in antiplatelet therapy. Prasugrel, cangrelor, ticagrelor, elinogrel and BX667 are some of these new generation platelet antagonists.

## Prasugrel

Prasugrel (CS-747) is an oral, irreversible and selective third generation thienopyridine that binds to P2Y12 receptors on the platelet surface (35). Prasugrel is a prodrug which converts to its active metabolite by hepatic cytochrome P450 system (36) Preclinical studies of prasugrel established potent, fast onset and longer antiplatelet effects in rat models (37-39). Studies conducted on human subjects validated that prasugrel is a more potent P2Y12 inhibitor and acts also faster than clopidogrel (40-42). A recent study assessed platelet function after loading dose showed that prasugrel inhibited platelets more effectively than clopidogrel at 30 min, 1 h and 2 h after the administration of loading dose (43). Prasugrel also inhibited more efficiently platelet function at maintenance doses compared to clopidogrel (78% versus 56%) (43).

Another phase Ib study compared prasugrel and clopidogrel in 110 stable coronary artery disease patients receiving aspirin. A 600-mg loading dose of clopidogrel followed by a 75 mg daily maintenance dose was compared to 60 mg loading dose of prasugrel followed by a 10 mg daily maintenance dose for 28 days (44). Prasugrel showed earlier and greater P2Y12 receptor inhibition than clopidogrel (p<0.001). The authors reported a significantly lower mean platelet aggregation with prasugrel both at 2 hours after administration of the loading dose (31% versus 55%, p<0.001) and at maintenance dose therapy (42% versus 54% p<0.001) (44). Prasugrel achieved greater and faster platelet inhibition in aspirin treated subjects with coronary artery disease and it was found to be related to higher and more efficient active metabolite generation (44).

The Joint Utilization of Medications to Block platelets Optimally-Thrombolysis In Myocardial Infarction 26 (JUMBO-TIMI 26) study aimed to investigate safety of prasugrel and to compare with clopidogrel in 904 patients undergoing PCI (45). Major adverse cardiac events in the first month after PCI were assessed. Major bleeding rate was found 0.5% for prasugrel versus 0.8% for clopidogrel while combined major and minor bleedings appeared to be slightly higher in the prasugrel group than in the clopidogrel group (1.7% versus 1.2%) but the difference did not reach statistically significant levels. Major adverse cardiac events occurred more frequently in the clopidogrel group as compared with prasugrel (9.4% versus 7.2%) (45).

'The prasugrel in comparison with clopidogrel for inhibition of platelet activation and aggregation-Thrombolysis In Myocardial Infarction 44' (PRINCIPLE-TIMI 44) trial compared loading dose of 60 mg prasugrel and 600 mg clopidogrel in patients undergoing cardiac catheterization for PCI (46). Patients were randomized to 60 mg prasugrel or 600 mg clopidogrel loading doses 1 h before PCI. Maintenance therapy was consisted of 10 mg prasugrel or 150 mg clopidogrel once daily for 14 days after PCI. Subjects directly switched to the alternate maintenance therapy for another 14 days without waiting a wash-out period. PRINCIPLE-TIMI 44 established that a loading dose of 60 mg prasugrel resulted in greater platelet inhibition than a 600-mg clopidogrel loading dose and also similarly a maintenance therapy of 10 mg/d prasugrel inhibited platelets more efficiently than 150 mg/d clopidogrel (46).

The TRITON–TIMI 38 (Trial to Assess Improvement in Therapeutic Outcomes by Optimizing Platelet Inhibition with Prasugrel – Thrombolysis In Myocardial Infarction 38) study aimed to compare prasugrel with clopidogrel in 13,608 patients with moderate to high risk ACS (%74 NSTEMI, %26 STEMI) with scheduled PCI (47). Death from cardiovascular causes, nonfatal MI and nonfatal stroke were primary efficacy end points. The study investigated also major bleeding as a safety end point. The primary efficacy end point occurred in 12.1% and 9.9% of the patients receiving clopidogrel and prasugrel respectively (hazard ratio (HR) for prasugrel versus clopidogrel, 0.81; 95% CI, 0.73 to 0.90; $p<0.001$). Prasugrel reduced significantly the rates of myocardial infarction (9.7% for clopidogrel versus 7.4% for prasugrel; $p<0.001$), urgent target-vessel revascularization (3.7% versus 2.5%; $p<0.001$), and stent thrombosis (2.4% vs. 1.1%; $p<0.001$). On the other hand at the site of safety evaluation, major bleeding was determined in 2.4% and 1.8% of the participants in prasugrel and clopidogrel groups respectively (HR, 1.32; 95% CI, 1.03 to 1.68; $p=0.03$). Life-threatening bleeding (1.4% versus 0.9%; $p=0.01$), nonfatal bleeding (1.1% versus 0.9%; HR, 1.25; $p=0.23$) and fatal bleeding (0.4% vs. 0.1%; $p=0.002$) were higher in the prasugrel group. As a conclusion TRITON-TIMI38 established that prasugrel reduces the risk of cardiovascular death, myocardial infarction and stroke more efficiently than clopidogrel in patients with ACS undergoing PCI but at the cost of increased bleeding (47).

In TRITON-TIMI38 study prasugrel provided greater risk reduction for cardiovascular death, myocardial infarction and stroke benefit in patients with diabetes compared with non diabetics (12.2% versus 17.0% in prasugrel and clopidogrel groups respectively). This relatively greater risk reduction combined with similar major bleeding risk compared with non-diabetics consolidated the benefit of prasugrel in diabetics (48).

Despite the increased bleeding risk both major and life threathening, a prespecified analysis of net clinical benefit, showed that the findings still favored prasugrel (13.9% of patients in the clopidogrel group vs 12.2% in the prasugrel group, HR 0.87, 95% CI 0.79-0.95, $p=0.004$). However, TRITON-TIMI38 established that three patient groups could not profit from prasugrel therapy; patients older than 75 years, lightweight patients (less than 60 kg) and subjects who had a history of cerebrovascular events (47, 49).

Curent available data suggest that prasugrel is a potent antiplatelet that acts faster and longer than clopidogrel at the cost of increased bleeding. However, statistical analyses reveal that the net clinical benefit is still better in patients treated with prasugrel compared to those treated with clopidogrel. Prasugrel may also be a good option to accomplish antiplatelet response variability and resistance. Prasugrel is shown to be more effective in patients with diabetes but failed in elder, lightweighted patients and patients with a stroke history. Further studies are needed to determine prasugrel's position in antiplatelet therapy.

## Cangrelor (ARC-69931MX)

Cangrelor is the first non-thienopyridine, reversible, direct P2Y12 receptor inhibitor that is administered intravenously. Its effect starts in seconds after administration. Cangrelor is a potent and active drug due to its adenosine triphosphate chain. When administered intravenously it has a short half life (approximately 3 minutes) that permits clinicians to avoid prolonged antiplatelet activity in case of bleeding. Its clearance is independent of renal or hepatic function with complete platelet recovery within 1 hour. Cangrelor's clinical effects are similar to those of intravenous glycoprotein IIb/IIIa inhibitors. Platelet function recovery is fast and it returns to baseline within one hour when cangrelor infusion is stopped (50-52).

A recent study established that cangrelor produced profound and stable platelet inhibition (>95%) and was well tolerated during a prolonged infusion of up to 72 hours in patients with ACS (50).

Animal models assessed cangrelor's efficacy and established that it is a potent antiplatelet drug. The dose of cangrelor that inhibits platelets completely extends bleeding time less than twofold while GpIIb/IIIa antagonists achieve the same effect by the cost of six to sevenfold increased bleeding times (53).

Recently, the influence of cangrelor was also assessed in conjunction with thrombolytic therapy, on the prevention of platelet aggregation and thrombus formation in a canine thrombosis model (54). The adjunctive administration of cangrelor inhibited platelet aggregation and thrombosis, resulted with prolongation of reperfusion time. Cangrelor provided decreases in reocclusion and cyclic flow variations and improved myocardial tissue perfusion (54).

It is not clear that cangrelor and clopidogrel have additive or competitive effects when used together because there are conflicting study results. A recent study with a small sample size suggested that cangrelor and clopidogrel acts competitively in healthy volunteers and therefore clopidogrel administration should be started after the termination of cangrelor infusion in order to achieve sustained platelet P2Y12 inhibition (55). However, another recent study conducted in patients with ischemic heart disease stated that cangrelor and clopidogrel have additive inhibitory effects on platelet aggregation (56).

The safety profile, tolerability, and plasma concentrations at steady state of intravenous cangrelor therapy were assessed in patients with ACS. Cangrelor, when used as an adjunctive therapy to aspirin and low molecular weight heparin in patients with unstable angina or non-Q-wave MI, showed no increased major bleeding in 91 patients but a slightly increased minor bleeding compared with placebo (57). 'STEP-AMI' trial investigated both safety and efficacy of cangrelor as an adjunctive therapy to fibrinolytics in patients with acute myocardial infarction (58). The combination of cangrelor and half-dose t-PA established similar 60 minute coronary patency rates as full-dose t-PA alone (55% versus 50%, p = not significant) and greater arterial patency than with cangrelor alone (55% versus 18%, p < .05). At the safety site, bleeding and adverse clinical events were found comparable among the groups (58).

'Cangrelor versus Standard Therapy to Achieve Optimal Management of Platelet Inhibition (CHAMPION) PCI' aimed to compare cangrelor with 600 mg of oral clopidogrel administered before PCI in patients with ACS (59). The study investigated as primary efficacy end point; a composite of death from any cause, myocardial infarction or ischemia driven revascularization at 48 hours. CHAMPION-PCI enrolled 8877 patients, and 8716 of these subjects underwent PCI. At 48 hours, the primary composite end point occured in 7.5% of patients in the cangrelor group and 7.1% of patients in the clopidogrel group (odds ratio, 1.05; 95% CI, 0.88 to 1.24; p=0.59). Cangrelor was not found superior to clopidogrel at 30 days. Major bleeding was slightly increased in the cangrelor arm however it did not reach a statistically significant level (3.6% vs. 2.9%, OR; 1.26, 95% CI, 0.99 to 1.60, p=0.06). This large and randomized trial established that cangrelor did not achieve to provide superior primary end points when administered intravenously 30 minutes before PCI and continued for 2 hours after PCI in comparison with standard clopidogrel therapy administered 30 minutes before PCI (59).

'CHAMPION PLATFORM' trial was a double-blind, placebo-controlled study that investigated efficacy and safety of cangrelor and compared with placebo in 5362 patients who had not been treated with clopidogrel at the time of PCI (60). Loading dose of clopidogrel was administered after PCI. The primary end point was the same as 'CHAMPION-PCI' trial; a composite of death, myocardial infarction or ischemia driven revascularization at 48 hours. However, enrollment was stopped after an interim analysis which revealed that cangrelor did not achieve to show superiority for the primary end point. The primary end point occurred in 185 of 2654 patients receiving cangrelor (7.0%) and in 210 of 2641 patients receiving placebo (8.0%) (OR; 0.87, 95% CI, 0.71 to 1.07, p=0.17). Cangrelor reduced the rate of stent thrombosis and death from any cause at 48 hours from 0.6% to 0.2% (OR; 0.31, 95% CI, 0.11 to 0.85, p=0.02), and from 0.7% to 0.2% (OR; 0.33, 95% CI, 0.13 to 0.83, p=0.02) respectively. Although major bleeding was found significantly increased in the cangelor group transfusion requirements were similar in both cangrelor and placebo groups (60).

CHAMPION trials demonstrated that intravenous cangrelor administration at the time of PCI did not overcome standard clopidogrel loading procedure in patients with ACS. Although CHAMPION trials results were disappointing it should not be interpreted as cangrelor is worthless. As shown in secondary special end points (stent thrombosis and death) of CHAMPION-PLATFORM cangrelor may be beneficial in special situations. With its unique pharmacological properties and succesful preclinical studies, cangrelor does merit further clinical investigations.

## Ticagrelor (AZD6140)

Ticagrelor is the first oral, reversible cyclopentyl trialzolopyrimidine P2Y12 receptor antagonist. Ticagrelor is a direct acting drug that contains an adenosine triphosphate chain and it does not require in vivo metabolic biotransformation. Ticagrelor binds reversibly to another site on the P2Y12 receptor from the ADP binding site and blocks receptor activation through allosteric modulation of the receptor function (61). Ticagrelor is quickly absorbed from gastrointestinal system after oral administration, it reachs to peak plasma concentration after a single dose of 100 to 400 mg within 2 hours and inhibit platelets completely. Ticagrelor's elimination half-life was reported as 6-12 h (62).

'The DISPERSE' study established greater platelet inhibition by ticagrelor compared to clopidogrel in patients with stable atherosclerotic coronary artery disease (63). Ticagrelor achieved rapid and near complete inhibition of platelet aggregation when used ≥100 mg daily. The DISPERSE trial reported only few minor or moderate bleeding episodes and one major gastrointestinal bleeding in the higher dose (400 mg/d) ticagrelor group (63).

The DISPERSE-2 study aimed to confirm dose related effects of ticagrelor and to compare with clopidogrel in 990 patients with non-ST segment elevation MI (64, 65). Patients were randomized to receive either clopidogrel (300 mg loading dose and 75 mg/d maintenance dose) or twice daily ticagrelor (90 or 180 mg with or without a loading dose of 270 mg) for up to 3 month follow-up (64). Bleeding rates were similar between the clopidogrel and ticagrelor groups. Decreased bleeding rates were noted in ticagrelor treated patients who underwent coronary artery bypass graft surgery within 1-5 days that the study drug was stopped. However, in the ticagrelor group, patients experienced some respiratory symptoms including dyspnoea and cough more frequently than those in the clopidogrel group. This effect was explained in part by the adenosine triphospate's bronchoconstrictive effects (66).

A multicenter, double-blind, randomized clinical trial, the PLATO trial, compared ticagrelor and clopidogrel in the prevention of cardiovascular events in 18,624 patients with an ACS (67). In the ticagrelor arm of the PLATO trial patients were treated by a 180-mg loading dose and 90 mg twice daily maintenance dose while the therapy regimen of the clopidogrel arm was consisted of 300-to-600-mg loading dose and 75 mg/d maintenance dose. The primary end point; a composite of death from vascular causes, myocardial infarction or stroke had occurred in 9.8% of patients receiving ticagrelor as compared with 11.7% of those receiving clopidogrel (HR; 0.84, 95% CI, 0.77 to 0.92, p<0.001) at 12 months (67). Ticagrelor reduced also the rate of death from any cause (4.5%, versus 5.9% with clopidogrel; p<0.001). Of note, PLATO trial did not determine a significant difference at the site of bleeding rates between the ticagrelor and clopidogrel groups (11.6% and 11.2%, respectively; p=0.43). However, ticagrelor was found to be associated with a higher rate of major bleeding episodes including fatal intracranial bleeding. PLATO investigators concluded that ticagrelor when compared to clopidogrel achieved a significantly reduction in primary end points of vascular death, MI and stroke but at the cost of increased non-procedure related bleeding in patients with ACS (67).

PLATO trial demonstrated us a new and powerful antiplatelet agent with reversible activities, had better clinical benefits and similar safety profile when compared to standard clopidogrel therapy regimens. Ticagrelor's reversible activity is important and will improve our control on antiplatelet therapy. Using an antiplatelet agent with reversible activity is an advantage for clinicians because it can provide benefits at the site of bleeding in some special situations (eg, urgent needs for surgery). However, the spectrum of antiplatelets' side effects seems to be enlarged by the addition of dyspnoea, bradyarrhythmia, and increased serum levels of uric acid and creatinine. Fortunately none of these side effects were reported to be life threatening.

## Elinogrel

Elinogrel (PRT060128) is a direct-acting, reversible P2Y12 receptor inhibitor that can be administered both intravenously and orally. This property allows elinogrel to provide prompt antiplatelet activity with an IV infusion and also an oral maintenance choice for long term therapy (68, 69). Mice studies demonstrated that elinogrel has a dose proportional antithrombotic activity in vivo at plasma concentrations which has minimal effect on tail bleeding times in mice (70). Elinogrel achieved also a superior inhibition of thrombosis in mice when compared with clopidogrel (70).

A recent study established that single oral dose of elinogrel overcame high platelet reactivity in clopidogrel resistant patients undergoing PCI (71). The major metabolic route of elimination of elinogrel was determined as 'demethylation' to form PRT060301 which is also the prominent circulating metabolite of elinogrel in plasma and the only major metabolite in urine and faeces (22.4% of the dose) (72).

'The ERASE-MI' pilot phase IIA study aimed to investigate the safety and tolerability of escalating doses (10, 20, 40 and 60 mg) of elinogrel versus placebo when administered to STEMI patients before primary PCI (73). In this randomized, double blind, placebo controlled, dose escalation study elinogrel was administered as a single intravenous bolus before the start of the diagnostic angiogram preceding primary PCI. Patients were randomized to either elinogrel or placebo within each dosing groups. All the patients received 600-mg clopidogrel loading dose, followed by a second 300-mg clopidogrel loading dose 4 hours after PCI. As a measure of major outcome bleeding was assessed with two different scales; the TIMI and Global Strategies to Open Occluded Coronary Arteries bleeding scales. A total of 70 patients were randomized in the dose escalation study then the trial was prematurely terminated for administrative reasons. This pilot study provided preliminary data on the feasibility and tolerability of escalating doses elinogrel as an adjunctive therapy for primary PCI for STEMI despite its small sample size (73).

Another recent study investigated the effect of elinogrel (PRT060128) and the relationship between cytochrome P450 (CYP) polymorphisms and high platelet reactivity in patients receiving standard dual antiplatelet therapy (74). Platelet reactivity fell within 4 h of dosing, the earliest time point evaluated as measured by the following assays; maximum 5 and 10 μM ADP LTA ($p<0.001$ for both vs. predosing); maximum 20 μM ADP LTA ($p<0.05$); VerifyNow ($p<0.001$); thrombelastography ($p<0.05$); VASP phosphorylation ($p<0.01$); and perfusion chamber assay ($p<0.05$). 'CYP2C19*2' polymorphism was determined in 44% of all patients but it was more frequently seen in patients with high platelet reactivity (77% vs. 16%, $p=0.0004$). The authors concluded that 60 mg single dose elinogrel might reversibly accomplish high platelet reactivity which was also found to be associated with CYP2C19*2 polymorphism (74).

'The INNOVATE-PCI' trial is a multi-center, randomized, double-blind, triple-dummy, clopidogrel-controlled study of IV and oral elinogrel (PRT060128) compared to clopidogrel in patients undergoing non-urgent (including elective) PCI. After diagnostic angiography, patients scheduled for non-urgent PCI are randomized to clopidogrel or to one of three dose of PRT060128. The aim of the study is to provide information on clinical efficacy, biological activity, tolerability and safety of PRT060128 in patients undergoing non-urgent PCI. The developer of elinogrel states that the design of INNOVATE-PCI is not powered to examine a pre-specified endpoint. The study is ongoing but not recruiting patients (NCT00751231, http://clinicaltrials.gov/ct2/show/study/NCT00751231?show_locs=Y#locn).

Current available data suggest that elinogrel have a potential to become an important instrument in prevention of atherothrombosis but there is still need for further large scale clinical randomized trials.

## Table 1. Brief summary of clinical trials performed with P2Y12 antagonists

| Investigational drug | Trial | Patient population | Efficacy | Safety |
|---|---|---|---|---|
| Prasugrel | JUMBO-TIMI (45) | 904 patients undergoing PCI for MI | Prasugrel reduced MACE compared with clopidogrel (7.2% versus 9.4%) | No increase in major bleeding with prasugrel |
| Prasugrel | TRITON-TIMI38 (47) | 13,608 patients with moderate to high risk ACS | Prasugrel reduced MI (7.4% vs 9.7%, p<0.001), urgent TVR (2.5% vs 3.7%, p<0.001), and stent thrombosis (11.% vs 2.4%, p<0.001) in comparison to clopidogrel | Prasugrel increased major (2.4% vs 1.8%), life-threatening (1.4% vs 0.9%, p=0.01), nonfatal (1.1% versus 0.9%, p=0.23) and fatal bleedings (0.4% vs. 0.1%, p=0.002) compared to clopidogrel |
| Prasugrel | PRINCIPLE-TIMI44 (46) | 201 patients undergoing PCI | 60 mg LD and 10 mg MD of prasugrel provided greater platelet inhibition than 600-mg LD and 150 mg/d MD of clopidogrel | NA |
| Cangrelor | CHAMPION-PCI (59) | 8,877 patients with ACS undergoing PCI | At the 48th hour primary composite end point occured in 7.5% and 7.1% of patients receiving cangrelor and clopidogrel (OR, 1.05; 95% CI, 0.88 to 1.24; p=0.59). Cangrelor was not found superior to clopidogrel at 30 days. | Major bleeding increased slightly but not statistically significant |
| Cangrelor | CHAMPION-PLATFORM (60) | 5362 patients undergoing PCI | Primary end point occurred in 185 (7.0%) and 210 (8.0%) patients cangrelor and placebo (p=0.17). Cangrelor reduced ST and death from any cause at 48 hours from 0.6% to 0.2% (p=0.02), and from 0.7% to 0.2% (p=0.02) | Major bleeding was significantly increased in cangelor group but transfusion requirements were similar in cangrelor and placebo groups |
| Ticagrelor | DISPERSE (63) | 200 patients with CAD | Ticagrelor provided greater inhibition of platelets compared to clopidogrel | NA |
| Ticagrelor | DISPERSE-2 (64) | 990 patients with non-STEMI | NA | Ticagrelor did not increase bleeding events |
| Ticagrelor | PLATO (67) | 18,624 patients with ACS | Composite end point of death from vascular causes, MI, or stroke occurred in 9.8% and 11.7% of patients receiving ticagrelor and clopidogrel (HR, 0.84; 95% CI, 0.77 to 0.92; p<0.001) at 12 months. | No significant difference in bleeding between ticagrelor and clopidogrel (11.6% and 11.2%, p=0.43). |
| Elinogrel | ERASE-MI# (73) | 70 patients with STEMI | Safety and tolerability of escalating doses of elinogrel was tested | Elinogrel was generally well tolerated |
| Elinogrel | INNOVATE-PCI* | Patients undergoing non urgent PCI | NA | NA |

*The study is ongoing and the results are not published yet. #; the study was prematurely terminated for administrative reasons.

ACS; acute coronary syndrome, CAD; coronary artery disease, HR; hazard ratio, LD; loading dose, MACE; major cardiac adverse event, MD; maintenance dose, MI; myocardial infarction, NA; not available, PCI; percutanous coronary intervention, ST; stent thrombosis, STEMI; ST elevation myocardial infarction, TVR; target vessel revascularization.

## Bx667

Another novel, reversibly acting, orally administrated P2Y12 receptor antagonist is BX 667. This is a prodrug that rapidly converts to an active metabolite called 'BX 048'. A recent study used different animal models in order to assess the therapeutic index of BX 667 and to compare with clopidogrel (75). When administered orally, BX 667 and clopidogrel showed similar efficacy, but BX 667 caused less bleeding than clopidogrel. The experimental models of thrombosis demonstrated that BX 667 had a wider therapeutic index than clopidogrel (75). BX 667 and its active metabolite BX 048 block the binding of 2MeSADP to platelets and antagonize ADP-induced platelet aggregation reversibly in human, dog and rat washed platelets. BX 048 blocks ADP-induced reduction of intracellular cAMP in a concentration-dependent manner. The specificity of BX 667 and BX 048 was demonstrated against cell lines expressing P2Y1 and P2Y6. BX 048 and BX 667 are potent P2Y12 antagonists with high specificity (76). BX 667 blocks ADP-induced platelet aggregation in human, dog and rat blood (IC50=97, 317 and 3000 nM respectively). BX 667 have nominal effects on collagen-induced aggregation and weakly inhibits arachidonic acid-induced aggregation. The bioavailability of BX 667 is high in both dog and rat unlike BX 048. Administration of BX 667 results with a rapid and sustained inhibition of platelet aggregation where the extent and duration of platelet inhibition was directly proportional to circulating plasma levels (77).

BX 677 and its active metabolite are new compounds and there are so few available data. Further clinical evidence is needed to determine whether these molecules may have a position in current antiplatelet regimens.

## THROMBOXANE RECEPTOR ANTAGONISTS

Thromboxane receptor inhibitors are another novel group of antiplatelet agents that can inhibit $TxA_2$ on platelets as well as aspirin, additionally endoperoxidase, prostanoids and isoprostanes. The effect of thromboxane receptor antagonist is not limited to platelets but it blocks thromboxane receptors expressed by different cells such as monocytes and vascular cells. Thromboxane receptor antagonists preserve also the production of prostacyclin which limits platelet aggregation and produces vasodilation (78).

## Terutroban (S18886)

Terutroban (S18886) is an orally administered thromboxane receptor antagonist that acts reversibly. It reaches to peak plasma levels within 2 hours and has a terminal half life of 5.8–10 hours. A recent study showed that maximal inhibition of platelet aggregation has been achieved within 1 h with all oral doses of terutroban and maintained for at least 12 hours. Furthermore, terutroban did not increase rates of adverse event (78).

Terutroban blocks thromboxane $A_2$ and under shear conditions it decreases fibrinogen deposition (79). Experimental studies suggested that terutroban can inhibit stent thrombosis as well as standard dual antiplatelet therapy consisted of aspirin and clopidogrel. Terutroban showed also reduced bleeding rates compared to aspirin and clopidogrel combination (80).

Furthermore, terutroban have some antiatherosclerotic properties and may provide atherosclerotic plaque regression (81, 82).

Another coronary arterial thrombosis and myocardial ischemia-reperfusion study performed in canines established that terutroban and clopidogrel combination achieved to prevent occlusive thrombus formation at the cost of a moderate increase in tongue bleeding time (83). Furthermore, terutroban has renoprotective effects, attenuates renal oxydative stress (84, 85).

A recent study showed that even a single dose of 10mg terutroban improved endothelial function (both flow mediated and acetylcholine mediated vasodilatation) in 12 patients with coronary artery disease (86).

A double-blind, parallel-group, 10 day study investigated the efficacy and safety of terutroban in 48 patients with cerebral ischemic events and/or carotid stenosis. At the 10th day of therapy, the mean cross sectional surface of dense thrombus was found significantly reduced in the terutroban group compared with aspirin group ($p < 0.01$). Terutroban achieved an antithrombotic activity that is superior to aspirin and similar to clopidogrel-aspirin combination. Terutroban provided significant reduction in endothelial and platelet activation with an acceptable safety and tolerability profile (87).

An ongoing double blind, randomized, controlled, phase III clinical trial, 'the PERFORM study' (Prevention of cerebrovascular and cardiovascular Events of ischemic origin with teRutroban in patients with a history oF ischemic strOke or tRansient ischeMic attack) aims to investigate the superiority of terutroban (30 mg/day) over aspirin (100 mg/day), in reducing cerebrovascular and cardiovascular events in patients with a recent history of ischemic stroke or transient ischemic attack. The primary efficacy endpoint is set as a composite of ischemic stroke (fatal or nonfatal), myocardial infarction (fatal or nonfatal) or other vascular death (excluding hemorrhagic death of any origin). Safety is being evaluated by assessing hemorrhagic events in the trial. Follow-up is expected to last for 2-4 years. The randomization of 19,119 patients is been realized and follow-up period is still ongoing (88, 89).

The PERFORM study may provide important findings and potentially terutroban may replace aspirin in our clinical practise in future. The trial seems to have enough statistical power to test the superiority of terutroban over aspirin in the secondary prevention of cerebrovascular and cardiovascular events in patients with a recent history of ischemic stroke or transient ischemic attack. Final results are expected in 2011.

## von Willebrand Factor Inhibitors

von Willebrand factor (vWF) binds to subendothelial collagen via its A3 domain and binds to platelets via its A1 or C3 domain to form homotypic multimers between matrix bound and soluble vWF molecules (90). In the arterial circulation under high shear condition vWF becomes activated and binds to the platelet glycoprotein (GP) Ib receptor (91). To obtain antithrombotic effects researchers designed monoclonal antibodies against human vWF. AJW200, ARC1779 and ALX0081 are human monoclonal vWF antagonists and are under investigation.

## Ajw200

AJW200 is an IgG$_4$ monoclonal antibody that binds human vWF. The inhibitory effect of AJW200 on vWF mediated platelet adhesion, aggregation and activation at comparative concentrations to parent monoclonal antibody are shown recently (92). A single parenteral administration of AJW200 blocked ristocetin induced platelet aggregation in cynomolgus monkeys (92).

The antithrombotic effect of AJW200 and its effect on bleeding time were also investigated in a canine coronary artery thrombosis model. The pharmacological blockade of platelet glycoprotein (GP) Ib-vWF interaction with AJW200 resulted with a succesfull and safer antithrombotic profile than abciximab in dogs (93).

## Arc1779

ARC1779 is a therapeutic aptamer antagonist of the A1 domain of vWF. A randomized, double-blind, placebo controlled study investigated its pharmacokinetics and pharmacodynamics in 47 healthy volunteers (94). ARC1779 established dose and concentration dependent inhibition of vWF activity and platelet function. ARC1779 was well tolerated and no bleeding was observed in the study (94).

The ARC1779 aptamer was assessed for inhibition of vWF induced platelet aggregation in another study. ARC1779 inhibited both botrocetin and shear force induced platelet aggregation. ARC1779 also inhibited the formation of occlusive thrombi in cynomolgus monkeys (95).

Another study investigated ex vivo dose response curves of ARC1779 on vWF activity, shear-dependent platelet function and agonist induced platelet aggregation. Up to two fold increased plasma vWF levels were determined in patients with acute MI in comparison with controls. ARC1779 inhibited vWF activity, platelet function measured by PFA-100 and Cone and Plate Analyzer in all groups. However, ARC1779 did not inhibit platelet aggregation induced by ADP, collagen or arachidonic acid. The authors conclude that ARC1779 potently and specifically inhibits vWF dependent platelet function in patients with acute MI (96).

This study established an important finding that ARC1779 specifically inhibits vWF mediated platelet aggregation but does not affect platelets activated by other important activators (eg, ADP, arachidonic acid). This means that vWF inhibitor ARC1779 may have a restricted clinical indication in future and almost always would be used together with another antiplatelet agent.

Recent studies showed that ARC1779 may provide benefits in patients with thrombotic thrombocytopenic purpura (97, 98).

## Alx-0081

ALX-0081 is the first nanobody antithrombotic that specifically targets the GPIb binding site of vWF. There is so few available data about this compound (99).

## DIRECT THROMBIN INHIBITORS (PAR-1 INHIBITORS)

Direct acting thrombin inhibitors bind to the protease-activated receptor 1 (PAR-1) which is essentially the main platelet receptor for thrombin. This new group of antiplatelets include; SCH 205831, SCH 602539, SCH 530348 and E 5555.

**Table 2. Summary of clinical trials performed with direct thrombin inhibitors (PAR-1), vWF antagonists and thromboxane inhibitors**

| Investigational drug | Trial | Patient population | Efficacy | Safety |
|---|---|---|---|---|
| SCH 530348 | TRA-PCI (101) | 1,030 patients with ACS undergoing non-urgent PCI | NA | No statistical difference in bleeding rates between SCH 530348 and placebo |
| SCH 530 348 | TRA 2°P-TIMI 50* (103) | Patients with atherosclerotic vascular disease | Priamry efficacy en point is MACE | NA |
| SCH 530348 | TRA-CER* (102) | 10,000 patients with non-STEMI | Primary efficacy end point is MACE | NA |
| E 5555 | LANCELOT* | 600 patients with non-STEMI | NA | Safety and tolerability is under assessment |
| ARC 1779 | VITAL-1 (96) | 300 patients with MI | ARC 1779 inhibited vWF activity, platelet function measured by PFA-100 and Cone and Plate Analyzer but not platelet aggregation induced by ADP, collagen or arachidonic acid. | NA |
| Terutoban | PERFORM* (88, 89) | 19,119 patients with a recent history of ischemic stroke or TIA | The superiority of terutroban (30 mg/day) over aspirin (100 mg/day), in reducing cerebrovascular and cardiovascular events is under investigation | Safety is being evaluated by assessing hemorrhagic events in the trial |

*The study is ongoing and the results are not published yet. ACS; acute coronary syndrome, MACE; major cardiac adverse event, MI; myocardial infarction, NA; not available, PCI; percutanous coronary intervention, STEMI; ST elevation myocardial infarction, TIA; transient ischemic attack.

## Sch 530348

SCH 530348 is a potent and highly selective platelet thrombin receptor (PAR-1) antagonist that acts by directly blocking thrombin mediated platelet activation without interfering with other pathways (100).

The tolerability and safety of SCH 530348 were assessed in patients aged 45 years or older and undergoing non-urgent PCI or coronary angiography with planned PCI. The primary endpoint of clinically significant major or minor bleeding according to the TIMI scale occurred in 2 (2%) of 129, 3 (3%) of 120, and 7 (4%) of 173 patients, respectively, in the SCH 530348 10 mg, 20 mg and 40 mg groups compared with 5 (3%) of 151 patients in the placebo group (p=0.5786). This study established that SCH 530348 was well tolerated and did not cause increased TIMI bleeding even when administered together with aspirin and clopidogrel (101).

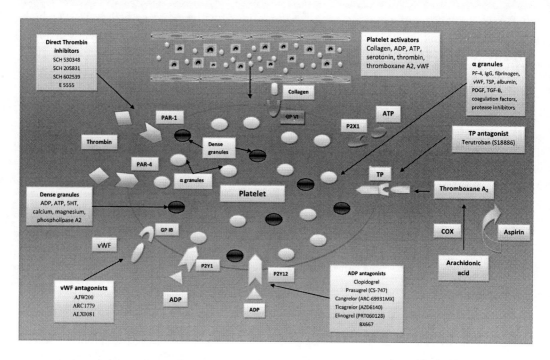

Figure: Platelet activation and inhibitors. Potential activators of platelets include; collagen, vWF, thrombin, thromboxane A2, serotonin, ADP, and ATP. Once platelets are activated they release dense granules ingredients (ADP, ATP, serotonin, phospholipase A2). Stimulation of P2Y12 receptors by ADP and GPIIbIIIa receptor activation increase platelet aggregation. Many steps of platelet activation and aggregation are targets for antiplatelet therapy. ADP; adenosine diphosphate, ATP; adenosine triphosphate, COX; cyclooxygenase, GP Ib; glycoprotein Ib, GP VI; glycoprotein VI, IgG; immunglobulin gamma, PAR-1; protease activated receptor-1, PAR-4; protease activated receptor-4, PDGF; platelet derived growth factor, PF-4; platelet factor-4, TGF-B; transforming growth factor beta, TP; thromboxane receptor, TSP; thrombospondin, vWF; von Willebrand factor, 5HT; 5 hydroxytryptamine (serotonin).

SCH 530348 is a selective, competitive PAR-1 antagonist that is administered orally. The efficacy and safety of SCH 530348 are under investigation in a prospective, randomized, double blind, multicentric, phase III trial in patients with non ST segment elevation ACS (the TRACER trial) (102). Primary efficacy end points are consisted of a composite of cardiovascular death, MI, stroke, recurrent ischemia with rehospitalization and urgent coronary revascularization compared with standard of care alone. Safety end points include the composite of moderate and severe GUSTO bleeding and clinically significant TIMI bleeding (102).

The 'Thrombin-Receptor Antagonist in Secondary Prevention of Atherothrombotic Ischemic Events' (TRA 2°P)-TIMI 50 trial is a phase III, randomized, double blind, placebo controlled clinical trial that aimed to evaluate the efficacy and safety of SCH 530348 during long term treatment of patients with atherosclerotic disease. The primary end point of the trial is a composite of cardiovascular death, MI, stroke, or urgent coronary revascularization. Long term safety investigation is based on bleeding rates defined by the GUSTO and TIMI criteria. TRA 2°P-TIMI 50 is supposed to establish whether a new antithrombotic approach by PAR-1 antagonism reduces major cardiovascular events with acceptable safety profile in patients with atherosclerotic vascular disease (103).

The results of 'TRACER' and 'TRA 2°P-TIMI 50' trials will provide pivotal findings and will determine the position of SCH 530348 in current antiplatelet therapy spectrum.

## E5555

E5555 is another potent PAR-1 antagonist that targets the G coupled receptor and modulates thrombin platelet-endothelial interactions. A recent study investigated the in vitro effects of E5555 on platelet function in healthy volunteers and patients with coronary artery disease receiving aspirin with or without clopidogrel. E5555 inhibited selectively platelet activity. The authors suggested that E5555 may enhance potenciate aspirin or aspirin-clopidogrel combination (104).

## CONCLUSION

In recent years, researchs in cardiovascular medicine are mostly focused on pathogenesis of atherosclerosis and cardiovascular risk modification. Atherothrombosis, one of the crucial and latest complications of atherosclerotic vascular disease became the most studied stage of the disease. Understanding the physiology of platelets allowed us to develop novel antiplatelet agents acting via different receptors and mechanisms. In the last two decades, advances in antiplatelet therapy extended the spectrum of therapeutics. Aspirin was the first clinically aproved antithrombotic agent and still protects its position. However, new generation thromboxane antagonists (eg, terutroban) or nitric oxide releasing aspirin may replace it in near future. In the last decade advances in percutaneous coronary interventions and stenting increased the importance of double antiplatelet therapy and ADP receptor antagonists, thus clopidogrel became the most prescribed antiplatelet after aspirin. Prasugrel and ticagrelor are new candidates which already overcame clopidogrel's antiplatelet effect with a similar safety profile or increased bleeding rates. vWF antagonists and direct thrombin inhibitors with different acting sites are under investigation and in some special patient groups or clinical situations these agents may provide benefits and may be useful. In any case, having many therapeutic options will facilitate management of atherothrombosis. Thus, we may yield more efficient and safer antithrombotic therapy. The next step in antiplatelet management may be a personalized and unique therapeutic regimen that depends on patient needs, current clinical situation and drug sensitivity profile.

## REFERENCES

[1] Rosamond W, Flegal K, Friday G, Furie K, Go A, Greenlund K, et al. American Heart Association Statistics Committee and Stroke Statistics Subcommittee. Heart disease and stroke statistics-2007 update: a report from the American Heart Association Statistics Committee and Stroke Statistics Subcommittee. *Circulation* 2007; 115: e69–e171.

[2] Langer HF, Gawaz M. Platelet–vessel wall interactions in atherosclerotic disease. *Thromb Haemost* 2008; 99: 480–6.

[3] Meadows TA, Bhatt DL. Clinical aspects of platelet inhibitors and thrombus formation. *Circ Res* 2007; 100: 1261-75.

[4] Ridker PM. Evaluating novel cardiovascular risk factors: can we better predict heart attacks? *Ann Intern Med* 1999; 130: 933–7.

[5] Libby P, Simon DI. Inflammation and thrombosis: the clot thickens. *Circulation* 2001; 103: 1718-20.

[6] Lindemann S, Tolley ND, Dixon DA, McIntyre TM, Prescott SM, Zimmerman GA, Weyrich AS. Activated platelets mediate inflammatory signaling by regulated interleukin-1 beta synthesis. *J Cell Biol* 2001; 154: 485–90.

[7] McNicol A, Israels SJ. Platelets and anti-platelet therapy. *J Pharmacol Sci* 2003; 93: 381-96.

[8] Ruggeri ZM. Platelets in atherothrombosis. *Nat Med* 2002; 8: 1227-34.

[9] Massberg S, Gawaz M, Gruner S, Schulte V, Konrad I, Zohlnhöfer D, Heinzmann U, Nieswandt B. A crucial role of glycoprotein VI for platelet recruitment to the injured arterial wall in vivo. *J Exp Med* 2003; 197: 41-9.

[10] Raju NC, Eikelboom JW, Hirsh J. Platelet ADP-receptor antagonists for cardiovascular disease: past, present and future. *Nat Clin Pract Cardiovasc Med* 2008; 5: 766-80.

[11] Arya M, Lopez JA, Romo GM, Cruz MA, Kasirer-Friede A, Shattil SJ, Anvari B. Glycoprotein Ib-IX-mediated activation of integrin alpha(IIb)beta(3): effects of receptor clustering and von Willebrand factor adhesion. *J Thromb Haemost* 2003; 1: 1150-7.

[12] Craven LL. Experiences with aspirin (acetylsalicylic acid) in the non-specific prophylaxis of coronary thrombosis. *Miss Valley Med J* 1953; 75: 38-44.

[13] Vane JR. Inhibition of prostaglandin synthesis as a mechanism of action for aspirin-like drugs. *Nature* 1971; 231: 232-5.

[14] Lewis HD Jr, Davis JW, Archibald DG, Steinke WE, Smitherman TC, Doherty JE 3rd et al. Protective effects of aspirin against acute myocardial infarction and death in men with unstable angina. Results of a Veterans Administration Cooperative Study. *N Engl J Med* 1983; 309: 396-403.

[15] Lewis HD Jr. Unstable angina: status of aspirin and other forms of therapy. *Circulation*. 1985; 72: V155-60.

[16] Ridker PM, Manson JE, Buring JE, Goldhaber SZ, Hennekens CH. The effect of chronic platelet inhibition with low dose aspirin on atherosclerotic progression and acute thrombosis:clinical evidence from Physicians Health Study. *Am Heart J* 1991; 122: 1588-92.

[17] Antithrombotic Trialists' Collaboration. Collaborative meta-analysis of randomised trials of antiplatelet therapy for prevention of death, myocardial infarction, and stroke in high risk patients. *BMJ* 2002; 324: 71–86.

[18] Randomised trial of intravenous streptokinase, oral aspirin, both, or neither among 17,187 cases of suspected acute myocardial infarction: ISIS-2. ISIS-2 (Second International Study of Infarct Survival) Collaborative Group. *Lancet* 1988; 2(8607): 349-60.

[19] ISIS-3 (Third International Study of Infarct Survival) Collaborative Group. ISIS-3: A randomised trial of streptokinase vs tissue plasminogene activator vs antistreplase and of aspirin plus heparin vs aspirin alone among 41,299 cases of suspected acute myocardial infarction. *Lancet* 1992; 339: 753-70.

[20] Patrono C, Coller B, Dalen JE, FitzGerald GA, Fuster V, Gent M et al. Platelet-active drugs: The relationships among dose, effectiveness and side effects. *Chest* 2001; 119 (1 Suppl): 39S-63S.

[21] Patrono C. Aspirin as an antiplatelet drug. *N Engl J Med* 1994; 330: 1287-94.

[22] ten Berg JM, Gerritsen WB, Haas FJ, Kelder HC, Verheugt FW, Plokker HW. High-dose aspirin in addition to daily low-dose aspirin decreases platelet activation in patients before and after percutaneous coronary intervention. *Thromb Res* 2002; 105: 385-90.

Pamukcu B. A review of aspirin resistance; definition, possible mechanisms, detection with platelet function tests and its clinical outcomes. *J Thromb Thrombolysis* 2007; 23: 213-22.

[23] Panak E, Maffrand JP, Picard-Fraire C, Vallée E, Blanchard J, Roncucci R. Ticlopidine: A promise for the prevention and treatment of thrombosis and its complications. *Haemostasis* 1983; 13(suppl 1): 1-54.

[24] Balsano F, Rizzon P, Violi F, Scrutinio D, Cimminiello C, Aguglia F et al. Antiplatelet treatment with ticlopidine in unstable angina. A controlled multicenter clinical trial. The Studio della Ticlopidina nell'Angina Instabile Group. *Circulation* 1990; 82: 17-26.

[25] Gill S, Majumdar S, Brown NE, Armstrong PW. Ticlopidineassociated pancytopenia: implications of an acetylsalicytic acid alternative. *Can J Cardiol* 1997; 13: 909-13.

[26] Fukushima K, Kobayashi Y, Okuno T, Nakamura Y, Sakakibara M, Nakayama T, et al. Incidence of side-effects of ticlopidine after sirolimus-eluting stent implantation. *Circ J* 2007; 71: 617-9.

[27] The CAPRIE Steering Committee. A randomised, blinded, trial of clopidogrel versus aspirin in patients at risk of ischaemic events. *Lancet* 1996; 348: 1329-39.

[28] The CURE Investigators. Effects of clopidogrel in addition to aspirin in patients with acute coronary syndromes without ST segment elevation. *N Engl J Med* 2001; 345: 494-502.

[29] Mehta SR, Yusuf S, Peters RJG, Bertrand ME, Lewis BS, Natarajan MK et al, on behalf of the CURE Investigators. Effects of pretreatment with clopidogrel and aspirin followed by long-term therapy in patients undergoing percutaneous coronary intervention: the PCI-CURE study. *Lancet* 2001; 358: 527-33.

[30] Steinhubl SR, Berger PB, Mann JT 3rd, Fry ET, DeLago A, Wilmer C, Topol EJ; CREDO Investigators. Clopidogrel for the Reduction of Events During Observation. Early and sustained dual oral antiplatelet therapy following percutaneous coronary intervention: a randomized controlled trial. *JAMA* 2002; 288: 2411-20. Erratum in: JAMA 2003; 289: 987.

[31] Chen ZM, Jiang LX, Chen YP, Xie JX, Pan HC, Peto R et al. COMMIT (ClOpidogrel and Metoprolol in Myocardial Infarction Trial) collaborative group.Addition of clopidogrel to aspirin in 45,852 patients with acute myocardial infarction: randomised placebo-controlled trial. *Lancet* 2005; 366: 1607-21.

[32] Sabatine MS, Cannon CP, Gibson CM, Lopez-Sendon JL, Montalescot G, Theroux P, et al. Addition of clopidogrel to aspirin and fibrinolytic therapy for myocardial infarction with ST-segment elevation. *N Engl J Med* 2005; 352: 1179-89.

[33] Sabatine MS, Cannon CP, Gibson CM, López-Sendón JL, Montalescot G, Theroux P, et al; Clopidogrel as Adjunctive Reperfusion Therapy (CLARITY)-Thrombolysis in Myocardial Infarction (TIMI) 28 Investigators. Effect of clopidogrel pretreatment before percutaneous coronary intervention in patients with ST-elevation myocardial infarction treated with fibrinolytics: the PCI-CLARITY study. *JAMA* 2005; 294: 1224-32.

[34] Storey RF, Newby LJ, Heptinstall S. Effects of P2Y(1) and P2Y(12) receptor antagonists on platelet aggregation induced by different agonists in human whole blood. *Platelets* 2001; 12: 443–7.

[35] Farid NA, Payne CD, Small DS, Winters KJ, Ernest CS, 2nd, Brandt JT et al. Cytochrome P450 3A inhibition by ketoconazole affects prasugrel and clopidogrel pharmacokinetics and pharmacodynamics differently. *Clin Pharmacol Ther* 2007; 81: 735-41.

[36] Sugidachi A, Asai F, Ogawa T, Inoue T, Koike H. The in vivo pharmacological profile of CS-747, a novel antiplatelet agent with platelet ADP receptor antagonist properties. *Br J Pharmacol* 2000; 129: 1439-46.

[37] Niitsu Y, Jakubowski JA, Sugidachi A, Asai F. Pharmacology of CS-747 (prasugrel, LY640315), a novel, potent antiplatelet agent with in vivo P2Y12 receptor antagonist activity. *Semin Thromb Hemost* 2005; 31: 184-94.

[38] Sugidachi A, Ogawa T, Kurihara A, Hagihara K, Jakubowski JA, Hashimoto M et al. The greater in vivo antiplatelet effects of prasugrel as compared to clopidogrel reflect more efficient generation of its active metabolite with similar antiplatelet activity to that of clopidogrel's active metabolite. *J Thromb Haemost* 2007; 5: 1545-51.

[39] Asai F, Jakubowski JA, Naganuma H, Brandt JT, Matsushima N, Hirota T, et al. Platelet inhibitory activity and pharmacokinetics of prasugrel (CS-747) a novel thienopyridine P2Y12 inhibitor: a single ascending dose study in healthy humans. *Platelets* 2006; 17: 209-17.

[40] Jernberg T, Payne CD, Winters KJ, Darstein C, Brandt JT, Jakubowski JA, et al. Prasugrel achieves greater inhibition of platelet aggregation and a lower rate of non-responders compared with clopidogrel in aspirin-treated patients with stable coronary artery disease. *Eur Heart J* 2006; 27: 1166-73.

[41] Brandt JT, Payne CD, Wiviott SD, Weerakkody G, Farid NA, Small DS, et al. A comparison of prasugrel and clopidogrel loading doses on platelet function: magnitude of platelet inhibition is related to active metabolite formation. *Am Heart J* 2007; 153: 66.e9 –16.

[42] Payne CD, Li YG, Small DS, Ernest CS, 2nd, Farid NA, Jakubowski JA et al. Increased active metabolite formation explains the greater platelet inhibition with prasugrel compared to high-dose clopidogrel. *J Cardiovasc Pharmacol* 2007; 50: 555-62.

[43] Wallentin L, Varenhorst C, James S, Erlinge D, Braun OO, Jakubowski JA, et al. Prasugrel achieves greater and faster P2Y12 receptor mediated platelet function than clopidogrel due to more efficient generation of its active metabolite in aspirin treated patients with coronary artery disease. *Eur Heart J* 2008; 29: 21-30.

[44] Wiviott SD, Antman EM, Winters KJ, Weerakkody G, Murphy SA, Behounek BD et al. Randomized comparison of prasugrel (CS-747, LY640315), a novel thienopyridine P2Y12 antagonist, with clopidogrel in percutaneous coronary intervention: results of the Joint Utilization of Medications to Block Platelets Optimally (JUMBO)-TIMI 26 trial. *Circulation* 2005; 111: 3366–73.

[45] Wiviott SD, Trenk D, Frelinger AL, O'Donoghue M, Neumann FJ, Michelson AD et al. Prasugrel compared with high loading and maintenance-dose clopidogrel in patients with planned percutaneous coronary intervention: the Prasugrel in Comparison to Clopidogrel for Inhibition of Platelet Activation and Aggregation-Thrombolysis in Myocardial Infarction 44 trial. *Circulation* 2007; 116: 2923–32.

[46] Wiviott SD, Braunwald E, McCabe CH, Montalescot G, Ruzyllo W, Gottlieb S, et al. Prasugrel versus clopidogrel in patients with acute coronary syndromes. *N Engl J Med* 2007; 357: 2001–15.

[47] Wiviott SD, Braunwald E, Angiolillo DJ, Meisel S, Dalby AJ, Verheugt FW et al. Greater clinical benefit of more intensive oral antiplatelet therapy with prasugrel in patients with diabetes mellitus in the trial to assess improvement in therapeutic outcomes by optimizing platelet inhibition with prasugrel-Thrombolysis in Myocardial Infarction 38. *Circulation* 2008; 118: 1626-36.

[48] Montalescot G, Wiviott SD, Braunwald E, Murphy SA, Gibson CM, McCabe CH et al. Prasugrel compared with clopidogrel in patients undergoing percutaneous coronary intervention for ST-elevation myocardial infarction (TRITON-TIMI 38): doubleblind, randomised controlled trial. *Lancet* 2009; 373: 723–31.

[49] Storey RF, Oldroyd KG, Wilcox RG. Open multicentre study of the P2T receptor antagonist AR-C69931MX assessing safety, tolerability and activity in patients with acute coronary syndromes. *Thromb Haemost* 2001; 85: 401-7.

[50] van Giezen JJ, Humphries RG. Preclinical and clinical studies with selective reversible direct P2Y12 antagonists. *Semin Thromb Hemost* 2005; 31: 195–204.

[51] Angiolillo DJ, Bhatt DL, Gurbel PA, Jennings LK. Advances in antiplatelet therapy: agents in clinical development. *Am J Cardiol* 2009; 103: 40A–51A (suppl).

[52] Ingall AH, Dixon J, Bailey A, Coombs ME, Cox D, McInally JI, et al. Antagonists of the platelet P2T receptor: a novel approach to antithrombotic therapy. *J Med Chem* 1999; 42: 213-20.

[53] Wang K, Zhou X, Zhou Z, Tarakji K, Carneiro M, Penn MS et al. Blockade of the platelet P2Y12 receptor by AR-C69931MX sustains coronary artery recanalization and improves the myocardial tissue perfusion in a canine thrombosis model. *Arterioscler Thromb Vasc Biol* 2003; 23: 357-62.

[54] Steinhubl SR, Oh JJ, Oestreich JH, Ferraris S, Charnigo R, Akers WS. Transitioning patients from cangrelor to clopidogrel: pharmacodynamic evidence of a competitive effect. *Thromb Res* 2008; 121: 527-34.

[55] Storey RF, Wilcox RG, Heptinstall S. Comparison of the pharmacodynamic effects of the platelet ADP receptor antagonists clopidogrel and AR-C69931MX in patients with ischaemic heart disease. *Platelets* 2002; 13: 407-13.

[56] Jacobsson F, Swahn E, Wallentin L, Ellborg M. Safety profile and tolerability of intravenous AR-C69931MX, a new antiplatelet drug, in unstable angina pectoris and non-Q-wave myocardial infarction. *Clin Ther* 2002; 24: 752-65.

[57] Greenbaum AB, Ohman EM, Gibson CM, Borzak S, Stebbins AL, Lu M et al. Preliminary experience with intravenous P2Y12 platelet receptor inhibition as an adjunct to reduced-dose alteplase during acute myocardial infarction: results of the Safety, Tolerability and Effect on Patency in Acute Myocardial Infarction (STEP-AMI) angiographic trial. *Am Heart J* 2007; 154: 702–9.

[58] Harrington RA, Stone GW, McNulty S, White HD, Lincoff AM, Gibson CM, et al. Platelet Inhibition with Cangrelor in Patients Undergoing PCI. *N Engl J Med* 2009; 361; 2318-29.

[59] Bhatt DL, Lincoff AM, Gibson CM, Stone GW, McNulty S, Montalescot G, et al for the CHAMPION PLATFORM Investigators. Intravenous Platelet Blockade with Cangrelor during PCI. *N Engl J Med* 2009; 361; 2330-41.

[60] Storey RF, Thornton SM, Lawrance R, Husted S, Wickens M, Emanuelsson H, et al. Ticagrelor yields consistent dose-dependent inhibition of ADP-induced platelet aggregation in patients with atherosclerotic disease regardless of genotypic variations in P2RY12, P2RY1, and ITGB3. *Platelets* 2009; 20: 341-8.

[61] Tantry US, Bliden KP, Gurbel PA. Azd6140. *Expert Opin Investig Drugs* 2007; 16: 225-9.

[62] Husted S, Emanuelsson H, Heptinstall S, Sandset PM, Wickens M, Peters G. Pharmacodynamics, pharmacokinetics, and safety of the oral reversible P2Y12 antagonist AZD6140 with aspirin in patients with atherosclerosis: A double-blind comparison to clopidogrel with aspirin. *Eur Heart J* 2006; 27: 1038-47.

[63] Cannon CP, Husted S, Harrington RA, Scirica BM, Emanuelsson H, Peters G, Storey RF. Safety, tolerability, and initial efficacy of AZD6140, the first reversible oral adenosine diphosphate receptor antagonist, compared with clopidogrel, in patients with non-ST-segment elevation acute coronary syndrome: Primary results of the DISPERSE-2 trial. *J Am Coll Cardiol* 2007; 50: 1844-51.

[64] Storey RF, Husted S, Harrington RA, Heptinstall S, Wilcox RG, Peters G, et al. Inhibition of platelet aggregation by AZD6140, a reversible oral P2Y12 receptor antagonist, compared with clopidogrel in patients with acute coronary syndromes. *J Am Coll Cardiol* 2007; 50: 1852-6.

[65] Doggrell SA. Ticagrelor, a platelet aggregation inhibitor for the potential prevention and treatment of arterial thrombosis and acute coronary syndromes. *IDrugs* 2009; 12: 309-17.

[66] Wallentin L, Becker RC, Budaj A, Cannon CP, Emanuelsson H, Held C, et al for the PLATO Investigators. Ticagrelor versus clopidogrel in patients with acute coronary syndromes. *N Engl J Med* 2009; 361: 1045-57.

[67] Gretler DD, Conley PB, Andre P, Jurek M, Pandey A, Romanko K, et al. First in human experience with PRT060128, a new direct-acting, reversible, P2Y12 inhibitor for IV and oral use. *J Am Coll Cardiol* 2007; 49: 326A.

[68] Lieu HD, Conley PB, Andre P, Leese PT, Romanko K, Phillips DR, et al. Initial intravenous experience with PRT060128 (PRT128), an orally-available, directacting, and reversible P2Y12 inhibitor. *J Thromb Haemost* 2007; 5 Suppl. 2: P-T-292.

[69] Andre P, Jurek M, Sim D, Deguzman F, Hollenbach S, Phillips DR et al. PRT060128, a novel, direct-acting orally available P2Y12 antagonist, confers superior antithrombotic activity over clopidogrel in a mice thrombosis model. *J Thromb Haemost* 2007; 5: O-W-031.

[70] Gurbel PA, Conley PB, Andre P, Stephens G, Gretler DD, Jurek MM et al. Oral Dosing of PRT060128, a Novel Direct-acting, Reversible P2Y12 Antagonist Overcomes High Platelet Reactivity in Patients Non-responsive to Clopidogrel Therapy. *Circulation* 2008; 118: S-972.

[71] Cattaneo M. New P2Y12 inhibitors. *Circulation* 2010; 121: 171-9.

[72] Berger JS, Roe MT, Gibson CM, Kilaru R, Green CL, Melton L, et al. Safety and feasibility of adjunctive antiplatelet therapy with intravenous elinogrel, a direct-acting and reversible P2Y12 ADP-receptor antagonist, before primary percutaneous intervention in patients with ST-elevation myocardial infarction: The Early Rapid ReversAl of Platelet ThromboSis with Intravenous Elinogrel before PCI to Optimize REperfusion in Acute Myocardial Infarction (ERASE MI) pilot trial. *Am Heart J* 2009; 158: 998-1004.

[73] Gurbel PA, Bliden KP, Antonino MJ, Stephens G, Gretler DD, Jurek MM, et al. The effect of elinogrel on high platelet reactivity during dual antiplatelet therapy and the relation to cyp 2c19*2 genotype: first experience in patients. *J Thromb Haemost* 2010; 8: 43-53.

[74] Wang YX, Vincelette J, da Cunha V, Martin-McNulty B, Mallari C, Fitch RM, Alexander S, et al. A novel P2Y(12) adenosine diphosphate receptor antagonist that inhibits platelet aggregation and thrombus formation in rat and dog models. *Thromb Haemost* 2007; 97: 847-55.

[75] Bryant J, Post JM, Alexander S, Wang YX, Kent L, Schirm S, et al. Novel P2Y12 adenosine diphosphate receptor antagonists for inhibition of platelet aggregation (I): In vitro effects on platelets. *Thrombosis Research* 2008; 122: 523-32.

[76] Post JM, Alexander S, Wang YX, Vincelette J, Vergona R, Kent L, et al. Novel P2Y12 adenosine diphosphate receptor antagonists for inhibition of platelet aggregation (II): Pharmacodynamic and pharmacokinetic characterization. *Thrombosis Research* 2008; 122: 533-40.

[77] Gaussem P, Reny JL, Thalamas C, Chatelain N, Kroumova M, Jude B, et al. The specific thromboxane receptor antagonist S18886: pharmacokinetic and pharmacodynamic studies. *J Thromb Haemost* 2005; 3: 1437-45.

[78] Osende JI, Shimbo D, Fuster V, Dubar M, Badimon JJ. Antithrombotic effects of S 18886, a novel orally active thromboxane A2 receptor antagonist. *J Thromb Haemost* 2004; 2: 492-8.

[79] Vilahur G, Casani L, Badimon L. A thromboxane A2/prostaglandin H2 receptor antagonist (S18886) shows high antithrombotic efficacy in an experimental model of stent-induced thrombosis. *Thromb Haemost* 2007; 98: 662-9.

[80] Worth NF, Berry CL, Thomas AC, Campbell JH. S18886, a selective TP receptor antagonist, inhibits development of atherosclerosis in rabbits. *Atherosclerosis* 2005; 183: 65-73.

[81] Chamorro A. TP receptor antagonism: a new concept in atherothrombosis and stroke prevention. *Cerebrovasc Dis* 2009; Suppl 3: 20-7.

[82] Hong TT, Huang J, Driscoll E, Lucchesi BR. Preclinical evaluation of S18886 in an experimental model of coronary arterial thrombosis. *J Cardiovasc Pharmacol* 2006; 48: 239-48.

[83] Sebekova K, Ramuscak A, Boor P, Heidland A, Amann K. The selective TP receptor antagonist, S18886 (terutroban), attenuates renal damage in the double transgenic rat model of hypertension. *Am J Nephrol* 2008; 28: 47-53.

[84] Xu S, Jiang B, Maitland KA, Bayat H, Gu J, Nadler JL et al. The thromboxane receptor antagonist S18886 attenuates renal oxidant stress and proteinuria in diabetic apolipoprotein E-deficient mice. *Diabetes* 2006; 55: 110-9.

[85] Belhassen L, Pelle G, Dubois-Rande JL, Adnot S. Improved endothelial function by the thromboxane A2 receptor antagonist S 18886 in patients with coronary artery disease treated with aspirin. *J Am Coll Cardiol* 2003; 41: 1198-1204.

[86] Bal Dit Sollier C, Crassard I, Simoneau G, Bergmann JF, Bousser MG, Drouet L. Effect of the thromboxane prostaglandin receptor antagonist terutroban on arterial thrombogenesis after repeated administration in patients treated for the prevention of ischemic stroke. *Cerebrovasc Dis* 2009; 28: 505-13.

[87] Bousser MG, Amarenco P, Chamorro A, Fisher M, Ford I, Fox K, et al; PERFORM Study Investigators. Rationale and design of a randomized, double-blind, parallel-group study of terutroban 30 mg/day versus aspirin 100 mg/day in stroke patients: the prevention of cerebrovascular and cardiovascular events of ischemic origin with terutroban in patients with a history of ischemic stroke or transient ischemic attack (PERFORM) study. *Cerebrovasc Dis* 2009; 27: 509-18.

[88] Bousser MG, Amarenco P, Chamorro A, Fisher M, Ford I, Fox K, et al; PERFORM Study Investigators. The Prevention of cerebrovascular and cardiovascular Events of ischemic origin with teRutroban in patients with a history oF ischemic strOke or tRansient ischeMic attack (PERFORM) study: baseline characteristics of the population. *Cerebrovasc Dis* 2009; 27: 608-13.

[89] Savage B, Sixma JJ, Ruggeri ZM. *Functional self-association of von Willebrand factor during platelet adhesion under flow.* Proc Natl Acad Sci U S A 2002; 99: 425-30.

[90] Siedlecki CA, Lestini BJ, Kottke-Marchant KK, Eppell SJ, Wilson DL, Marchant RE. Shear-dependent changes in the three-dimensional structure of human von Willebrand factor. *Blood* 1996; 88: 2939-50.

[91] Kageyama S, Yamamoto H, Nakazawa H, Matsushita J, Kouyama T, Gonsho A, et al. Pharmacokinetics and pharmacodynamics of AJW200, a humanized monoclonal antibody to von Willebrand factor, in monkeys. *Arterioscler Thromb Vasc Biol* 2002; 22: 187- 92.

[92] Kageyama S, Matsushita J, Yamamoto H. Effect of a humanized monoclonal antibody to von Willebrand factor in a canine model of coronary arterial thrombosis. *European Journal of Pharmacology* 2002; 443: 143-9.

[93] Gilbert JC, DeFeo-Fraulini T, Hutabarat RM, Horvath CJ, Merlino PG, Marsh HN, et al. First in human evaluation of anti–von willebrand factor therapeutic aptamer ARC1779 in healthy volunteers. *Circulation* 2007; 116: 2678-86.

[94] Diener JL, Daniel Lagasse HA, Duerschmied D, Merhi Y, Tanguay JF, Hutabarat R et al. Inhibition of von Willebrand factormediated platelet activation and thrombosis by the anti-von Willebrand factor A1-domain aptamer ARC1779. *J Thromb Haemost* 2009; 7: 1155-62.

[95] Spiel AO, Mayr FB, Ladani1 N, Wagner PG, Schaub RG, Gilbert JC, Jilma B. The aptamer ARC1779 is a potent and specific inhibitor of von Willebrand factor mediated ex vivo platelet function in acute myocardial infarction. *Platelets* 2009; 20: 334-40.

[96] Knöbl P, Jilma B, Gilbert JC, Hutabarat RM, Wagner PG, Jilma-Stohlawetz P. Anti von Willebrand factor aptamer ARC1779 for refractory thrombotic thrombocytopenic purpura. *Transfusion* 2009; 49: 2181-85.

[97] Jilma B, Jilma P, Gilbert JC, Hutabarat R, Siller J, Spiel A et al. Safety, pharmacokinetics and pharmacodynamics of the anti von Willebrand factor aptamer ARC1779 in patients with acute thrombotic thrombocytopenic purpura TTP. *J Thromb Haemost* 2009; 7 (Suppl.1): AS-WE-014.

[98] Siller-Matula JM, Krumphuber J, Jilma B. Pharmacokinetic, pharmacodynamic and clinical profile of novel antiplatelet drugs targeting vascular diseases. *Br J Pharmacol* 2009 Dec 24. [Epub ahead of print] PubMed PMID: 20050853.

[99] Bhatt DL, Topol EJ. Scientific and therapeutic advances in antiplatelet therapy. *Nat Rev Drug Discov* 2003; 2: 15-28.

[100] Becker RC, Moliterno DJ, Jennings LK, Pieper KS, Pei J, Niederman A, et al for the TRA-PCI Investigators. Safety and tolerability of SCH 530348 in patients undergoing non-urgent percutaneous coronary intervention: a randomised, double-blind, placebo-controlled phase II study. *Lancet* 2009; 373: 919-28.

[101] The TRACER Executive and Steering Committees. The Thrombin Receptor Antagonist for Clinical Event Reduction in Acute Coronary Syndrome (TRACER) trial: study design and rationale. *Am Heart J* 2009; 158: 327-34.

[102] Morrow DA, Scirica BM, Fox KAA, Berman G, Strony J, Veltri E, et al for the TRA 2-P-TIMI 50 Investigators. Evaluation of a novel antiplatelet agent for secondary prevention in patients with a history of atherosclerotic disease: Design and rationale for the Thrombin-Receptor Antagonist in Secondary Prevention of Atherothrombotic Ischemic Events (TRA 2°P)-TIMI 50 trial. *Am Heart J* 2009; 158: 335-41.

[103] Serebruany VL, Kogushi M, Pitei DD, Flather M, Bhatt DL. The in vitro effects of E5555, a protease-activated receptor (PAR)-1 antagonist, on platelet biomarkers in healthy volunteers and patients with coronary artery disease. *Thromb Haemost* 2009; 102: 111-9.

*Chapter V*

# UNCONTROLLED IMMUNE RESPONSE IN ACUTE MYOCARDIAL INFARCTION

## *Vicente Bodí Peris[1] and María José Forteza de los Reyes[2]*
[1]Cardiology Department, Hospital Clinico Universitario, Valencia, Spain
[2]Physiology Department, Universidad de Valencia, Valencia, Spain

### ABSTRACT

Recently, the theory that hyperinflammation is the body's primary response to potent stimulus has been challenged. Indeed, a deregulation of the immune system could be the cause of multiple organ failure. So far, clinicians have focused on the last steps of the inflammatory cascade. However, little attention has been paid to lymphocytes, which play an important role as strategists of the inflammatory response. Experimental evidence suggests a crucial role of T lymphocytes in the pathophysiology of atherosclerosis and acute myocardial infarction (AMI). In summary, from the bottom of an imaginary inverted pyramid, a few regulatory T-cells control the upper parts represented by the wide spectrum of the inflammatory cascade. In AMI, a loss of regulation of the inflammatory system occurs in patients with a decreased activity of regulatory T-cells. As a consequence, aggressive T-cells boost and anti-inflammatory T-cells drop. A pleiotropic proinflammatory imbalance with damaging effects in terms of left ventricular performance and patient outcome is the result of this uncontrolled immune response.

Nowadays, in order to reduce infarct size and microvascular obstruction, a broad range of innovative therapeutic approaches have been proposed, i.e.: cell therapy with regulatory T-cells, inhibition of pro-inflammatory cytokines (TNF-α antagonists), anti-inflammatory cytokines (IL-10 therapy), vaccination with antigens responsables of the immune response in atherosclerosis (vaccination with LDLox or vaccination with Heat Shock Protein 60 HSP60), or the use of gene therapy. The aim of this review is to get an insight into the pathophysiology of the role of the immune system in AMI as well as to describe new therapeutic options on the basis of the regulation of the immune system.

## INTRODUCTION

Infection and trauma have been the most important causes of death in human history (1). Nonsurprisingly, potent innate immunity and inflammatory response have been needed to ward off infection and survive trauma. However, our ancestors, who lived a short physically demanding life, did not die of atherosclerosis or acute myocardial infarction (AMI). From an evolutionary point of view, it would be possible that an adaptative pattern could become, in specific circumstances, a maladaptative response (1,2). In our modern life, atherosclerosis has resulted to be the main cause of death, and inflammation plays a crucial role from the early stages of the disease to the most severe forms (1-7). Moreover, in the context of AMI, a deregulated immune system is being recognized not only as a trigger factor but also as a decisive factor amplifying an excessive and unnecessary inflammatory response (8-10).

For prognostic purposes, clinicians have focused on the last steps of a complex chain of mechanisms, for example, white blood cells (WBC) as a whole, neutrophils or downstream products such as C-reactive protein (CRP). However, little is known regarding the role of lymphocytes, which play an important role in the control of the inflammatory system and in the pathophysiology of AMI. Furthermore, pro- and anti-inflammatory T lymphocytes as well as regulatory T-cells (Treg) have been barely analyzed in this scenario.

The purpose of this work is to move a step forward to unravel the thread of the inflammatory cells in AMI. We propose an "inverted pyramid" model: from the bottom, a few Treg control the upper parts represented by the wide spectrum of the inflammatory cascade. First, we will address the outer parts of this imaginary inverted pyramid, namely, WBC as a whole, neutrophils, and monocytes. Afterward, we will focus on effector T lymphocytes and on the deepest part of the inverted pyramid, Treg. Finally, on the basis of this alternative pathophysiological model, several innovative and potentially beneficial therapeutic options will be analyzed.

## LEUKOCYTES

The leukocyte response during AMI has been traditionally considered as expression of acute-phase reactant. This response is triggered by the necrotic insult and considered a central component of the reparative process. A correlation exists between the degree of leukocytosis and the extension of the infarcted area (11,12).

Apart from necrosis, a higher WBC count has also been related to a worse coronary perfusion. Barron et al, (13) in the context of ST-elevation AMI, reported an association of leukocytosis upon admission with more deteriorated coronary and microvascular perfusion. The availability of reliable imaging techniques such as cardiovascular magnetic resonance, which permits in a single session a comprehensive characterization of the structural consequences of AMI (Figure 1), will allow in the near future a better understanding of the pathophysiological implications of WBC in this scenario (14,15).

Nonsurprisingly, leukocytosis has emerged as a powerful predictor of death in patients with AMI (12,13). The fact that WBC count is inexpensive and commonly measured makes it a potentially helpful prognostic marker (11). Its usefulness has been confirmed in the entire spectrum of AMI both in a short-term (12) and in a long-term perspective (16). We followed up a cohort of 515 consecutive patients admitted to a university hospital from October 2000 to June 2003 for ST-elevation AMI. Patients with cancer, chronic inflammatory disease, or any systemic infection were excluded. During 3 years median follow- up, 106 deaths were documented. We observed that a WBC count >10,000 cells/mL independently doubled the risk of death in 1 year (12).

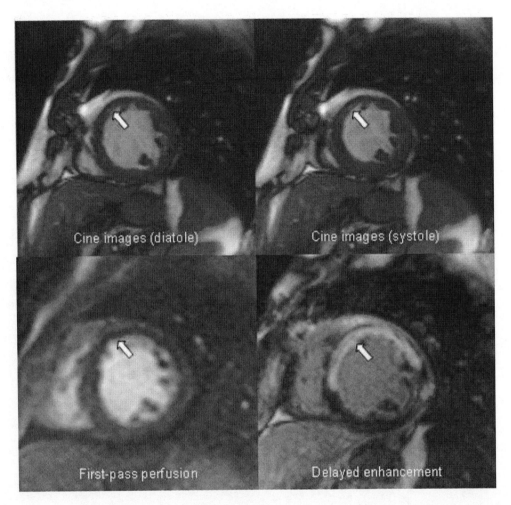

Figure 1. Cardiovascular magnetic resonance imaging allows a comprehensive analysis of patients after myocardial infarction. Arrows show areas of hypokinesia in cine images (upper panels), microvascular obstruction in first-pass perfusion imaging (lower panel, left) and a large infarcted area in delayed enhancement imaging (lower panel, right).

The WBC count could also represent a potential prognostic marker in patients with non–ST-elevation AMI (16,17). In 634 patients who presented to the emergency department with non–ST-elevation chest pain and increased troponin, WBC count >10,000 cells/mL associated to higher mortality (26% vs 10%, P = .0001) and added independent information to predict death beyond troponin (hazard ratio 2.2, P b .0001) (16). Therefore, WBC count could be helpful to further stratify risk in this high- risk population.

Despite the evidence associating total WBC count with cardiovascular outcomes in patients with AMI, little has been published about the predictive ability of specific differential

WBC counts. Recent studies demonstrate different associations of WBC subtypes and prognosis (18). Neutrophilia (19) and, to a lesser extent, monocytosis (20) and lymphopenia (21) have been related to worse prognosis in patients with AMI. In the end, WBC count is a result of all the individual courses of each cell subtype.

## NEUTROPHILS

The most dramatic and pathologically significant abnormalities associated with neutrophil accumulation in AMI are microvascular obstruction and myocardial injury. Neutrophils are large, and stiff cells and may adhere to capillary endothelium preventing reperfusion of capillaries after thrombolysis or primary angioplasty (19).

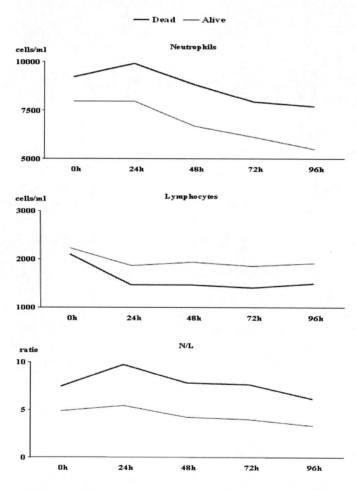

Figure 2. Temporal evolution of inflammatory cells in a series of 515 consecutive patients admitted for ST-segment elevation myocardial infarction (reference 12). More neutrophils, less lymphocytes and a higher neutrophil to lymphocyte ratio during the acute phase related to a higher risk of death during follow-up. Abbreviations: N/L = neutrophil to lymphocyte ratio.

In the absence of inflammation, leukocytes are rarely seen to interact with the vessel wall (19). After the inflammatory stimulus is applied, distinct sets of adhesion molecules, namely, L-selectin, E-selectin, and P- selectin, promote leukocyte rolling and attachment at postcapillary venules and entry into tissues (22). For neutrophils, firm adhesion requires activation of the β2 (CD18) integrins and binding to intercellular adhesion mollecule-1. Transendothelial migration follows and leads to direct injury on parenchymal cells through release of specific toxic products (11,19).

In patients with ST-segment elevation AMI, neutrophilia at baseline predicts a large infarct size and an altered coronary perfusion (11,19). In our series of 515 patients with clinical follow-up, (12) neutrophilia and a larger neutrophil to lymphocyte ratio were predictors of death during the subsequent months (Figure 2).

## MONOCYTES

Neutrophils are the first leukocytes to be found in the damaged myocardial area and are removed from myocardial tissue after phagocytosing the debris. In contrast, monocytes migrate from capillaries to extra- vascular space and are transformed into macrophages and outnumber neutrophils 2 to 3 days after the acute episode. Macrophage-secreted cytokines stimulate fibroblast proliferation and collagen production and promote monocytosis (20).

Macrophages and monocytes synthesize and secrete a variety of humoral factors including interleukin (IL)-6, the main stimulus for CRP production in the liver. Among the various inflammatory markers tested in patients with acute coronary syndromes, CRP is the most widely investigated (23,24).

Mariani et al, (25) in a group of 238 patients treated with primary angioplasty after acute ST-segment elevation AMI, sequentially measured WBC subtypes count and quantified systolic function using echocardiography at baseline and at 6 months. They observed that monocytosis related to failed or incomplete myocardial reperfusion. Moreover, monocyte count was independently associated with less systolic recovery in 6 months (25). This course suggests the participation of monocytes in the reparative process once the hyperacute phase has been completed.

Although neutrophilia and monocytosis are associated with poorer angiographic and clinical outcomes, it remains unclear whether they are simply a causal markers of the extent of necrosis or whether elevations of these cells are causally related to greater reperfusion injury. Perhaps, the association is actually bidirectional (20). It is notable that pharmacotherapies directed against the inflammatory cascade such as corticoids treatment, anticomplement antibodies, or neutrophil blockade have failed in human studies (11,20). This would suggest that WBC elevations are a marker rather than a causative agent in adverse outcomes. It is, however, also possible that the targeted specific ligand may not be relevant. Exploration of alternative routes is needed to understand the directionality of causation and the potential targets for future pharmacotherapy.

# LYMPHOCYTES

## Rationale and Clinical Evidence

The most powerful protective tool that we have is inflammation, a genetic response pattern that allows the immune system to rapidly recognize threats, mobilize cells to injury sites, remove instigators, and heal wounds (9). Although neutrophils live only for hours and generate no memory of their engagement, which is carried out through inherited receptors that are similar in all hosts, lymphocytes are long-lived cells that can survive for decades, and the lymphocyte repertoire is tailored for each individual.9 When mobilized in immune responses, lymphocytes undergo clonal burst, differentiate into distinct types of effector cells, and memorize information about the antigen (8,9,26). Genetics, age, sex, infections, and environmental exposures mold the individual's lymphocyte pool (27).

An increased incidence of cardiovascular events has been reported in diseases with lymphopenia-mediated immunosuppression. Situations such as acquired immu- nodeficiency syndrome, posttransplant-induced immunosuppression, or atomic bomb survivors relate to a significant decrease in CD4 cells and to an accelerated atherosclerotic process (26). This evidence fueled the thought that a loss of lymphocytes could be involved in the genesis and outcome of ischemic heart disease.

Recently, the theory that hyperinflammation is the body's primary response in stress situations such as sepsis was challenged. Indeed, a deregulation of the immune system could be the cause of multiple organ failure (27). In this line, severe lymphopenia occurs during the initial stages of sepsis. Massive lymphocyte apoptosis, may be as a philogenetically inherited self-protective response in front of an overshoot of proinflammatory cytokines, seems to be the main underlying mechanism. Patient survival goes along with lymphocyte count recovery (27).

Although acute lymphopenia also occurs in patients with AMI, its prognostic and pathophysiological implications have been barely explored so far. Studies analyzing patients without (21) and with (12,18) AMI demonstrated that a lower lymphocyte count and a higher neutrophil to lymphocyte ratio related to more cardiovascular events during the follow-up. Recently, Dragu et al, (18) in 1,037 patients with AMI (68% ST-elevation AMI), reported that a low lymphocyte count at baseline was an independent predictor of mortality over a 23-month median follow-up even after adjustment for baseline characteristics. In our series of 515 patients with ST- elevation AMI with clinical follow-up, not only did we confirm that lymphopenia was an usual finding in the acute phase of AMI but also that less lymphocytes and a higher neutrophil-to-lymphocyte ratio predicted a worse outcome (12) (Figure 2).

Whether this sort of association is causative or it merely represents a marker of myocardial and microvascular injury cannot be elucidated in clinical studies. However, these data open a window for alternative approaches in the understanding of the pathophysiology of AMI and in the research of innovative therapies such as those directed at stopping the deregulation of the immune response provoked by a predominance of the proinflammatory effector T-cells and cytokines by means of the expansion or mobilization of Treg (8,9).

## Effector T-Cells

Lymphocyte count appears as a useful, simple, and easy-to-obtain tool that can significantly improve risk prediction in AMI. However, it barely reflects the amazing complexity of cells and interactions embraced under this denomination. For pathophysiological and therapeutic purposes, a much deeper knowledge of lymphocyte subtypes and regulation is warranted.

T-cell–mediated immunodeficiency as reflected by CD4 lymphocytopenia is associated with atherosclerosis. Ducloux et al (26) observed in renal transplant recipients that CD4 cell count in the highest quartile (>663/mL) divided the risk of atherosclerotic events by 10. T-cells helper (CD4) and suppressor (CD8) subtypes are activated in AMI. In patients with AMI, the CD4/CD8 ratio is inverted on admission, and a prolonged depressed CD4/CD8 ratio is a poor prognostic factor (28).

Upon antigenic stimulation, CD4+ T-cells differentiate into T helper 1 (Th1) and T helper 2 (Th2) subsets characterized by the release of distinct cytokines. T helper 1 typically release proinflammatory cytokines such as interferon-γ, tumor necrosis factor-α, IL-2, IL-12, or IL-18. T helper 2 exhibit an opposed activity, mainly releasing anti-inflammatory cytokines such as IL-4, IL-5, IL-6, IL-9, IL-10, or IL-13. T helper 2–derived IL-10 can inhibit Th1 polarization (28,29). In unstable patients with angina, Th1 activity predominates. These cells seem to play a role not only in the formation and growth of the atherosclerotic plaque but also in its destabilization and in the onset of AMI (29,30).

T helper 1 stimulate the production of metalloproteinases by macrophages and induce apoptosis of smooth muscle cells; both actions weaken and thins the fibrous cap of atherosclerotic plaques, the preamble of plaque rupture and coronary thrombosis (3,4) Steppich et al, (29) Cheng et al, (31) and Methe et al (30) have consistently demonstrated in small groups of patients that a significant rise in Th1 numbers occurs in unstable patients with angina in comparison with control cases.

In patients with AMI, an acute deregulation of the immune system has been described, and it seems to bring about deleterious consequences. Cheng et al, in a group of 33 patients with AMI, sequentially measured Th1 and Th2 cells; a proinflammatory Th1/Th2 imbalance (in comparison with a control group) was detected in all measure- ments and it associated to left ventricular dilation, systolic dysfunction, and to a worse functional class (31). By means of proinflammatory cytokines, a pro-Th1 imbalance contributes to the activation of endothelial cells, induces adhesion molecules, and activates leukocytes (29,31). Moreover, reperfusion of the occluded artery with a proin- flammatory milieu could induce endothelial cells apoptosis and in turn aggravate microvascular obstruction (32,33). Therefore, a pro-Th1 imbalance is able to boost a pleiotropic and harmful inflammatory response.

Experimental studies support the idea of a causal role of a pro-Th1 imbalance in the pathophysiology of AMI. Interleukin-10 is a Th2-derived anti-inflammatory cytokine that suppresses Th1 activity (28,29) Yang et al (34) demonstrated that lack of IL-10 in genetically manipulated mice related to an enhanced inflammatory response, neutrophil infiltration, increased expression of tumor necrosis factor- α, and intercellular adhesion molecule-1 as well as to a larger infarct size and less survival. In patients with AMI, a higher proinflammatory–to–anti-inflammatory cytokines ratio predicts more cardiac events (35).

Apart from Th1 and Th2 cells, patients with AMI experience expression of a subset of CD4 cells that lack the CD28 marker. These cells, known as CD4+CD28null cells, express killer immunoglobulin-like receptors, a characteristic of the natural killers cells, and have cytolytic function (36,37). The fact that they are able to produce high levels of interferon-$\gamma$ together with the fact that they can be isolated from unstable plaques support the notion that CD4+CD28null cells have damaging effects in AMI. Zal et al (37) demonstrated that human heat- shock protein 60 is an antigen recognized by these cells. Liuzzo et al (36) have recently reported that patients with recurrence of acute coronary events present a higher CD4+CD28null T-cell frequency.

A perturbation of T-cell repertoire is strongly involved in the pathophysiology of AMI. Effector T-cells seem an attractive and experimentally well-rooted therapeutic target. Deeper and probably more transcendent parts of the inflammatory cascade can, however, be explored.

## Regulatory T-Cells

Without down-regulation, physiological processes are at high risk of becoming pathological. Hence, down-regulation is of utmost importance. This applies in particular to immune reactions (8-10), (38). Immunologic down-regulation brings immune responses to an end. The origin of the lymphocyte response in AMI has been a matter of debate in the last decade. The putative target antigenic stimuli evoked in AMI can also be found in patients with chronic atherosclerotic disease. This indicates that the repertoire of antigens targeted by the immune system cannot explain the deviant lymphocyte responses observed in acute coronary disease (8).

The cause of the pathological autoreactive immune response observed in AMI might reside in a tolerance break due to a defective regulation of the T lymphocyte compartment (8-10). Concepts of suppressor T-cells entered the immunologic landscape in the 1970s (39). However, at that time, neither the cells nor the postulated soluble factors released by these cells could be convincingly characterized, and the entire concept was criticized. In the mid-1980s, CD4+CD25+ Treg entered the stage and soon attracted deep interest (40). CD4+CD25+ T-cells constitutively express the surface receptors CTLA-4 and GITR and use the transcription factor Foxp3. They are naturally occurring suppressor cells, possibly arising as a separate thymic lineage (9). Activated by self-antigen or non–self-antigen, they suppress T-cells in an antigen- nonspecific manner. Cell membrane contact is necessary for this effect. Peripheral numbers of CD4+CD25+ T-cells appear to critically depend on IL-2 (8-10), (38).

CD4+CD25+ Treg are centrally involved in maintaining self-tolerance and suppress aberrant or excessive immune responses. Murine CD4+CD25+ T-cells can affect trypto- phan metabolism in dendritic cells resulting in tryptophan deficiency. Because tryptophan is an essential proliferative stimulus for effector T-cells, these cells undergo apoptosis (38). This could be one of the mechanisms involved in the severe lymphopenia occurring within the acute phase of AMI (Figure 2), and this way Treg would protect the organism from a boost of effector T-cells–derived proinflammatory cytokines. The relationship between CD4+CD25+ T-cells and dendritic cells seems to be bidirectional. Dendritic cells, as professional antigen-presenting cells, can induce and expand Treg, suggesting that accumulation of Treg depends on continuous peripheral stimulation, perhaps via tissue antigens presented by resident antigen presenting cells (38). Besides influencing dendritic cells, CD4+CD25+ T-cells can convey suppressor activity to conventional CD4+ T effector cells; this suppressor function is contact dependent and partially mediated by transforming growth factor-β (TGF-β) and IL-10 (38).

Apart from CD4+CD25+ T-cells, other Treg such as the Tr1 and Th3 regulatory T lymphocytes have been described (8,9,38). Tr1 exert their inhibitory function not only against the initial antigen but also against other antigens by secreting TGF-β and IL-10. The suppressor effects of Th3 cells are antigen-nonspecific and mediated as bystander inhibition, mainly via TGF-β. Th3 cells could suppress the activation of Th1 as well as Th2 clones, and they are a unique subset of T-cells induced by orally fed antigens (38). Experimental evidence suggests that activation of Treg is antigen specific, but that once activated, their suppressive activity is nonspecific (9,38). It seems that therapeutic strategies using Treg will be successful only if these cells home to the target organs (38).

Solid experimental data support the role of Treg in plaque inflammation and plaque development. Mallat et al (10) demonstrated that transfer of CD4+CD25+ Treg to genetically manipulated mice abrogated the induction of atherosclerosis and reduced the infiltration of T-cells and macrophages into plaques. Conversely, depletion of Treg resulted in an increase of lesion size, less accumulation of collagen, and more infiltration of T-cells and macrophages (10).

Preliminary clinical findings indicate that the autoaggressive lymphocyte response observed in AMI might derive from a flawed regulatory lymphocyte network. This could partially explain the difference between stable and acute atherosclerotic clinical manifestation, in spite of common plaque structure and antigenic content. Mor et al (41) were the first to demonstrate a defective Treg compartment in patients with AMI. Oxidized low-density lipoprotein (OxLDL)-specific T lymphocytes were activated in patients with unstable, but not in patients with, chronic stable angina. The number and the suppressor efficiency of Treg were reduced in unstable patients (41). This is a crucial finding in this research area with important implications for possible future therapeutic strategies.

The cause of the regulation malfunction remains to be discovered. However, regardless of the cause, lack of regulation commonly spawns deviant behavior. Given their role in T-cell–mediated immunity, CD4+CD25+ T-cells are now proposed as a panacea of immunomodulation and a unique opportunity to expand the knowledge about the pathophysiology of AMI as well as to explore promising therapeutic options (8,9).

## The Inverted Pyramid Model

Although important lessons in terms of pathophysiology and risk prediction have already been obtained, inflammatory parameters evaluated in clinical cardiology so far only represent the tip of an amazing variety of processes (8,9). For a better understanding of the pathophysiological implications of inflammation in AMI as well as for new therapeutic approaches, unraveling the thread of the inflammatory cascade is warranted.

We propose an "inverted pyramid" model to explain the damaging effects of an uncontrolled inflammatory response in AMI (Figure 3). Obviously, it is a simplistic view, but it briefly updates current knowledge derived from preliminary clinical data, (12,18,26-31) studies carried out in medical specialties apart from cardiology, (38) and a huge experimental research not assimilated by clinicians yet (8-10).

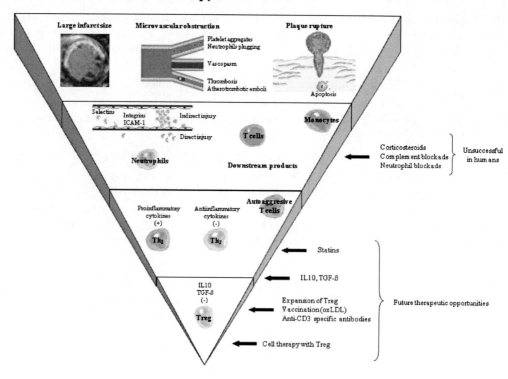

Figure 3. In patients with acute myocardial infarction, loss of regulation of the immune system by a few regulatory T cells located at the bottom of an imaginary inverted pyramid results in a pleiotropic inflammatory response. Loss of regulation of the immune system by Treg cells induces a proinflammatory imbalance by enhancing T helper 1 and autoaggresive cells and decreasing T helper 2 cells activity. This activates the upper parts of the inverted pyramid. An increased expression of selectins, integrins and adhesion molecules results in rolling, adhesion and migration of neutrophils through the endothelial wall and, as a consequence, direct and indirect injury (due to neutrophil plugging). Monocytes and T cells activation aggravate microvascular obstruction by promoting platelet aggregation, neutrophil plugging, vasospasm and thrombosis. Monocyte-derived proteases and T cells-induced apoptosis can weaken the fibrous cap of the atherosclerotic plaque and provoke future acute coronary syndromes. Some antiinflammatory therapies such as neutrophil blockade, corticosteroids or anti-complement have been already tested in humans without beneficial effects. The proposed model could be hypothesis generating to investigate several therapeutic options such as cell therapy with *in vitro* expanded Treg, *in vivo* expansion of Treg by means of specific anti-CD3 antibodies or OxLDL vaccination. Th1 blockade using IL-10, TGF-β or statins are other possible options trying to simulate the downregulatory effects of Treg. Abbreviations: ICAM-1 = intercellular adhesion molecule-1. IL-10 = interleukin 10. MVO = microvascular obstruction. OxLDL = oxidized low-density lipoproteins. Th = T helper cell. TGF-β = transforming growth factor- β. Treg = regulatory T cell.

In summary, at the bottom of the inverted pyramid would reside a few Treg (8-10). Using inhibitory messages, these cells are able to suppress proinflammatory Th1, enhance antiinflammatory Th2, and inhibit autoaggressive CD4 +CD28null cells (10,38). Failure of Treg to exert their suppressing function could boost a proinflammatory Th1/ Th2 state (8) as well as the expansion of CD4+CD28null cells (36) Moreover, Treg can induce apoptosis on effector T-cells as a defensive mechanism (38). In AMI, an acute deregulation of the immune system could provoke an indiscriminate loss not only of Th1 but also of Th2 cells, this exacerbating further the proinflammatory state. This pro- Th1 imbalance would boost, mainly by means of cytokines, the upper parts of the inverted pyramid represented by a pleiotropic inflammatory response, which includes monocytes, neutrophils, and downstream products (10). Microvascular obstruction, myocardial injury, and clinical events follow this uncontrolled immune response. A variety of bidirectional relationships and feedback processes among all the players of the inflammatory cascade along with interactions with parallel systems such as endothelium, platelets, or coagulation take place.

An unsolved question is the homeostasis of Treg. Older age, diabetes, or cumulative classical risk factors could reduce Treg activity (38) and, in case of AMI, provoke a hyperinflammatory response and a worse outcome. Moreover, similar to recent observations in infectious diseases, a genetically predetermined proinflammatory pattern could underlay the individual response in front of potent stimulus such as AMI. In this line, some polymorphisms have been associated with the severity of the systemic inflammatory response (42). Recently, de Servi et al (24) have proposed that those patients with a high baseline inflammatory state (in part, genetically predetermined) exhibit an exaggerated response in the context of AMI. It could be speculated that a chronically reduced Treg activity would explain why these patients present a bigger atherosclerotic burden and why they have a boost of inflammatory markers during AMI.

The proposed model can be helpful to better understand the pathophysiology of atherosclerosis, non–ST-elevation acute coronary syndromes, and ST-elevation AMI. Chronic atherosclerosis is a decades-long process that probably demands a much more comprehensive approach. In the case of non–ST-elevation acute coronary syndromes (this including unstable angina and small infarctions), a transitory Th1 predominance has been described, (29-31) which probably participates in the weakening and thinning of the fibrous cap of atherosclerotic plaques, the preamble of plaque rupture and coronary thrombosis. However, it seems that the most acute and severe immune deregulation takes place in the case of large ST-elevation AMI; in this scenario, severe lymphopenia, (12) a marked proinflammatory Th1/Th2 imbalance, (31) and a decrease and dysfunction of Treg (41) have been detected.

Enhancing Treg activity, the very bottom of the inverted pyramid, to stop the inflammatory cascade and, as a result, to reduce infarct size, to restore microvascular perfusion, and to improve patient outcome is an appealing but still unexplored route in the management of patients with AMI (10).

## THERAPEUTIC OPPORTUNITIES

### First Aims to Stop the Inflammatory Process Did Not Succeed in Patients with AIM

In patients with AMI, a variety of therapies aimed at combating the upper parts of the inverted pyramid have been tested. Unfortunately, in spite of their effectiveness in experimental studies, none of these attempts brought about beneficial results.

## Corticosteroids

Corticosteroids are potent anti-inflammatory agents that are used in the treatment of asthma, hypersensitivity reactions and autoimmune diseases. They inhibit the inflammatory response through binding to the glucocorticoid receptor (GR). In cardiovascular disease, corticosteroids exert both beneficial and harmful effects. As early as 1953 Johnson et al (51) reported the cardioprotective effects of cortisone by its ability to limit myocardial damage after an AIM induced in dogs. Subsequently, other animal experiments (52-54) showed that corticosteroids provided positive results in reducing infarct size and attenuating myocardial necrosis (Table 1).

**Table 1. Some therapeutic options have succeeded in animal experimentation.**

| THERAPY | ANIMAL | REFERENCE | RESULTS |
|---|---|---|---|
| Corticosteroids | Cats | Spath et al. (1974) [53] | Reduction of Infarct size |
| | Dogs | Johnson et al. (1953) [51], Libby et al. (1973) [52] | Reduction of fibrosis |
| | Mice | Hafezi-Moghadam et al. (2000) [54] | Reduction of infarct size and vascular inflammation |
| Complement inhibition | Rats | Vakeva et al. (1998) [43] | Inhibition of cell apoptosis and necrosis |
| | Pigs | Amsterdam et al. (1995) [58] | Reduction of Infarct size |
| Neutrophil depletion | Dogs | Litt et al. (1989) [60] | Reduction of Infarct size |
| | Rats | Kin et al. (2006) [61] | Reduction of myocardial apoptosis |

Nevertheless, several clinical trials that followed the animal studies, resulted in inconclusive results, even increased infarct size and mortality (Table 2). Corticosteroids indiscriminately inhibit the inflammatory process: they decrease the number of infiltrating leukocytes, but they can also increase damage and collagen deposition (19). The subsequent development of cardiac rupture has been attributed mainly to the genomic inhibitory effects of GR on wound healing and cardiomyocyte remodelling. Because of these negative effects on wound healing and scar tissue formation, corticosteroids were considered inappropriate for the treatment of AIM in humans (55), (90, 91).

**Table 2. Therapies that have not succeeded in humans.**

| THERAPY | REFERENCE | RESULTS |
|---|---|---|
| Corticosteroids | Giugliano et al. (2003) [55], LeGal et al. (1990) [90] | No beneficial effects |
| | Roberts et al. (1976) [91] | Increase of Mortality |
| Complement blockade | Granger et al. (2003) [44] | No reduction of infarct size. |
| Neutrophil depletion | Faxon et al. (2002) [45] | No beneficial effects |

## Complement Inhibition

Complement activation may have an important role in the initiation of the inflammatory response by means of neutrophil and monocyte recruitment in the injured myocardium. Complement can be activated through three different pathways: the classical, the alternative, and the lectin pathway. During reperfusion, complement may be activated by exposure to intracellular components such as mitochondrial membranes or intermediate filaments. Two elements of the activated complement contribute directly or indirectly to damage: anaphylatoxins (C3a and C5a) and the membrane attack complex (MAC). Hill and Ward (56) first demonstrated that complement activation occurs during myocardial ischemia and it is responsible for the infiltration of neutrophils. Plasma levels of activated complement components were found after an AIM in animals and humans (57). In an experimental study, Vakeva et al (43) demonstrated that anti-C5 antibodies administered in rats, in which an anterior infarction had been induced, significantly reduced infarct size, neutrophil infiltration and apoptosis. Administration of an antibody that specifically inhibits the activity of C5a resulted in improved hemodynamic parameters and less tissue injury after ischemia-reperfusion (58) (Table 1).

However, clinical trials such as the COMMA trial in which they used Pexelizumab, an anti-C5 complement antibody, as an adjunctive therapy to primary percutaneus coronary intervention, did not reduce infarct size in randomized studies in 960 patients with ST-segment elevation AMI (44). In AMI patients, the complement cascade shoots up rapidly, but anticomplement therapy cannot be administered until a few hours after myocardial infarction onset, a time when the beneficial effects are probably reduced (Table 2).

## *Neutrophil Depletion*

During AMI, neutrophils infiltrate, accumulate, and degranulate in the infarcted parts of the myocardium. The inflammatory-like response that follows the onset of reperfusion involves intense interactions with the coronary vascular endothelium, arterial wall and cardiomyocytes. Results from animal studies suggest an important role for neutrophils in the inflammatory reactions during AMI (59). The involvement of these cells in the pathogenesis of lethal myocardial injury has been inferred from: their presence and accumulation in reperfused myocardium in temporal agreement with injury induced, the release of proteases and oxidants by neutrophils in the infracted myocardium, and inhibition of lethal post-ischemic myocyte or endothelial cell injury by strategies that interdict neutrophil interactions at any number of stages (60). Reduction, depletion or inactivation of neutrophils during AMI indeed resulted in a significant reduction in myocardial necrosis in several animal models of AMI (Table 1). Also depletion of neutrophils into the infarcted myocardium significantly reduced myocardial apoptosis and attenuates activation of nuclear factor kappa B (NFκB) mediated by the release of the inflammatory cytokine tumor necrosis factor alpha (TNFα) in the myocardium in ischemia-reperfusion experiments (61).

Despite the strong scientific data supporting a role for anti-neutrophil therapy, the translation of this therapeutic potential to the clinical field has not been carried out. Even anti-neutrophil strategies with very strong experimental support have not shown consistent clinical benefit.

In randomized studies in patients with ST-segment elevation AMI, the blockade of CD11/CD18 integrin receptor did not reduce infarct size nor improve coronary perfusion (45). This probably reflects the fact that neutrophils act in a very rapid and difficult-to-stop manner in the context of AMI (Figure 2).

These negative results are necessary and useful steps in research, but they also indicate the need for exploring different mechanisms of the inflammatory cascade.

## Future Therapeutic Approaches in AMI

Immunotherapy is a type of treatment that uses immunological tools, such as monoclonal antibodies, receptor-immunoglobulin proteins, vaccines and immune cells. Such therapeutic options are now increasingly being used to tackle a wide spectrum of human diseases.

The failure of the majority of immunological approaches that are effective in animal models to modulate autoimmune disease in humans suggests that we do not understand many of the principles behind the pathogenic mechanisms of these diseases (62).

Targeting various critical molecules involved in pathological pathways has led to the modulation of disease in animal models (67). Components of the pathological cascade that have received most attention are: factors involved in lymphocyte homing to target tissues (chemokine receptors and adhesion molecules) (63, 65); enzymes that are critical for the penetration of blood vessels and the extracellular matrix by immune cells (metalloproteinases (MMPs) and cathepsin) (88), cytokines that mediate pathology within the tissues (TNFα, IL-1, IL-12) (74, 75), various cell types that mediate the adaptive response at the site of disease (lymphocytes) (70, 71), as well as the antigen specific response (OxLDL and Heat Shock proteins) (49, 82).

Nowadays there is a wide range of emerging therapeutics strategies for chronic inflammatory diseases (Table 3) which modulate immune response.

Table 3. Emergent therapeutic strategies for chronic inflammatory diseases.

| CHRONIC INFLAMMATORY DISEASE | TARGETS | MODE OF ACTION | THERAPY | REFERENCE |
|---|---|---|---|---|
| Rheumatoid arthritis | CD3 | Inhibition of T cell activation | CTLA 4Ig | Kremer et al. (2003) [68] |
| Crohn's disease | IL-12 | IL-12 inhibition: decrease of pro-inflammatory mediators | Antigen-specific therapies | Cascieri et al. [63] |
| Multiple sclerosis | IL-2 | IL-2 receptor inhibition. Decrease of NK cells | Daclizumab | Lopez-Diego et al. (2008) [64] |
| | VLA-4 | Blockade of T cell-endothelium adhesion | Natalizumab | |

Table 4. Future therapeutic approaches in AMI.

| THERAPY | REFERENCE | RESULTS |
|---|---|---|
| Statins | Vilahur et al. (2009) [92] | Reduction of infarct size in pigs |
| Citokines | Krishnamurty et al (2009) [93] | Atenuates remodeling in mice |
| LDLox | Van Puijvelde et al. (2006) [49] | Reduction of plaque size in mice |
| HSP 60 | Van Puijvelde et al. (2007) [82] | Reduction of plaque formation in mice |
| Antagonists of MMPs | Hu et al. (2007) [88] | MMPs as indicator of ventricular remodelling |
| Tregs | Brusko et al. (2009) [71] | Proposed therapy for inflammatory diseases. |

## Therapies That Inhibit Adhesion Molecules

The immunoglobulin-like adhesion molecules vascular cell-adhesion molecule 1 (VCAM-1) and intercellular adhesion molecule 1 (ICAM-1) are both expressed in early and late lesions in hypercholesterolaemic rabbits, in ApoE knockout (-/-) mice, and in humans. These adhesion molecules are expressed on endothelial cells, and interact with leukocyte cell-surface integrins. Deletion of ICAM-1 has a modest and variable effect on lesion size and pathology in the ApoE -/- mouse. However, a synthetic peptide antagonist of the leukocyte $\alpha_4\beta_1$-integrin, (also known as the very late activation antigen 4; VLA-4) which is the cognate ligand for VCAM-1, delays monocyte and lipid accumulation in lesions in low-density lipoprotein receptor knockout (Ldlr -/-) mice (63).

Studies in multiple sclerosis (MS) with Natalizumab, a humanized monoclonal antibody that is directed against the $\alpha_4$ subunit of the integrin VLA-4 adhesion complex, which is normally expressed on activated lymphocytes, monocytes and other cell types, demonstrated its beneficial effects in acute MS relapses (64). In addition, VLA-4 seems to be involved in T-cell co-stimulation, and anti-VLA-4 signals can modulate immune-cell proliferation and disrupt T-cell activation by blocking the interaction of VLA-4 with the extracellular matrix.

## Therapies That Inhibit Chemokine-Receptors

The chemokines are a large family of proteins that have diverse biological roles in the development of homeostatic control and activation of the immune system. Many chemokines are expressed in vascular lesions, but the most highly studied so far is monocyte chemoattractant protein 1 (MCP-1). MCP-1 is highly expressed in most inflammatory sites, and delection of MCP-1 or its receptor, chemokine (CC) motif receptor 2 (CCR2), results in marked attenuation of monocyte recruitment to several inflammatory challenges (65).

Chemokine induction seems to be a prominent response to myocardial injury in a variety of situations. In myocardial infarcts, cellular necrosis may trigger several chemokines inducing pathways regulated through NFκ-B activation, TNF-α release, and complement activation. Both CC (CCL2/ MCP-1 and CCL3 macrophage inflammatory protein – MIP-1) are markedly induced in the infracted myocardium (66).

## Targeting T Cells

The efficacy of CD3 specific monoclonal antibody therapy in mice and humans stems from its ability to re-establish immune homeostasis in treated individuals. This occurs through modulation of the T-cell receptor (TCR)-CD3 complex and/or induction of apoptosis of activated autoreactive T cells, survival and expansion of adaptative regulatory T cells, which establishes long-term tolerance (69).

Steffens et al (50) reported persuasive results from experiments in which they administered nonmitogenic antibodies targeting the CD3 molecule. Anti-CD3 treatment reduced atherosclerotic lesion size in the aortas of LDL receptor knockout mice fed a high-cholesterol diet.

Targeting T cells response in patients with rheumatoid arthritis has obtained positive results with drugs such as cytotoxic T-lymphocyte antigen 4-Immunoglobulin fusion protein (CTLA 4Ig) that blocks interactions with CD28 and inhibits T cell activation (68).

## *Modulating T Reg Cells Response*

The study of Treg, the deepest part of the inverted pyramid, is progressing to a new level where the need to demonstrate their existence has been replaced by the need to understand their biology so that therapeutic use will become reality (38) (Figure 3). The ability to induce or expand Treg in vitro or in vivo may have important implications in the field of autoimmunity and inflammation. An important advantage of using Treg therapeutically would be that these cells can exert bystander suppression in an antigen-nonspecific fashion, which means that Treg do not necessarily need to recognize the antigen that is the subject of immune attack (73).

In vitro expanded Treg cells maintain their lineage markers and phenotype and are, in general, more suppressive than freshly isolated Tregs (70). Expanded Tregs stay at $FOXP3^+$ and $CD25^{hi}$ when compared with similarly expanded Th cells. Other molecules implicated in Treg function such as CTLA-4 and programmed death1 (PD-1), remain highly expressed on the cell surface of expanded Treg cells. In some settings, but not all, enhanced production of TGFβ and IL-10 was observed after expansion. Importantly, secretion of IL-2 and INFγ by the cells remains low, suggesting minimal contamination of potentially pathogenic Th cells. Importantly even after extensive expansion, Tregs continue to express CD62L and CCR7 and maintain their ability to home peripheral lymph nodes and further expand in vivo (71).

These options could be valid in chronic disorders, but one important question that needs to be addressed in more detail is whether Treg can down-regulate ongoing (auto-) immune responses such as AMI. To down-regulate already ongoing inflammatory responses, Treg are required to migrate into the areas where the inflammation takes place. If the cells are injected directly in the area of inflammation, they perfectly suppress inflammation. Therefore, a crucial question is whether it would be possible to manipulate Treg in such a way that they express homing receptors for the periphery (72). It could be speculated that in patients with AMI treated with primary angioplasty, this issue would be overcome by direct administration of previously expanded Treg into the infarct related artery.

## *Immunomodulation With Cytokines*

Cytokines are short-range protein mediators with a wide range of actions. They are important in all biological processes, including T-cell grown (IL-2, IL-12), inflammation (TNFα, IL-1, IL-6 and INF-γ) as well as the inhibition of inflammation (IL-10, TGF-β, and IL-4). As extracellular molecules, there are accessible to protein therapies such as antibodies or soluble receptors. But one problem is the redundancy in their biological properties.

The existence of TNF-inhibiting biological antibodies and receptors has been successful in the treatment of many inflammatory diseases, such as rheumatoid arthritis, and it is showing itself to be a promising approach in treating AMI patients. TNFα is released by macrophages and monocytes after and AMI (74) and the concentration of TNFα in serum increases along with the area in risk. A high concentration of TNFα is found in the adjacent area of infarction if the ischemia persists. An experimental study with rabbits (75) showed that anti-TNFα antibodies are as effective as ischemic preconditioning in reducing infarct size.

In many inflammatory diseases, such as rheumatoid arthritis and psoriasis, antibodies or fusion receptor protein of TNFα (TNFR) that inhibit TNFα are widely used and they are effective.

Other therapies have investigated the role of the blockade of proliferating cytokines, daclizumab is a drug that inhibits IL-2 and it has a successful effect in diseases such as multiple sclerosis. In Crohn's disease the inhibition of IL-12, results in decrease of pro-inflammatory mediators (62). A recent experimental study has shown that exogenous administration of a recombinant human interleukin 1 (IL-1) receptor antagonist (anakira) can reduce cardiomiocyte apoptosis and left ventricle remodelling after AMI (76).

The regulatory cytokine IL-10 has been studied in several scenarios as a candidate for immune therapy (77, 93). Its main biological function seems to be the limitation and termination of inflammatory responses and the regulation of differentiation and proliferation of several immune cells such as T cells, B cells, natural killer cells, antigen-presenting cells, mast cells and granulocytes. Recombinant human IL-10 has been produced and is currently being tested in clinical trials. This includes rheumatoid arthritis; inflammatory bowel disease, psoriasis, organ transplantation, and hepatitis C. Stumpf et al (78) demonstrated that the administration of repeated intravenous doses of recombinant human IL-10 in an experimental model of myocardial infarction in rats improves left ventricular function.

Transforming Growth Factor beta (TGF-β) is markedly induced and rapidly activated in the infarcted myocardium. Experimental studies suggest that TGF-β signalling may be crucial for repression of inflammatory gene synthesis in healing infarcts mediating resolution of the inflammatory infiltrate. TGF-β is also a key mediator in the pathogenesis of hypertrophic and dilated ventricular remodelling by stimulating cardiomyocyte growth and by inducing interstitial fibrosis (79). Anti-TGF-β gene therapy within 24 h following infarction enhanced cytokine and chemokine synthesis and increased neutrophil infiltration resulting in exacerbated left ventricular dysfunction and increased mortality (79). However, late inhibition of TGF-β has beneficial actions through attenuation of hypertrophic remodelling. This contradiction can serve as an initial guide to frame future studies exploring the mechanistic basis of the TGF-β mediated effects in AMI.

Recently a new cytokine, Interleukin-33 (IL-33), has been discovered and studies have demonstrated that IL-33 is clearly a potential mediator of the diverse inflammatory diseases. Myocardial production of IL-33 can protect cardiac function in response to pressure overload, and may play a part in the progression of atherosclerotic vascular disease (80). Il-33 could induce a shift in balance Th1/Th2 towards a Th2 direction. ApoE knockout mice fed in a high-fat diet and who develop high serum cholesterol level, treated with IL-33 reduced aortic atherosclerotic plaque burden and lower levels of serum antibodies to LDLox compared with control mice (81).

## *Vaccination With Specific Antigens*

Recent data points to the possibility that immunomodulatory interventions to treat atherosclerotic diseases may function through vaccination by orally administering the antigen.

Van Puijvelde et al (49), building on the concept that OxLDL is critical for atherosclerotic lesion induction and progression, modulated anti-OxLDL immunity through vaccination by orally administering the antigen. Feeding mice with OxLDL, they mitigated plaque formation in the carotid arteries and aortas of LDL receptor knockout mice. On induction of oral tolerance, frequencies of CD4+CD25+ T-cells in the spleen and in mesenteric lymph nodes increased, CD25, Foxp3 and CTLA-4 mRNA increased in atherosclerotic plaques, suggesting Treg enrichment at the inflamed site.

Heat-Shock Protein 60 (HSP-60) has also been postulated as a candidate for antigen-specific vaccination. This protein is an antigen recognized by CD4$^+$CD28$^{null}$ T cells of patients with acute coronary syndrome (32), endothelial cells express HSP60 either constitutively or under stress conditions. Circulating HSP-60 specific CD4$^+$CD28$^{null}$ T cells may contribute to vascular damage in these patients. Oral administration of this antigen may prevent atherosclerotic plaque formation by means of T cell regulation (82).

Recently a nuclear protein has been discovered called high mobility group box 1 (HMGB1) which acts as a modifier of inflammation when released. The intramyocardial injection of HMGB1 in rats with experimentally induced AMI, modulated the local inflammation in the failing myocardium, particularly via reducing the accumulation of dendritic cells. This modulated inflammation attenuated ventricular remodelling, and improved cardiac performance of postinfarction (83).

## *Statins*

Although not totally understood yet, immunomodulation could mediate some of the benefits afforded by statins in patients with ischemic heart disease. These 3-hydroxy-3-methylglutaryl-coenzime A reductase inhibitors have anti-inflammatory properties, and recent clinical trials (46) have shown that high-dose statin therapy reduced cardiovascular events in patients with AMI. Link et al (47) demonstrated for the first time in patients with AMI that statins inhibit T-cell immune response by down-regulation of the proinflammatory intracellular cytokines and suppressing Th1 immune response, thereby targeting adaptive immunity of T lymphocytes. These effects appear rapidly at 72 hours. Whether this effect could mediate the reduction in the incidence of no-reflow recently reported among patients who were taking statins before primary angioplasty however, is unknown. Statins also show immunomodulatory effects (94) as previously reported. Statins selectively blocked leukocyte function antigen-1 (LFA-1). In other studies in pigs, HMG-CoA inhibition can reduce the extent of damaged myocardium and improve heart fuction after AMI. Major histocompatibility complex class II (MHC-II) molecules are expressed on specialized cells and are involved in directly controlling aspects of the immune response, such as activation of T cells, at this point statins have been shown to reduce INF-γ-mediated induction of MHC-II in endothelial cells and, as a consequence, to reduce T-cell activation (84).

The toll-like receptors (TLRs) are a class of transmembrane molecules that have important functions in both innate and acquired immunity. Activation of these receptors also plays a role in a variety of systemic inflammatory diseases such as atherosclerosis, acute coronary artery disease, and left ventricular remodelling. Patients with acute MI and unstable angina had significantly higher expression of TLR4+/CD14+ monocytes than stable angina or control patiens (89). When the level of TLR4′s endogenous ligand HSP60 was investigated, it was found to be significantly higher in patients with unstable angina and acute MI. It has been shown that statins can reduce TLR4 surface expression on monocytes both in vivo and ex vivo (84). There have some clinical trials in patients with sepsis using drugs that antagonize the TLR signalling system, but more studies need to be done and its use for AMI treatment is still far off.

Because of their potential in therapeutic approaches, metalloproteinases (MMPs) have been tested in many animal models of acute and chronic inflammation. Sudden death after myocardial infarction can occur by cardiac rupture, a process in which MMPs are involved. In mouse model studies the inhibition of MMP2 by means of an oral dosis, can reverse this pathology (88).

Gene therapy is proving likely to be a viable alternative to conventional therapies in coronary artery disease and heart failure. Gene transfer of plasmid DNA encoding vascular endothelial growth factor (VEGF) brought about clinical benefits, such as the abolition of rest pain, limb salvage and the healing of ischemic ulcers (85). Other approaches combine immunomodulation plus gene therapy, Watanabe et al (86) transferred successfully a plasmid contained IL-10 gene into the myocardium of rats with myocarditis. It significantly improved myocardial lesion and haemodinamic parameters. Recently, hydrodynamic gene delivery using a rapid injection of a relatively large volume of DNA solution has opened up a new avenue for gene therapy studies in vivo. This method is remarkable from the existing delivery systems because of its efficiency and versatility (87).

## CONCLUSION

Existing evidence clearly demonstrates that inflammation plays a decisive role in the pathophysiology of AMI. From the bottom of an imaginary inverted pyramid, a few Treg down-regulate the rest of the inflammatory cascade. In AMI, an acute loss of regulation of the immune system by Treg occurs and induces a pleiotropic and exaggerated inflammatory response. The alternative pathophysiological model presented in this review may be useful in updating our knowledge regarding the role of immunity and inflammation in unstable ischemic heart disease. More studies on this topic are warranted allowing a better understanding of the inverted pyramid model that might help the development of new treatments for this common disease. For that purpose, therapies based on regulating the immune response that have been successful in other inflammatory diseases might be a future approach for limiting infarct size and microvascular obstruction after an AMI.

## REFERENCES

[1] Ridker PM. Inflammatory biomarkers, statins, and the risk of stroke: cracking a clinical conundrum. *Circulation* 2002;105:2583-5.

[2] Fernández-Real JM, Ricart W. Insulin resistance and inflammation in an evolutionary perspective: the contribution of cytokine genotype/phenotype to thriftiness. *Diabetología* 1999;42:1367-74.

[3] Libby P. Current concepts of the pathogenesis of the acute coronary syndromes. *Circulation*. 2001;104:365-72.

[4] Hansson GK. Inflammation, atherosclerosis, and coronary artery disease. *N Engl J Med* 2005;352:1685-95.

[5] Michaels AD, Gibson CM, Barron HV. Microvascular dysfunction in acute myocardial infarction: Focus on the roles of platelet and inflammatory mediators in the no-reflow phenomenon. *Am J Cardiol* 2000;85:50B-60B.

[6] Camici PG, Crea F. Coronary Microvascular Dysfunction. *N Engl J Med.* 2007;356:830-40.

[7] Okuda M. A multidisciplinary overview of cardiogenic shock. *Shock* 2006;557-70.
[8] Caliguri G, Nicoletti A. Lymphocytes responses in acute coronary syndromes: lack of regulation spawns deviant behaviour. *Eur Heart J* 2006;27:2485-6.
[9] Goronzy JJ, Weyand CM. Immunosuppression in atherosclerosis. *Circulation* 2006;114:1901-4.
[10] Mallat Z, Ait-Oufella H, Salomon BL, Tedgui A. Regulatory T-cell immunity in atherosclerosis. *Trends Cardiovasc Med* 2007;17:113-8.
[11] Nunez J, Nunez E, Sanchis J, et al. Prognostic value of leukocytosis in acute coronary syndromes: the cinderella of the inflammatory markers. *Curr Med Chem.* 2006;13:2113-8.
[12] Nunez J, Nunez E, Bodi V, et al. Usefulness of the neutrophil to lymphocyte ratio in predicting long-term mortality in ST segment elevation myocardial infarction. *Am J Cardiol* 2008;101:747-52.
[13] Barron HV, Cannon CP, Murphy SA, et al. Association between white blood cell count, epicardial blood flow, myocardial perfusion, and clinical outcomes in the setting of acute myocardial infarction: a thrombolysis in myocardial infarction 10 substudy. *Circulation.* 2000;102:2329-34.
[14] Bodi V, Sanchis J, Lopez-Lereu MP, et al. Usefulness of a comprehensive cardiovascular magnetic resonance imaging assessment for predicting recovery of left ventricular wall thickening in the setting of myocardial stunning. *J Am Coll Cardiol* 2005;46:1747-52.
[15] Bodi V, Sanchis J, Lopez-Lereu MP, et al. Evolution of 5 cardiovascular magnetic resonance-derived viability indexes after reperfused myocardial infarction. *Am Heart J* 2007;153:649-55.
[16] Sanchis J, Bodi V, Núñez J, et al. Prognostic usefulness of white-blood cell count on admisión and one-year outcome in patients with non-ST elevation acute chest pain. *Am J Cardiol* 2006;98:885-889.
[17] Sanchis J, Bodi V, Núñez J, et al. New risk score for patients with acute chest pain, non-ST-segment deviations and normal troponin concentrations. A comparison with the TIMI risk score.*J Am Coll Cardiol* 2005;46;443-449.
[18] Dragu R, Zuckerman R, Suleiman M, et al. Predictive value of white blood cell subtypes for long-term outcome following myocardial infarction. *Atherosclerosis* 2008;196:405-12.
[19] Frangogiannis NG, Smith CW, Entman ML. The inflammatory response in myocardial infarction. *Cardiovasc Res* 2002;53:31-47.
[20] Gibson WJ, Gibson CM. The association of impaired myocardial perfusion and monocytosis with late recovery of left ventricular function following primary percutaneous coronary intervention. *Eur Heart J.* 2006;27:2487-8.
[21] Horne BD, Anderson JL, John JM, et al. Which white blood cell subtypes predict increased cardiovascular risk? *J Am Coll Cardiol.* 2005;45:1638-43.
[22] Tousoulis D, Charakida M, Stefanidis C. Endothelial function and inflammation in coronary artery disease. *Heart* 2006;92:441-4.
[23] Bodi V, Sanchis J, Llàcer A, al. Multimarker risk strategy for predicting one-month and one-year major events in non-ST elevation acute coronary syndromes. Assessment of troponin I, myoglobin, C-reactive protein, fibrinogen and homocysteine. *Am Heart J* 2005;149:268-74.

[24] De Servi S, Mariani M, Mariani G, et al. C-reactive protein increase in unstable coronary disease. Cause or effect? *J Am Coll Cardiol* 2005;46:1496-502.
[25] Mariani M, Fetiveau R, Rossetti E, et al. Significance of total and differential leucocyte count in patients with acute myocardial infarction treated with primary coronary angioplasty. *Eur Heart J.* 2006;27:2511-5.
[26] Ducloux D, Challier B, Saas P, et al. CD4 cell lymphopenia and atherosclerosis in renal transplant recipients. *J Am Soc Nephrol.* 2003;14:767-72.
[27] Hotchkiss RS, Karl IE. The pathophysiology and treatment of sepsis. *N Engl J Med.* 2003;348:138-50.
[28] Blum A, Yeganeh S. The role of T-lymphocyte subpopulations in acute myocardial infarction. *Eur J Intern Med.* 2003;14:407-410.
[29] Steppich BA, Moog P, Matissek C, et al. Cytokine profiles and T cell function in acute coronary syndromes. *Atherosclerosis.* 2007;190:443-51.
[30] Methe H, Brunner S, Wiegand D, et al. Enhanced T-helper-1 lymphocyte activation patterns in acute coronary syndromes. *J Am Coll Cardiol.* 2005;45:1939-45.
[31] Cheng X, Liao YH, Ge H, et al. TH1/TH2 functional imbalance after acute myocardial infarction: coronary arterial inflammation or myocardial inflammation. *J Clin Immunol.* 2005;25:246-53.
[32] Pasqui AL, Di Renzo M, Bova G, et al. T cell activation and enhanced apoptosis in non-ST elevation myocardial infarction. *Clin Exp Med* 2003;3:37-44.
[33] Rössig L, Flichtlscherer S, Heeschen C, et al. The pro-apoptotic serum activity is an independent mortality predictor of patients with heart failure. *Eur Heart J;*2004:25:1620-5.
[34] Yang Z, Zingarelli B, Szabo C. Crucial role of endogenous interleukin-10 production in myocardial ischemia/reperfusion injury. *Circulation.* 2000;101:1019-26.
[35] Kilic T, Ural D, Ural E, et al. Relation between proinflammatory to anti-inflammatory cytokine ratios and long-term prognosis in patients with non-ST elevation acute coronary syndrome. *Heart.* 2006;92:1041-6.
[36] Liuzzo G, Biasucci LM, Trotta G, et al. Unusual CD4+CD28null T lymphocytes and recurrence of acute coronary events. *J Am Coll Cardiol* 2007;50:1450-8.
[37] Zal B, Kaski JC, Arno G, et al. Heat-shock protein 60-reactive CD4+CD28null T cells in patients with acute coronary syndromes. *Circulation* 2004;109:1230-5.
[38] Beissert S, Schwarz A, Schwarz T. Regulatory T cells. *J Invest Dermatol* 2006;126:15-24.
[39] Gershon RK, Cohen P, Hencin R, et al. Suppressor T cells. *J Immunol* 1972;108:586-90
[40] Sakaguchi S. Naturally arising CD4+ regulatory T cells for immunologic self-tolerance and negative control of immune responses. *Annu Rev Immunol* 2004;22:531-62.
[41] Mor A, Luboshits G, Planer D, et al. Altered status of CD4+CD25+ regulatory T cells in patients with acute coronary syndromes. *Eur Heart J* 2006;27:2530-7.
[42] Gallagher PM, Lowe G, Fitzgerald T, et al. Association of IL-10 polymorphism with severity of illness in community acquired pneumonia. *Thorax.* 2003;58:154-6.
[43] Vakeva AP, Agah A, Rollins SA, et al, Myocardial infarction and apoptosis after myocardial ischemia and reperfusion: role of the terminal complement components and inhibition by anti-C5 therapy. *Circulation.* 1998;97:2259-67.

[44] Granger CB, Mahaffey KW, Weaver WD, et al. Pexelizumab, an anti-C5 complement antibody, as adjunctive therapy to primary percutaneous coronary intervention in acute myocardial infarction: the COMplement inhibition in Myocardial infarction treated with Angioplasty (COMMA) trial. *Circulation.* 2003;108:1184-90.

[45] Faxon DP, Gibbons RJ, Chronos NA, et al. HALT-MI Investigators. The effect of blockade of the CD11/CD18 integrin receptor on infarct size in patients with acute myocardial infarction treated with direct angioplasty: the results of the HALT-MI study. *J Am Coll Cardiol.* 2002;40:1199-204.

[46] Waters D, Schwartz GG, Olsson AG. The Myocardial Ischemia Reduction with Acute Cholesterol Lowering (MIRACL) trial: a new frontier for statins? *Curr Control Trials Cardiovasc Med.* 2001;2:111-4.

[47] Link A, Ayadhi T, Bohm M, et al. Rapid immunomodulation by rosuvastatin in patients with acute coronary syndrome. *Eur Heart J.* 2006;27:2945-55.

[48] Iwakura K, Ito H, Kawano S, et al. Chronic pre-treatment of statins is associated with the reduction of the no-reflow phenomenon in the patients with reperfused myocardial infarction. *Eur Heart J* 2006;27:534-9.

[49] Van Puijvelde GH, Hauer AD, de Vos P, et al. Induction of tolerance to oxidized low-density lipoprotein ameliorates atherosclerosis. *Circulation* 2006;114:1968-76.

[50] Steffens S, Burger F, Pelli G, et al. Short-term treatment with anti-CD3 antibody reduces the development and progression of atherosclerosis in mice. *Circulation.* 2006;114:1977-84.

[51] Jonhson AS, Scheinberg SR, et al. Effect of cortisone on the size of experimentally produced myocardial infarcts. *Circulation*; 1953:224-8.

[52] Libby P, Maroko PR, Bloor CM, et al. Reduction of experimental myocardial infarct size by corticosteroid administration. *J Clin Invest*; 1973:599-607.

[53] Spath JA, Lane DL, Lefer AM. Protective action of methylprednisoloneon the myocardium during experimental myocardial ischemia in the cat. *Circulation Research;* 1974:44-51.

[54] Hafezi-Moghadam A, Simoncini T, Yang Z, et al. Acute cardiovascular protective effects of corticosteroids are mediated by non-transcriptional activation of endothelial nitric oxide synthase. *Nat Med*; 2002:473-9.

[55] Giugliano GR, Giugliano RP, Gibson CM, et al. Meta-analysis of corticosteroid treatment in acute myocardial infarction. *Am J Cardiol*; 2003:1055-9.

[56] Hill JH, Ward PA. The phlogistic role of C3 leukotactic fragments in myocardial infarcts of rats. *J Exp Med*; 1971:885-900.

[57] Monsinjon T, Richard V, Fontaine M. Complement and its implications in cardiac ischemia/reperfusion: strategies to inhibit complement. *Fundam Clin Pharmacol*; 2001:293-306.

[58] Amsterdam EA, Stahl GL, Pan HL, et al. Limitation of reperfusion injury by a monoclonal antibody to C5a during myocardial infarction in pigs. *Am J Physiol* 1995;268:H448-57.

[59] Vinten-Johansen J. Involvement of neutrophils in the pathogenesis of lethal myocardial reperfusion injury. *Cardiovasc Res*; 2004:481-97.

[60] Litt MR, Jeremy RW, Weisman HF, et al. Neutrophil depletion limited to reperfusion reduces myocardial infarct size after 90 minutes of ischemia. Evidence for neutrophil-mediated reperfusion injury. *Circulation*; 1989:1816-27.

[61] Kin H, Wang NP, Halkos ME, et al. Neutrophil depletion reduces myocardial apoptosis and attenuates NFkappaB activation/TNFalpha release after ischemia and reperfusion. *J Surg Res* 2006;135:170-8.

[62] Feldmann M, Steinman L. Design of effective immunotherapy for human autoimmunity. *Nature*; 2005:612-9.

[63] Cascieri MA. The potential for novel anti-inflammatory therapies for coronary artery disease. *Nat Rev Drug Discov* 2002;1:122-30.

[64] Lopez-Diego RS, Weiner HL. Novel therapeutic strategies for multiple sclerosis--a multifaceted adversary. In: *Nat Rev Drug Discov*; 2008:909-25.

[65] Horuk R. Chemokine receptor antagonists: overcoming developmental hurdles. In: *Nat Rev Drug Discov*; 2009:23-33.

[66] Frangogiannis NG, Entman ML. Targeting the chemokines in myocardial inflammation. Circulation 2004;110:1341-2.

[67] Rader DJ, Daugherty A. Translating molecular discoveries into new therapies for atherosclerosis. In: *Nature*; 2008:904-13.

[68] Kremer JM, Westhovens R, Leon M, et al. Treatment of rheumatoid arthritis by selective inhibition of T-cell activation with fusion protein CTLA4Ig. In: *N Engl J Med;* 2003:1907-15.

[69] Chatenoud L, Bluestone JA. CD3-specific antibodies: a portal to the treatment of autoimmunity. *Nature Reviews Immunology* 2007;7:622-32.

[70] Tang Q, Bluestone JA. Regulatory T-cell physiology and application to treat autoimmunity. In: *Immunol Rev*; 2006:217-37.

[71] Brusko TM, Bluestone JA. *Regulatory T cells directed to the site of the action*. Proc Natl Acad Sci USA 2009.

[72] Bluestone JA. Regulatory T-cell therapy: is it ready for the clinic? *Nature Reviews Immunology* 2005;5:343-9.

[73] Ait-Oufella H, Salomon BL, Potteaux S, et al. Natural regulatory T cells control the development of atherosclerosis in mice. In: *Nat Med*; 2006:178-80.

[74] Schulz R, Aker S, Belosjorow S, et al. TNFalpha in ischemia/reperfusion injury and heart failure. In: *Basic Res Cardiol*; 2004:8-11.

[75] Belosjorow S, Bolle I, Duschin A, et al. TNF-alpha antibodies are as effective as ischemic preconditioning in reducing infarct size in rabbits. In: *Am J Physiol Heart Circ Physiol*; 2003:H927-30

[76] Landmesser U, Wollert KC, Drexler H. Potential novel pharmacological therapies for myocardial remodelling. In: *Cardiovascular Research*; 2009:519-27.

[77] Asadullah K, Sterry W, Volk HD. Interleukin-10 therapy--review of a new approach. *Pharmacol Rev* 2003;55:241-69.

[78] Stumpf C, Seybold K, Petzi S, et al. Interleukin-10 improves left ventricular function in rats with heart failure subsequent to myocardial infarction. In: *European Journal of Heart Failure*; 2008:733-9.

[79] Bujak M, Frangogiannis NG. The role of TGF-beta signaling in myocardial infarction and cardiac remodeling. *Cardiovascular Research* 2007;74:184-95.

[80] Kakkar R, Lee RT. The IL-33/ST2 pathway: therapeutic target and novel biomarker. In: *Nat Rev Drug Discov*; 2008:827-40.

[81] Miller AM, Xu D, Asquith DL, et al. IL-33 reduces the development of atherosclerosis. In: *J Exp Med*; 2008:339-46.

[82] van Puijvelde GHM, van Es T, van Wanrooij EJA, et al. Induction of oral tolerance to HSP60 or an HSP60-peptide activates T cell regulation and reduces atherosclerosis. In: *Arteriosclerosis, Thrombosis, and Vascular Biology*; 2007:2677-83.

[83] Takahashi K, Fukushima S, Yamahara K, et al. Modulated inflammation by injection of high-mobility group box 1 recovers post-infarction chronically failing heart. In: *Circulation*; 2008:S106-14.

[84] Jain MK, Ridker PM. Anti-inflammatory effects of statins: clinical evidence and basic mechanisms. In: *Nat Rev Drug Discov*; 2005:977-87.

[85] Isner JM. Myocardial gene therapy. In: *Nature*; 2002:234-9.

[86] Watanabe K, Nakazawa M, Fuse K, et al. Protection against autoimmune myocarditis by gene transfer of interleukin-10 by electroporation. In: *Circulation*; 2001:1098-100.

[87] Suda T, Liu D. Hydrodynamic gene delivery: its principles and applications. In: *Mol Ther;* 2007:2063-9.

[88] Hu J, Van den Steen PE, Sang Q-XA, Opdenakker G. Matrix metalloproteinase inhibitors as therapy for inflammatory and vascular diseases. In: *Nat Rev Drug Discov;* 2007:480-98.

[89] Erickson B, Sperber K, Frishman WH. Toll-like receptors: new therapeutic targets for the treatment of atherosclerosis, acute coronary syndromes, and myocrdial failure. In: *Cardiol Rev*; 2008:273-9.

[90] LeGal YM, Morrissey LL. Methylprednisolone interventions in myocardial infarction: a controversial subject. *Can J Cardiol* 1990;6:405-10.

[91] Roberts R, DeMello V, Sobel BE. Deleterious effects of methylprednisolone in patients with myocardial infarction. *Circulation* 1976;53:I204-6.

[92] Vilahur G, Casaní L, Peña E, et al. Induction of RISK by HMG-CoA reductase inhibition affords cardioprotection after myocardial infarction. *In: Atherosclerosis;* 2009:95-101.

[93] Krishnamurthy P, Rajasingh J, Lambers E, IL-10 Inhibits Inflammation and Attenuates Left Ventricular Remodeling After Myocardial Infarction via Activation of STAT3 and Suppression of HuR. In: *Circulation Research*; 2009:e9-e18.

[94] Weitz-Schmidt G, Welzenbach K, Brinkmann V, et al. Statins selectively inhibit leukocyte function antigen-1 by binding to a novel regulatory integrin site. *Nat Med* 2001;7:687-92.

*Chapter VI*

# TISSUE TRANSGLUTAMINASE ENZYME AND ANTI-TISSUE TRANSGLUTAMINASE ANTIBODIES: IMPLICATION FOR ACUTE CORONARY SYNDROME

*Marco Di Tola*[*] *and Antonio Picarelli*[#]

Center for Research and Study of Celiac Disease
Department of Clinical Sciences, Sapienza University, Rome, Italy

## ABSTRACT

The type II or tissue transglutaminase (TG2) is an ubiquitous enzyme involved in angiogenesis, fibrogenesis, wound healing, cell adhesion/migration, intracellular signaling pathways, respiratory chain assembly, cell proliferation/differentiation, neurite formation, apoptosis, and inflammation. Some years ago, an increased extracellular localization of TG2 has been demonstrated in damaged or inflamed portions of the small intestine from patients with celiac disease (CD). This antigenic overexpression is able to explain, at least in part, the anti-TG2 antibody induction observable in CD patients. On the other hand, anti-TG2 antibodies have been recently described in patients affected from disorders in which the target organ is located at a distance from the intestine, such as acute coronary syndrome (ACS), dilated cardiomyopathy (DCM), valvular heart disease and other causes of end-stage heart failure. In this regard, a cardiac TG2 overexpression has been described in some experimental models of heart failure and in occurrence of myocardial ischemia/reperfusion injury. In the arteries with or without minimal atherosclerosis, TG2 is detectable only in the medium and along the luminal endothelial border while in the atherosclerotic arteries, especially coronaries and carotid vessels, this enzyme is also evident in the fibrous cup and in shoulder regions of the plaque. Consequently, an anti-TG2 antibody-inducing mechanism similar to those taking part in the intestine of CD patients may also occur in the cardiovascular tissues affected

---

[*] Correspondence should be sent to: Marco Di Tola, Ph.D., Department of Clinical Sciences, Sapienza University - Policlinico Umberto I, Viale del Policlinico, 155, 00161 - Rome, Italy, e-mail: m.ditola@tiscali.it, Telephone +39649978369, Fax +39649970524

[#] Correspondence should be sent to: Antonio Picarelli, M.D., Department of Clinical Sciences, Sapienza University - Policlinico Umberto I, Viale del Policlinico, 155, 00161 - Rome, Italy, e-mail: antonio.picarelli @uniroma1.it, Telephone +39649978370, Fax +39649970524

from an acute or chronic disorder. Consistent with this hypothesis, anti-TG2 antibodies seem to be related to severity of the acute coronary event, as well as to extent of the myocardial tissue lesion occurring in ACS patients. Furthermore, since TG2 enzymatic activity may result in myocardial wound healing and stabilization of atherosclerotic plaque, anti-TG2 antibodies could have biological effects able to define a prognostic significance. In this light, vulnerable or ruptured atherosclerotic plaque, as well as injured myocardium (following an infarction, myocarditis, etc.) may be sources of TG2 antigen resulting in formation of anti-TG2 antibodies that in turn, by neutralizing TG2 enzymatic activity, could promote destabilization of the plaque or impaired myocardial wound healing, thereby contributing to a chronic disorder such as DCM. The finding that anti-TG2 antibodies are able to induce proliferation and inhibit differentiation of intestinal epithelial cell, increase epithelial permeability, activate monocytes, and disturb angiogenesis in CD patients suggests that they may have a functional role also in cardiovascular disorders. In the near future, these observations and related hypothesis could to become the subject of interesting researches.

## INTRODUCTION

By combining the keywords "transglutaminase" and "cardiovascular system" on PubMed platform appear 194 articles published over the last 32 years (from April 1979 to November 2009). Dividing these articles in 7 groups of 5 years each and studying their progress over time, it is possible to observe a steady increase in the number of publications from the first quinquennium onwards (Figure 1).

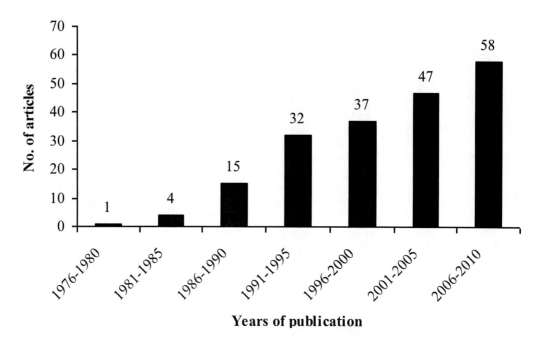

Figure 1. Articles related to the keywords "transglutaminase" and "cardiovascular system". The number of articles reported in the graph has been obtained by combining the afore mentioned keywords on PubMed platform (http://www.ncbi.nlm.nih.gov/sites/entrez). All columns refer to a publication period of 5 years.

While this finding suggests that the research in question is still young, on the other hand it testifies an increasing interest that, in the near future, could lead to unexpected advances both in basic and clinical science.

For duty to chronicle, the first half of this chapter describes features and functions of all the transglutaminases, as well as their implication for a wide variety of physiological and pathological human processes, including those occurring in the cardiovascular system. In the second part, attention is focused on the relationship among tissue transglutaminase, celiac disease, and the acute coronary syndrome, in order to clarify the common pathogenetic events and propose some operational tools that might be useful in both conditions.

## TRANSGLUTAMINASES: A MULTIFACED ENZYME FAMILY

The transglutaminases (acronym: TG or TGase; NC-IUBMB/IUPAC-IUBMB JCBN nomenclature: EC 2.3.2.13; systematic nomenclature: R-glutaminyl-peptide-aminase-gamma-glutamyltransferase) are a multifaced (both multiform and multifunctional) family of enzymes widely distributed in bacteria, animals, and plants. They catalyze post-translational modifications in proteins, mainly producing stable and proteolysis resistant covalent amide bonds between the $\varepsilon$-amino group of a lysine residue (amine donor) and the $\gamma$-carboxyamide group of a glutamine residue (amine receptor) [1]. Among the reactions catalyzed by TGs, the cross-linking of a glutamine residue in a protein/peptide substrate to a lysine residue in a protein/peptide co-substrate (transamidation), resulting in the formation of a N-$\varepsilon$-($\gamma$-L-glutamyl)-L-lysine (or simply $\gamma$-glutamyl-$\varepsilon$-lysine, GGEL) isopeptidic bond and concomitant release of ammonia, has historically generated a great interest because of its implications in both physiological and pathological human processes [1,2], as well as for its potential applications in various industrial fields (e.g. in biomedicine, food processing, polymer obtaining, etc.) [3].

The human TG family consists of a structural protein (protein 4.2) lacking of catalytic activity, and eight zymogens/enzymes (factor XIII-A and TG1-7) which overall, are able to catalyze the following reactions of post-translational protein modification: transamidation (or alternatively, deamidation), esterification, hydrolysis, phosphorylation, and disulfide bond formation. All human TG family members are comprised of four molecular domains (a NH$_2$-terminal $\beta$-sandwich, an $\alpha/\beta$ catalytic core, and two COOH-terminal $\beta$-barrel domains) that normally assume a compact conformation, thereby hiding the active site. Some family members have also a NH$_2$-terminal sequence that must be cleaved to generate the functional enzyme. The activation of TGs is associated with a conformational change from the compact form to an extended ellipsoid structure, which exposes the active site. With the exception of protein 4.2, the active site of TGs is comprised of a catalytic triad (a cysteine, histidine, and aspartate residue) indispensable for enzymatic activity, as well as a highly conserved tryptophan residue that stabilizes the transition state during catalysis. All the reactions catalyzed by TGs are essential for physiological processes such as blood coagulation, extracellular matrix (ECM) remodeling, and skin barrier formation but can also contribute to the pathogenesis of several inflammatory, autoimmune, and degenerative diseases [2].

## Protein 4.2

Given the striking amino acid sequence homology observed between various types of TG and the structural protein 4.2 [1], the latter is increasingly being considered as an effective member of the human TG family, irrespective of catalytic activity lacking. The protein 4.2 is one of the most abundant non-lipidic components of the erythrocyte membrane (band 4.2, as detected by electrophoresis) which, via interactions with band 3, CD47 and the cytoskeletal protein ankyrin, acts as a point of connection between the band 3 and Rhesus protein complexes, thus stabilizing the cell membrane structure. Consistently, its absence/reduction due to natural mutations in humans or gene knockout in mice has a detrimental effect on the erythrocyte membrane stability, resulting in hereditary spherocytosis which in turn is responsible for hemolytic anemia [4].

## Factor XIII-A

Also known as plasma TG, the factor XIII (FXIII) is a pro-enzyme circulating in blood as an $A_2B_2$ heterotetramer consisting of two catalytic subunits ($A_2$ dimeric enzyme or FXIII-A) and two non-catalytic subunits ($B_2$ dimeric carrier). This pro-enzyme is activated by thrombin cleavage of the A subunits, or through cleavage of the Arg37-Gly38 peptide bond by other serine proteases (e.g. endogenous platelet acid protease and calpain) in the presence of fibrin polymers at sites of blood coagulation, where it impedes blood loss by stabilizing the fibrin clot against physical and fibrinolytic disruption [1]. In detail, after thrombin cleavage of fibrinopeptide A from fibrinogen and consequent formation of fibrin monomers, both intra and intermolecular associations begin to create a clot network. This fibrin assembly facilitates the intermolecular alignment of adjacent chain pairs, which are then transamidated by FXIII-A to form molecular dimers up to complete polymerization, characterized by the conversion from soluble to insoluble fibrin (blood clot). The clot resistance to fibrinolysis is further secured by FXIII-mediated attachment of the plasmin inhibitor to fibrin polymers. Unlike the other clotting factors, neither FXIII nor fibrinogen are serine proteases, while the transamidase activity of FXIII-A is typically regulated by the calcium ions [5,6].

As a consequence of its main biological function, FXIII plays a significant role in hemostasis, wound healing, and maintenance of pregnancy. Accordingly, a chronic bleeding tendency up to intracranial blood loss (hemorrhagic diathesis), defective wound healing, and spontaneous miscarriage are typical manifestations of an uncommon, inherited disorder characterized by the congenital blood coagulation FXIII deficiency [7-9]. Common variations in FXIII genes, as well as elevated FXIII-A activity (e.g. in patients with anti-phospholipid syndrome) are further associated to altered risk profiles for thrombosis and atherosclerosis progression [5,9]. Finally, other findings suggest that an increased FXIII-A activity may contribute to development or exacerbation of elevated blood pressure [9].

Recent data show that in addition to its classical transamidase activity, FXIII-A may catalyze the phosphorylation of suitable protein substrates [10], as well as the formation of disulfide bonds [11]. The combined effect of transamidase and phosphorylase activities suggests a direct role of the plasma TG in angiogenesis and wound healing [10], while the biological impact of FXIII-catalyzed disulfide bond formation is not yet known.

Beyond the bloodstream and hemostasis area, FXIII is also present in bone marrow derived cells including platelets, monocytes, and macrophages. As intracellular enzyme, FXIII-A is indeed expressed during compartmentalisation of megakaryocyte/platelet precursors in the bone marrow, is packaged into budding platelets and is particularly abundant in circulating ones, where it plays an important role in the cytoskeletal remodelling associated with various platelet activation stages. FXIII-A is also present in monocytes and in all subsets of monocyte-derived macrophages in which, through association with cytoskeletal filaments, it participates to the phagocytic activity [9,12]. In addition, the expression of functional FXIII-A by monocytes/macrophages seems to play a crucial role in monocyte entry into the artery wall and consequently, in the progression of atherosclerotic plaque [9].

On the other hand, the occurrence of anti-FXIII atypical antibodies in serum of patients with celiac disease (CD) or Crohn's disease suggests that plasma TG may act as an autoantigen able to trigger secondary autoimmunity [13].

## TG1

The type I or keratinocyte TG (TG1 or kTG) is a plasma membrane-anchored enzyme confined in the squamous epithelium (to a lesser extent, also in the brain), where it is activated by calpain- and/or cathepsin D-catalyzed proteolysis during keratinocyte terminal differentiation. Once activated, TG1 catalyzes $Ca^{2+}$-dependent transamidation of suitable protein substrates and co-substrates (mainly involucrin and desmosomal proteins such as envoplakin and periplakin), as well as esterification of long chain ω-hydoxyceramides onto various structural proteins (mainly involucrin), thus contributing to form a cross-linked protein layer known as cornified cell envelope (CE). This protein stratus, in cooperation with intercellular lipid layers, keratin-filaggrin degradation products, and keratinocytes that have completed their cell differentiation, constitutes the stratum corneum (or skin barrier) designed to protect the body against dehydration, abrasion, and infection [1,14]. To date, more than 100 germline mutations have been identified in TG1 gene [15]. By destabilization of a hydrophobic pocket, some of these mutations distort the active site of the enzyme, resulting in loss of its transamidase activity. TG1 deficiency leads to impaired CE formation, with consequent defects in the stratum corneum and skin barrier function. These defects cause a clinical phenotype compatible with several forms of autosomal recessive ichthyosis, normally grouped as lamellar ichthyosis [14,15].

## TG2

The type II TG (TG2), also called tissue or cell TG (tTG or cTG), is a multifunctional enzyme typically expressed in a multitude of human cells (e.g. cardiomyocytes in subendocardial and subepicardial regions; endothelial and smooth muscle cells in blood vessels; chondrocytes in bones and within the arterial wall; erythrocytes, neutrophils, lymphocytes, monocytes, and platelets in the bloodstream; monocyte-derived macrophages throughout the body; pericryptal fibroblasts and smooth muscle cells in the intestine; β-cells in the pancreas; hepatocytes in the liver; mesangial and renomedullary interstitial cells in kidneys; astrocytes and neurons in the central nervous system; etc.), although it may be present in several ECMs [1,9,16]. Indeed, TG2 is predominantly a cytoplasmic protein, but depending on the state of cell proliferation or in response to increased intracellular calcium concentrations, it is dynamically translocated into various subcellular and ECM compartments. Within cells, this enzyme localizes in cytosol, plasma membrane, nucleus, mitochondria, and cell surface, where the presence or absence of suitable substrates and co-substrates, as well as the modulating effects of specific regulatory factors (calcium ions, nucleotides, redox potential, and pH) are key elements to switch on or off its biochemical activities. Additional subcellular compartments that may contain active TG2 are the external surface of synaptosomes, and probably the endoplasmic reticulum [16,17].

Under physiological conditions, low calcium (<1 mM) and high guanosine triphosphate (>9 µM) intracellular levels confine the transamidase activity in ECM compartment, in which TG2 catalyzes the formation of protein cross-links. Conversely, in response to various stressful and/or apoptotic stimuli, elevated intracellular calcium concentrations (>1 mM) potentiate the transamidase activity in cytosol, plasma membrane, nucleus, and mitochondria, where TG2 catalyzes the massive formation of protein cross-links. In ECM, the transamidase activity is operational also under pathological conditions [16]. As a rule, in a neutral microenvironment (pH ~7.4) rich in amine donors, TG2 catalyzes the cross-linking of protein substrates and co-substrates mainly by $Ca^{2+}$-dependent transamidation, while lowering the pH and/or the content of amine donors increases the reaction rate of TG2-catalysed $Ca^{2+}$-dependent deamidation. The latter consists in the conversion of glutamine in glutamic acid residues, and concomitant release of ammonia, after interaction of protein substrates with water instead of the missing co-substrates. Furthermore, the spacing between the targeted glutamine and neighbouring proline residues is particularly important for the specificity of both transamidase and deamidase TG2 activities (Gln-Xaa-Pro is a sequence preferred by TG2, whilst Gln-Pro and Gln-Xaa-Xaa-Pro are sequences not preferred by TG2) [17]. Besides its classical transamidase activity, TG2 possesses some other biochemical functions. Depending on subcellular compartment and its microenvironment, TG2 can indeed operate as a G protein (under physiological conditions, it shows both GTP-binding and GTP-hydrolytic activities limited to plasma membrane), protein kinase (under normal conditions, it presents a phosphorylase activity in association to plasma membrane and nucleus), protein disulfide isomerase (under physiological conditions, it catalyzes disulfide bond formation in mitochondria), DNA nuclease (under normal conditions, it exhibits a DNA-hydrolytic activity circumscribed to nucleus), and adaptor protein (under both physiological and pathological conditions, it shows a fibronectin-, integrin-, and syndecan-binding activity confined to cell surface) [16].

The multiple biochemical activities of TG2 account for its involvement in a wide variety of physiological and pathological processes, including:

- angiogenesis, fibrogenesis, wound healing;
- cell adhesion/migration, intracellular signaling pathways, respiratory chain assembly, cell proliferation/differentiation, neurite formation;
- programmed cell death, inflammation [9,16].

The extracellular TG2 is involved in ECM remodeling via formation of protein cross-links, thereby promoting angiogenesis, fibrogenesis, and wound healing. Conversely, the interaction of cell surface TG2 with the extracellular domains of several integrins does not require transamidase activity. In this interaction model, the cell surface TG2 acts as an integrin-binding coreceptor for fibronectin, thus promoting adhesion, spreading, and migration of cells. Also in association with the inner of plasma membrane, TG2 is able to modulate cell motility through its interaction with integrins. The plasma membrane TG2 can further act as a G protein, by mediating some intracellular signaling pathways. Last but not least, the G protein-like activity of TG2 contributes to cell survival. A loss of GTP-binding activity may indeed convert the plasma membrane TG2 into a cell death-promoting factor. In mitochondria, the protein disulfide isomerase-like activity of TG2 contributes to the correct assembly of respiratory chain complexes, while the nuclear TG2 ability to catalyze phosphorylation of specific protein substrates, including the cell cycle regulating factor p53, account for its involvement in both proliferation and differentiation cell processes. Instead, neurite formation is specifically promoted by the transamidase activity of TG2 expressed on the external surface of synaptosomes. In relation to programmed cell death, TG2 has both pro- and anti-apoptotic functions. This is because, depending on cell type, nature of cell death inducer, intensity of stimulus, TG2-splice variants and their subcellular location, TG2 can exert diverse downstream effects resulting in cell death or survival. The ability of TG2 to bind and transamidate some important regulators of apoptosis, such as nuclear retinoblastoma and mitochondrial Bax proteins, further confirms its role on cell death decision. Once cells undergo apoptotic cell death, part of the $Ca^{2+}$-activated TG2 is translocated into the nucleus, where it mediates the chromatin condensation by catalyzing the cross-linking of histone proteins. The remaining $Ca^{2+}$-activated TG2 is almost entirely committed to massively form protein cross-links, generating protective shells that reduce the leakage of harmful contents from the apoptotic cells. Finally, by acting in the dying cells as well as in macrophages, TG2 facilitates the phagocytosis of apoptotic bodies. Based on these observations, it is possible to affirm that TG2 is able to promote the apoptotic cell death, prevent the leakage of intracellular contents, and facilitate the removal of apoptotic bodies, lessening both inflammation and apparent tissue damage [16]. In contrast to this protective activity, TG2 participates to an inflammatory loop by promoting the translocation of the nuclear factor-kB (NF-kB) into the nucleus, which in turn induces TG2 by interacting with the specific gene promoter. Once in the nucleus, the transcription factor NF-kB acts as a master switch for inflammation, inducing a wide variety of pro-inflammatory proteins such as adhesion molecules, cytokines, and chemokines. Furthermore, IFN-γ pro- and TGF-β1 anti-inflammatory cytokines are able to up-regulate TG2, suggesting its involvement in diverse inflammatory processes. The inflammation-related TG2 activity is also suggested by the high rate of TG2-catalyzed transamidation, and consequent activation of phospholipases A2 (EC 3.1.1.4), NF-kB-induced enzymes that catalyze the release of arachadonic acid from cell membrane glycerophospholipids, resulting in the synthesis of inflammatory eicosanoids [9].

In addition to its role in modulating inflammation, TG2 is considered the dominant autoantigen of CD [18]. The occurrence of anti-TG2 specific antibodies in serum [19], gut lavage fluid [20], fecal supernatant [21], saliva [22], and culture medium of duodenal/oral biopsies from patients having this gastroenterological disorder [23,24] confirms the ability of TG2 to elicit autoimmunity. Furthermore, the presence of anti-TG2 atypical antibodies in serum and synovial fluid of patients with arthritic diseases (ankylosing spondylitis, osteoarthritis, psoriatic arthritis, rheumatoid arthritis) [25], in serum and fecal supernatant of patients with inflammatory bowel disease (IBD, including Crohn's disease and ulcerative colitis) [26], and in serum of patients with cardiovascular disorders (acute coronary syndrome, dilated cardiomyopathy, valvular heart disease and other causes of end-stage heart failure) [27,28] suggests that TG2 may act as an autoantigen able to trigger secondary autoimmunity.

Taking a step back, the proteins cross-linked by TG2 often result in highly insoluble compounds characterized by high-molecular masses [16,29]. According to this biochemical feature, some neurodegenerative disorders such as Alzheimer's disease, Huntington's disease, Parkinson's disease, and supranuclear palsy are associated with an aberrant TG2 activity, resulting in increased cross-linked proteins in the affected brain [29,30].

In synergy (or antagonism) with the biochemical activities of FXIII-A, TG2 participates in a wide variety of physiopathological processes occurring in the cardiovascular system. In relation to blood coagulation cascade, TG2 may act in concert with FXIII-A to favor platelet adhesion, as well as the formation of coated platelets. These activated platelets have high surface content of pro-coagulant proteins, resulting in enhanced ability to promote thrombin generation. Inside as well outside the atheroma, TG2 activity can lead to plaque progression by various mechanisms, including TGF-β1 activation and consequent deposition of ECM proteins, formation of elafin-ECM cross-links or fibrous cap stabilization against metalloproteinase-mediated rupture, endothelial barrier stabilization and ensuing reduction in endothelial permeability, enhancement of angiogenesis with atheroma neovascularization. Given that TG2 promotes the arteriolar remodeling in response to blood flow reduction, an increased expression of this ubiquitous enzyme may enhance the vascular tone, which in turn could favor hypertension. In relation to myocardium, it has been shown that an increase in TG2 activity is associated with left ventricular hypertrophy, myocardial fibrosis, and reduced left ventricular ejection fraction in transgenic mice [9].

An aberrant TG2 activity is implicated in the pathogenesis of several other illnesses, such as diabetes and cancer [9,16]. In detail, TG2 plays a role in the insulin release from pancreatic β-cells, as well as in intracellular processing of the insulin receptor. According to these biological functions, at least three missense mutations of TG2 gene (c.989T>G, p.M330R; c.992T>A, p.I331N; c.998A>G, p.N333S) have been described in patients with maturity-onset diabetes of the young (MODY) or early-onset type 2 diabetes. Since these mutations reduce in vitro the enzymatic activity of TG2, they may contribute to diabetes via an impairment of insulin secretion and/or intracellular insulin signaling [9,31,32]. Conversely, TG2 is up-regulated in a number of cancer cell types, where it inhibits the apoptotic cell death, promotes drug resistance, and favors metastatic spread. In order to enhance the therapeutic efficacy of anti-cancer drugs, and contemporarily inhibit metastatic tumor spread, the use of TG2-specific interfering RNA or enzymatic inhibitors is currently under discussion [16,33]. Finally, TG2 plays an important role in the pathogenesis of some chronic liver diseases. In relation to alcoholic steatohepatitis, TG2-catalyzed cross-linking of keratin 8 is essential for the formation of Mallory-Denk bodies, while intracellular TG2 translocates into the nucleus and provokes hepatocyte death, which in turn is associated with liver fibrosis [34].

## TG3

The type III or epidermal TG (TG3 or eTG) is a cytoplasmic enzyme mainly expressed in the epidermis and hair follicles, where it is activated by cathepsins L and/or S-catalyzed proteolysis during keratinocyte differentiation. Once activated, TG3 catalyzes $Ca^{2+}$-dependent transamidation of suitable protein substrates and co-substrates (mainly loricrin and small proline-rich proteins), thus contributing to CE formation [1,14]. Despite the close relationships existing between TG1 and TG3 enzymatic isoforms, no defect in the skin barrier function has yet been linked to mutations in the gene encoding TG3 [2]. On the other hand, the epidermal TG is considered the dominant autoantigen of dermatitis herpetiformis. The occurrence of anti-TG3 circulating antibodies, as well as TG3-targeted IgA skin deposits in patients having this illness confirms the ability of TG3 to elicit autoimmunity [35].

## TG4

The type IV or prostate TG (TG4 or pTG) is an enzyme uniquely expressed in prostate tissues. The functional role of TG4 has been well characterized in prostatic secretion of rodents, where it catalyzes $Ca^{2+}$-dependent transamidation of suitable protein substrates and co-substrates, resulting in semen coagulation [36,37]. In humans, TG4 probably has additional functions in ECM compartment. Recent investigations have shown that TG4 is associated with the invasive potential of prostate cancer cells [38], and also plays a role in the interaction between cancerous cells and the vascular endothelium [39]. Furthermore, four alternative splicing variants of TG4 (TG4-L, -M1, -M2, and -S) have been variously associated to prostate cancer and benign prostate hyperplasia [40].

## TG5

The type V or x TG (TG5 or TGx) is an intracellular enzyme expressed ubiquitously, except in the brain. In epithelial cells, the proteolytically-activated TG5 catalyzes Ca2+-dependent transamidation of suitable protein substrates and co-substrates (mainly involucrin, loricrin, and small proline-rich proteins), thereby contributing to CE formation [14,41]. In addition, TG5 overexpression is able to induce apoptotic cell death in a similar fashion to TG2 [42]. A missense mutation in the gene encoding TG5 totally abolishes its activity, leading to an autosomal recessive genodermatosis known as acral peeling skin syndrome (APSS) [43]. As a secondary effect, TG5 contributes to the hyperkeratotic phenotype in psoriasis and ichthyosis (both vulgaris and lamellar), while its local expression is strongly altered in Darier's disease [44].

## TG6

The type VI or y TG (TG6 or TGy) is a newly identified enzyme [45], which is predominantly expressed by a subset of neurons in the central nervous system (CNS). It is able to catalyze $Ca^{2+}$-dependent transamidation of protein substrates and co-substrates, although its functions in humans remain to be elucidated. The preferential expression of TG6 in neural tissue, as well as its close homology to TG2 suggest that this enzyme could be involved in the pathogenesis of several neurological dysfunctions. On the other hand, the presence of anti-TG6 specific antibodies in serum of patients with gluten ataxia implies that TG6 may act as an autoantigen able to elicit autoimmunity [46]. The intrathecal synthesis of anti-TG2 antibodies, as well as their presence in cerebrospinal fluid have been further demonstrated [47], suggesting the possibility that a cell-mediated immune response against any cerebral TG can take shape directly in CNS.

## TG7

The type VII or z TG (TG7 or TGz) is a newly identified enzyme expressed ubiquitously [45]. Although TG7 is able to catalyze $Ca^{2+}$-dependent transamidation of protein substrates and co-substrates, neither its functions nor its pathological implications are yet known.

## Overview on TGs

The amino acid sequences of protein 4.2, FXIII-A, TG1, TG2, TG3, TG4, TG5, TG6, and TG7 establish them as a homologous gene family (EPB42 on 15q15.2, F13A1 on 6p24-25, TGM1 on 14q11.2, TGM2 on 20q11-12, TGM3 on 20q11-12, TGM4 on 3p21-22, TGM5 on 15q15.2, TGM6 on 20q11, and TGM7 on 15q15.2), which members mainly catalyze the formation of protein cross-links, as well as the incorporation of polyamines (primary amines) into suitable protein substrates by transamidation of available glutamine/lysine residues, thereby increasing the resistance of tissues to chemical, enzymatic, and mechanical disruption [1]. However, this enzymatic activity not only enhances the original functions of protein substrates, but also adds new functions that may cause pathological conditions [2]. For each human TG family member, a summary about its localization, reactions catalyzed, biological functions, and associated disorders is reported in table 1.

## TG2 AND ANTI-TG2 IN CELIAC DISEASE

CD is a chronic inflammatory disorder resulting from the interaction among dietary gluten (gliadins and glutenins), genetic pattern (HLA-DQ2 and/or -DQ8 alleles), and immune system (T cell-driven immunity) that in turn, initiates a cascade of events leading to intestinal damage. A proper diagnosis of CD initially requires clinician's attention to evaluate the wide spectrum of symptoms, as well as the presence of anti-endomysial (EMA) and/or anti-TG2 antibodies in patient's serum. Thereafter, the diagnosis is defined by the histological evidence of duodenal villous atrophy, crypt hyperplasia, and intraepithelial lymphocytosis, which recover after a suitable period of gluten withdrawal. The clinical remission, together with the disappearance of circulating EMA and anti-TG2 antibodies after a gluten-free diet, confirm the diagnosis [48].

## Table 1. Main features of each human TG family member

| TG type | Localization | Reactions catalyzed | Biological functions | Associated disorders |
|---|---|---|---|---|
| Protein 4.2 | Erythrocyte membrane | None | Membrane stabilization | Hereditary spherocytosis<br>Hemolytic anemia |
| FXIII-A | Blood clotting sites Intracellular (platelets, macrophages, and monocytes) | Transamidation Phosphorylation S-S bond formation | Blood clot stabilization Angiogenesis Wound healing Cytoskeletal remodelling | Hemorrhagic diathesis Defective wound healing Spontaneous miscarriage Thrombosis (altered risk) Atherosclerosis Arterial hypertension Celiac disease Crohn's disease |
| TG1 (kTG) | Intracellular (squamous epithelium and brain) | Transamidation Esterification | CE formation | Lamellar ichthyosis |
| TG2 (tTG) | Intracellular ubiquitous Several ECMs | Transamidation Deamidation Hydrolysis Phosphorylation S-S bond formation | Angiogenesis Fibrogenesis Wound healing Cell adhesion/migration Signal transduction Respiratory chain assembly Cell proliferation Cell differentiation Neurite formation Apoptosis Inflammation | Celiac disease Arthritic diseases IBD Cardiovascular disorders Neurological diseases Diabetes Cancer Chronic liver diseases |
| TG3 (eTG) | Intracellular (epidermis and hair follicles) | Transamidation | CE formation | Dermatitis herpetiformis |
| TG4 (pTG) | Prostate tissues | Transamidation | Seminal fluid coagulation (only in rodents) | Prostate cancer Prostate hyperplasia |
| TG5 (TGx) | Intracellular ubiquitous (except in the brain) | Transamidation | CE formation Apoptosis | APSS Psoriasis Ichthyosis Darier's disease |
| TG6 (TGy) | CNS | Transamidation | – | Gluten ataxia |
| TG7 (TGz) | Ubiquitous | Transamidation | – | – |

Legend: TG = transglutaminase; Protein 4.2 = electrophoretic band 4.2 of the erythrocyte membrane; FXIII-A = A-subunit of the blood coagulation factor XIII; kTG = keratinocyte TG; tTG = tissue TG; eTG = epidermal TG; pTG = prostate TG; ECMs = extracellular matrices; CNS = central nervous system; S-S = disulfide; CE = cornified cell envelope; IBD = inflammatory bowel disease; APSS = acral peeling skin syndrome.

Given the current knowledge on CD, it is possible to affirm that:

- both the primary antigen (gluten peptides) and dominant autoantigen (TG2) are known;
- the primary antigen can be removed and reintroduced in a controlled manner;
- HLA alleles predisposing to disease (HLA-DQ2 and -DQ8) are also known;
- to perform studies on duodenal mucosa or isolated cell populations, access to the target organ (small intestine) is relatively simple.

These findings make CD an optimal study model that has been already used to clarify the pathogenesis of rheumatoid arthritis [49], an autoimmune condition often associated to the presence of anti-TG2 atypical antibodies in diverse biological fluids [25].

## From TG2 to Anti-TG2: A Pathogenetic Pathway

In CD patients, the gliadin epitopes are deamidate (and thus acidified) by TG2 in the slightly acidic environment of the small intestine (pH ~6.6). In this new molecular form, they are presented to T lymphocytes by means of HLA-DQ2, which needs residues negatively charged at P4, P6, and P7 anchor positions, or through HLA-DQ8, which requires residues negatively charged at P1, P4, and P9 anchor positions, resulting in activation of gliadin-specific T and B cell clones [50]. This mechanism starts, increases, and self nourishes the immunological response against gluten peptides, emphasizing the role of TG2 in the pathogenesis of CD. At the same time, an increased extracellular localization of TG2 is observable in damaged or inflamed intestine of CD patients [51]. This antigenic overexpression can explain the afore mentioned mechanism, as well as the anti-TG2 antibody induction observable in CD patients. In detail, the intestinal TG2 can act through two way: deamidate the gliadin epitopes or cross-link these peptides to itself [50]. When gliadin and TG2 antigens are bound, the gliadin-specific T lymphocytes already present in the intestine can provide help for B cells that in meantime have encountered the new antigen complex, promoting local production of anti-gliadin and/or anti-TG2 antibodies by a mechanism known as hapten-carrier model [52,53].

An epitope spreading-based theory has been recently enrolled to explain the occurrence of anti-FXIII, anti-TG3, and anti-TG6 circulating antibodies in patients with CD, dermatitis herpetiformis, and gluten ataxia [54]. The epitope spreading is another immunological model, in which some lymphocyte clones adapt their specificity to changing environmental conditions, such as a decrease in concentration ratio of primary antigen (TG2) to any of its isoforms (FXIII, TG3, or TG6). In a different pathway, the intestinal TG2 can deamidate or cross-link external agents (e.g. bacteria, viruses, or food proteins) as well as self antigens (e.g. intracellular or ECM proteins), creating more potent antigens or antigenic neoepitopes. The new antigens can elicit an immune response that in turn, may cause a wide antibody production or disseminated tissue destruction (secondary autoimmunity) [55]. The latter mechanism, in concert with the epitope spreading theory, provides a possible explanation for both extraintestinal symptoms and autoimmune conditions frequently seen in CD patients.

## Anti-TG2: Implication for Celiac Disease

For a long time, the scientific community has classified the occurrence of circulating EMA and anti-TG2 antibodies as an epiphenomenon useful to diagnose, monitor, or exclude CD. Conversely, it has been recently demonstrated that anti-TG2 are able to inhibit intestinal epithelial cell differentiation, induce intestinal epithelial cell proliferation, increase epithelial permeability, activate monocytes, and disturb angiogenesis, suggesting that these antibodies may also have a functional role in the pathogenesis of CD [54,56].

## TG2 AND ANTI-TG2 IN ACUTE CORONARY SYNDROME

Acute coronary syndrome (ACS) is a clinical condition encompassing angina pectoris (also known as unstable angina) and myocardial infarction, which result from thrombus formation subsequent to the disruption of a vulnerable atherosclerotic plaque. The proper identification, as well as differential diagnosis of ACS are based on the following criteria:

- presence of typical symptoms (e.g. chest discomfort, dyspnea, nausea, and light-headedness);
- evidence of electrocardiographic (ECG) myocardial ischemia (ST-T segment wave changes);
- typical rise and gradual fall (troponin I), or more rapid rise and fall (CK-MB mass and myoglobin) of the biochemical markers of myocardial necrosis;
- loss of electrically functioning cardiac tissue (development of pathologic Q waves on ECG tracing).

After diagnosis of ACS, further interventions including risk stratification, selection of therapy, monitoring of disease progression and treatment efficacy need to be carefully performed [57].

Recently, Di Tola and Peracchi have identified anti-TG2 circulating antibodies in patients affected from disorders in which the target organ is located at a distance from the intestine, such as ACS, dilated cardiomyopathy (DCM), valvular heart disease and other causes of end-stage heart failure [27,28]. In this regard, other authors have suggested that the occurrence of anti-TG2 positive results in patients without CD can be method-dependent (e.g. use of kits prepared with guinea pig extractive antigen rather than human recombinant TG2, presence of minor impurities in the antigenic mixture used to sow the solid phase) or alternatively, can be due to an increase in immunoglobulin serum levels, commonly found in many pathological conditions [58-61]. However, Di Tola's and Peracchi's studies have been performed by using kits prepared with human recombinant TG2 [27,28], while the real presence of anti-TG2 circulating antibodies in patients with diverse cardiac disorders has been demonstrated by enzyme-linked immunosorbent assay-blocking experiments and western blot analysis [27].

## From TG2 to Anti-TG2: A Pathogenetic Pathway

TG2 is predominantly a cytoplasmic enzyme present in many cells, including cardiomyocytes and some cell types in the blood vessel wall [1]. In cardiovascular system, it acts mainly to stabilize intra and/or extracellular molecules in a wide variety of physiological and pathological processes (table 2) [9].

**Table 2. Biological functions and pathological implications of TG2 in cardiovascular system**

| Cardiovascular district | Mechanisms of action | Functions/implications |
|---|---|---|
| Arterial lumen | Platelet adhesion<br>Formation of coated platelet | Stabilization of the thrombus |
| Endothelial barrier | Endothelial barrier stabilization<br>Reduction of endothelial permeability | Plaque progression<br>Myocardial edema<br>Pleural effusions |
| Atheroma | TGF-β1 activation<br>Deposition of ECM proteins<br>Formation of elafin-ECM cross-links<br>Fibrous cap stabilization | Plaque progression |
| Blood vessels | Enhancement of angiogenesis | Plaque progression and stability<br>Coronary collateral formation<br>Would healing after myocardial infarction |
| Bloodstream | Arteriolar remodeling<br>Increasing of vascular tone | Hypertension |
| Myocardium | Abnormal enzymatic activity | Left ventricular hypertrophy<br>Myocardial fibrosis<br>Reduced left ventricular ejection fraction |

Legend: TGF-β1 = transforming growth factor-β1; ECM = extracellular matrix.

Increased TG2 activity is a common feature of several human diseases [2]. Consistently, a cardiac TG2 overexpression has been described in some experimental models of heart failure and in occurrence of myocardial ischemia/reperfusion injury. In the arteries with or without minimal atherosclerosis, TG2 is detectable only in the medium and along the luminal endothelial border while in the atherosclerotic arteries, especially coronaries and carotid vessels, this enzyme is also evident in the fibrous cup and in shoulder regions of the plaque [9,62]. On the other hand, it has been recently hypothesized that an aberrant induction of TG2 activity in tissues may contribute to a variety of diseases via formation of inappropriate protein aggregates, which can trigger inflammation, apoptosis, and several other pathological processes [63]. Since this hypothesis brings to mind the immunological model used to explain humoral response in CD (hapten-carrier model) [52,53], a similar if not the same anti-TG2 antibody-inducing mechanism could also occur in damaged or inflamed non-intestinal tissues, such as the cardiovascular tissues affected from an acute or chronic disorder.

## Anti-TG2: Implication for Acute Coronary Syndrome

Several studies have shown an increased prevalence of CD in patients having a chronic cardiac disorder, such as DCM (up to 5.7%) or myocarditis (4.4%). In order to explain this finding, it has been postulated that TG2 can act as an autoantigen shared by multiple organs, so that patients who develop anti-TG2 antibodies (e.g. CD patients) may also develop a cardiac disorder [9,55]. However, since Di Tola's and Peracchi's studies refer to patients for whom CD had been previously excluded [27,28], it is not the case.

In relation to ACS, Di Tola's study [28] has revealed a dose-response effect with higher anti-TG2 antibody concentrations in patients with recurrent events and larger infarcts. Another finding that emerges from this study is the correlation between anti-TG2 antibody levels and the biochemical markers of myocardial necrosis (troponin I, CK, CK-MB mass, and myoglobin). All these data suggest that anti-TG2 antibodies are related to severity of the acute coronary event, as well as to extent of the myocardial tissue lesion occurring in ACS patients. On the other hand, the finding that anti-TG2 titre reaches a peak at 30 days and returns to baseline after 150 days confirms the association between these antibodies and the acute coronary event, and suggests a possible use of anti-TG2 in the long-term follow-up of ACS patients, for which a reliable marker does not exist yet.

Recently, Sane has proposed an interaction model that considers all possible relations among TG2 enzymatic activity, anti-TG2 biological effects (as well as their possible prognostic significance), and the resulting cardiovascular disturbances (figure 2) [64].

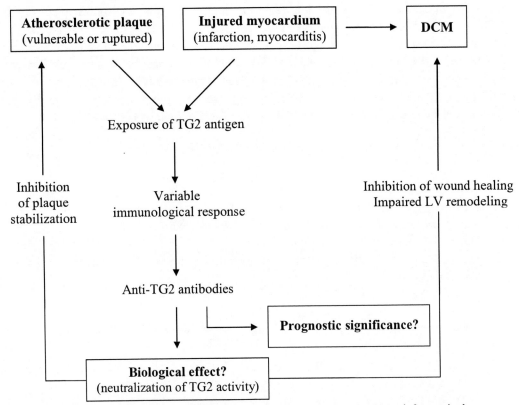

Legend: DCM = dilated cardiomyopathy; TG2 = type 2 transglutaminase; LV = left ventricular.

Figure 2. Sane's model on TG2, anti-TG2, and cardiovascular disturbances

Given that TG2 enzymatic activity may result in myocardial wound healing and stabilization of atherosclerotic plaque [9,64], the Sane's model hypothesizes that anti-TG2 antibodies could have biological effects able to define a prognostic significance [64]. In detail, vulnerable or ruptured atherosclerotic plaque, as well as injured myocardium (following an infarction, myocarditis, etc.) may be sources of TG2 antigen resulting in formation of anti-TG2 antibodies that in turn, by neutralizing TG2 enzymatic activity, could promote destabilization of the plaque or impaired myocardial wound healing, thereby contributing to a chronic disorder such as DCM. The finding that anti-TG2 antibodies have biological effects in patients with CD [54,56], including inhibition of angiogenesis, suggests that they may have a functional role also in cardiovascular disorders.

## CONCLUSION

TG2 is a pivotal enzyme widely distributed in cardiovascular system, where it contributes to a variety of physiological and pathological processes [1,9,64]. Following an acute coronary event, TG2 overexpression may result in formation of anti-TG2 antibodies that in turn, by neutralizing its enzymatic activity, could have biological effects able to define a prognostic significance [28,64]. On the other hand, if anti-TG2 antibodies can really contribute to the onset and/or evolution of a chronic cardiac disorder such as DCM [64], additional therapies targeted to obtain antibody inhibition (e.g. immunosuppression and plasmapheresis) or enzymatic stimulation (e.g. administration/infusion of TG2) should be taken into consideration. Despite their potentially adverse effects on human health, these antibodies could be useful as long-term marker in ACS patients, for whom the presence of disorders already known to be associated to anti-TG2 positive results (e.g. CD, arthritic diseases, and IBD) [19,25,26] has been previously excluded. In the near future, these observations and related hypothesis could to become the subject of interesting researches.

## REFERENCES

[1] Greenberg CS, Birckbichler PJ, Rice RH. Transglutaminases: multifunctional cross-linking enzymes that stabilize tissues. *FASEB J* 1991;5:3071-7.

[2] Iismaa SE, Mearns BM, Lorand L, Graham RM. Transglutaminases and disease: lessons from genetically engineered mouse models and inherited disorders. *Physiol Rev* 2009;89:991-1023.

[3] Santos M, Torné JM. Recent patents on transglutaminase production and applications: a brief review. *Recent Pat Biotechnol* 2009;3:166-74.

[4] Satchwell TJ, Shoemark DK, Sessions RB, Toye AM. Protein 4.2: a complex linker. *Blood Cells Mol Dis* 2009;42:201-10.

[5] Ariëns RA, Lai TS, Weisel JW, Greenberg CS, Grant PJ. Role of factor XIII in fibrin clot formation and effects of genetic polymorphisms. *Blood* 2002;100:743-54.

[6] Mosesson MW. Fibrinogen and fibrin structure and functions. *J Thromb Haemost* 2005;3:1894-904.

[7] Ichinose A, Asahina T, Kobayashi T. Congenital blood coagulation factor XIII deficiency and perinatal management. *Curr Drug Targets* 2005;6:541-9.

[8] Asahina T, Kobayashi T, Takeuchi K, Kanayama N. Congenital blood coagulation factor XIII deficiency and successful deliveries: a review of the literature. *Obstet Gynecol Surv* 2007;62:255-60.

[9] Sane DC, Kontos JL, Greenberg CS. Roles of transglutaminases in cardiac and vascular diseases. *Front Biosci* 2007;12:2530-45.

[10] Dardik R, Loscalzo J, Eskaraev R, Inbal A. Molecular mechanisms underlying the proangiogenic effect of factor XIII. *Arterioscler Thromb Vasc Biol* 2005;25:526-32.

[11] Lahav J, Karniel E, Bagoly Z, Sheptovitsky V, Dardik R, Inbal A. Coagulation factor XIII serves as protein disulfide isomerase. *Thromb Haemost* 2009;101:840-4.

[12] Adány R, Bárdos H. Factor XIII subunit A as an intracellular transglutaminase. *Cell Mol Life Sci* 2003;60:1049-60.

[13] Sjöber K, Eriksson S, Tenngart B, Roth EB, Leffler H, Stenberg P. Factor XIII and tissue transglutaminase antibodies in celiac and inflammatory bowel disease. *Autoimmunity* 2002;35:357-64.

[14] Hitomi K. Transglutaminases in skin epidermis. *Eur J Dermatol* 2005;15:313-9.

[15] Herman ML, Farasat S, Steinbach PJ, Wei MH, Toure O, Fleckman P, Blake P, Bale SJ, Toro JR. Transglutaminase-1 gene mutations in autosomal recessive congenital ichthyosis: summary of mutations (including 23 novel) and modeling of TGase-1. *Hum Mutat* 2009;30:537-47.

[16] Park D, Choi SS, Ha KS. Transglutaminase 2: a multi-functional protein in multiple subcellular compartments. *Amino Acids* 2010 [Epub ahead of print].

[17] Fleckenstein B, Molberg Ø, Qiao SW, Schmid DG, von der Mülbe F, Elgstøen K, Jung G, Sollid LM. Gliadin T cell epitope selection by tissue transglutaminase in celiac disease. Role of enzyme specificity and pH influence on the transamidation versus deamidation process. *J Biol Chem* 2002;277:34109-16.

[18] Dieterich W, Ehnis T, Bauer M, Donner P, Volta U, Riecken EO, Schuppan D. Identification of tissue transglutaminase as the autoantigen of celiac disease. *Nat Med* 1997;7:797-801.

[19] Alaedini A, Green PH. Autoantibodies in celiac disease. *Autoimmunity* 2008;41:19-26.

[20] Dahele A, Aldhous MC, Kingstone K, Humphreys K, Bode J, McIntyre M, Ghosh S. Gut mucosal immunity to tissue transglutaminase in untreated celiac disease and other gastrointestinal disorders. *Dig Dis Sci* 2002;47:2325-35.

[21] Picarelli A, Sabbatella L, Di Tola M, Di Cello T, Vetrano S, Anania MC. Antiendomysial antibody detection in fecal supernatants. In vivo proof that small bowel mucosa is the site of antiendomysial antibody production. *Am J Gastroenterol* 2002;97:95-8.

[22] Bonamico M, Ferri M, Nenna R, Verrienti A, Di Mario U, Tiberti C. Tissue transglutaminase autoantibody detection in human saliva: a powerful method for celiac disease screening. *J Pediatr* 2004;144:632-6.

[23] Carroccio A, Di Prima L, Pirrone G, Scalici C, Florena AM, Gasparin M, Tolazzi G, Gucciardi A, Sciumè C, Iacono G. Anti-transglutaminase antibody assay of the culture medium of intestinal biopsy specimens can improve the accuracy of celiac disease diagnosis. *Clin Chem* 2006;52:1175-80.

[24] Vetrano S, Zampaletta U, Anania MC, Di Tola M, Sabbatella L, Passarelli F, Maffia C, Sanjust MG, Lettieri F, De Pità O, Picarelli A. Detection of anti-endomysial and anti-tissue transglutaminase autoantibodies in media following culture of oral biopsies from patients with untreated celiac disease. *Dig Liver Dis* 2007;39:911-6.

[25] Picarelli A, Di Tola M, Sabbatella L, Vetrano S, Anania MC, Spadaro A, Sorgi ML, Taccari E. Anti-tissue transglutaminase antibodies in arthritic patients: a disease-specific finding? *Clin Chem* 2003;49:2091-4.

[26] Di Tola M, Sabbatella L, Anania MC, Viscido A, Caprilli R, Pica R, Paoluzi P, Picarelli A. Anti-tissue transglutaminase antibodies in inflammatory bowel disease: new evidence. *Clin Chem Lab Med* 2004;42:1092-7.

[27] Peracchi M, Trovato C, Longhi M, Gasparin M, Conte D, Tarantino C, Prati D, Bardella MT. Tissue transglutaminase antibodies in patients with end-stage heart failure. *Am J Gastroenterol* 2002;97:2850-4.

[28] Di Tola M, Barillà F, Trappolini M, Palumbo HF, Gaudio C, Picarelli A. Antitissue transglutaminase antibodies in acute coronary syndrome: an alert signal of myocardial tissue lesion? *J Intern Med* 2008;263:43-51.

[29] Martin A, Romito G, Pepe I, De Vivo G, Merola MR, Limatola A, Gentile V. Transglutaminase-catalyzed reactions responsible for the pathogenesis of celiac disease and neurodegenerative diseases: from basic biochemistry to clinic. *Curr Med Chem* 2006;13:1895-902.

[30] De Vivo G, Gentile V. Transglutaminase-catalyzed post-translational modifications of proteins in the nervous system and their possible involvement in neurodegenerative diseases. *CNS Neurol Disord Drug Targets* 2008;7:370-5.

[31] Bernassola F, Federici M, Corazzari M, Terrinoni A, Hribal ML, De Laurenzi V, Ranalli M, Massa O, Sesti G, McLean WH, Citro G, Barbetti F, Melino G. Role of transglutaminase 2 in glucose tolerance: knockout mice studies and a putative mutation in a MODY patient. *FASEB J* 2002;16:1371-8.

[32] Porzio O, Massa O, Cunsolo V, Colombo C, Malaponti M, Bertuzzi F, Hansen T, Johansen A, Pedersen O, Meschi F, Terrinoni A, Melino G, Federici M, Decarlo N, Menicagli M, Campani D, Marchetti P, Ferdaoussi M, Froguel P, Federici G, Vaxillaire M, Barbetti F. Missense mutations in the TGM2 gene encoding transglutaminase 2 are found in patients with early-onset type 2 diabetes. Mutation in brief no. 982. Online. *Hum Mutat* 2007;28:1150.

[33] Chhabra A, Verma A, Mehta K. Tissue transglutaminase promotes or suppresses tumors depending on cell context. *Anticancer Res* 2009;29:1909-19.

[34] Tatsukawa H, Kojima S. Recent advances in understanding the roles of transglutaminase 2 in alcoholic steatohepatitis. *Cell Biol Int* 2010;34:325-34.

[35] Sárdy M, Kárpáti S, Merkl B, Paulsson M, Smyth N. Epidermal transglutaminase (TGase 3) is the autoantigen of dermatitis herpetiformis. *J Exp Med* 2002;195:747-57.

[36] Tseng HC, Lin HJ, Sudhakar Gandhi PS, Wang CY, Chen YH. Purification and identification of transglutaminase from mouse coagulating gland and its cross-linking activity among seminal vesicle secretion proteins. *J Chromatogr B Analyt Technol Biomed Life Sci* 2008;876:198-202.

[37] Tseng HC, Lin HJ, Tang JB, Gandhi PS, Chang WC, Chen YH. Identification of the major TG4 cross-linking sites in the androgen-dependent SVS I exclusively expressed in mouse seminal vesicle. *J Cell Biochem* 2009;107:899-907.

[38] Davies G, Ablin RJ, Mason MD, Jiang WG. Expression of the prostate transglutaminase (TGase-4) in prostate cancer cells and its impact on the invasiveness of prostate cancer. *J Exp Ther Oncol* 2007;6:257-64.

[39] Jiang WG, Ablin RJ, Kynaston HG, Mason MD. The prostate transglutaminase (TGase-4, TGaseP) regulates the interaction of prostate cancer and vascular endothelial cells, a potential role for the ROCK pathway. *Microvasc Res* 2009;77:150-7.

[40] Cho SY, Choi K, Jeon JH, Kim CW, Shin DM, Lee JB, Lee SE, Kim CS, Park JS, Jeong EM, Jang GY, Song KY, Kim IG. Differential alternative splicing of human transglutaminase 4 in benign prostate hyperplasia and prostate cancer. *Exp Mol Med* 2010 [Epub ahead of print].

[41] Pietroni V, Di Giorgi S, Paradisi A, Ahvazi B, Candi E, Melino G. Inactive and highly active, proteolytically processed transglutaminase-5 in epithelial cells. *J Invest Dermatol* 2008;128:2760-6.

[42] Cadot B, Rufini A, Pietroni V, Ramadan S, Guerrieri P, Melino G, Candi E. Overexpressed transglutaminase 5 triggers cell death. *Amino Acids* 2004;26:405-8.

[43] Cassidy AJ, van Steensel MA, Steijlen PM, van Geel M, van der Velden J, Morley SM, Terrinoni A, Melino G, Candi E, McLean WH. A homozygous missense mutation in TGM5 abolishes epidermal transglutaminase 5 activity and causes acral peeling skin syndrome. *Am J Hum Genet* 2005;77:909-17.

[44] Candi E, Oddi S, Paradisi A, Terrinoni A, Ranalli M, Teofoli P, Citro G, Scarpato S, Puddu P, Melino G. Expression of transglutaminase 5 in normal and pathologic human epidermis. *J Invest Dermatol* 2002;119:670-7.

[45] Grenard P, Bates MK, Aeschlimann D. Evolution of transglutaminase genes: identification of a transglutaminase gene cluster on human chromosome 15q15. Structure of the gene encoding transglutaminase X and a novel gene family member, transglutaminase Z. *J Biol Chem* 2001;276:33066-78.

[46] Hadjivassiliou M, Aeschlimann P, Strigun A, Sanders DS, Woodroofe N, Aeschlimann D. Autoantibodies in gluten ataxia recognize a novel neuronal transglutaminase. *Ann Neurol* 2008;64:332-43.

[47] Schrödl D, Kahlenberg F, Peter-Zimmer K, Hermann W, Kühn HJ, Mothes T. Intrathecal synthesis of autoantibodies against tissue transglutaminase. *J Autoimmun* 2004;22:335-40.

[48] Di Sabatino A, Corazza GR. Celiac disease. *Lancet* 2009;373:1480-93.

[49] Molberg Ø, Sollid LM. A gut feeling for joint inflammation - using celiac disease to understand rheumatoid arthritis. *Trends Immunol* 2006;27:188-94.

[50] Sollid LM. Celiac disease: dissetting a complex inflammatory disorder. *Nat Rev Immunol* 2002;2:647-55.

[51] Farrace MG, Picarelli A, Di Tola M, Sabbatella L, Marchione OP, Ippolito G, Piacentini M. Presence of anti-"tissue" transglutaminase antibodies in inflammatory intestinal diseases: an apoptosis-associated event? *Cell Death Differ* 2001;8:767-70.

[52] Sollid LM, Molberg O, McAdam S, Lundin KE. Autoantibodies in celiac disease: tissue transglutaminase-guilt by association? *Gut* 1997;41:851-2.

[53] Fleckenstein B, Qiao SW, Larsen MR, Jung G, Roepstorff P, Sollid LM. Molecular characterization of covalent complexes between tissue transglutaminase and gliadin peptides. *J Biol Chem* 2004;279:17607-16.

[54] Lindfors K, Kaukinen K, Mäki M. A role for anti-transglutaminase 2 autoantibodies in the pathogenesis of celiac disease? *Amino Acids* 2009;36:685-91.
[55] Schuppan D, Ciccocioppo R. Celiac disease and secondary autoimmunity. *Dig Liver Dis* 2002;34:13-5.
[56] Caputo I, Barone MV, Martucciello S, Lepretti M, Esposito C. Tissue transglutaminase in celiac disease: role of autoantibodies. *Amino Acids* 2009;36:693-9.
[57] No authors listed. Myocardial infarction redefined - a consensus document of the joint european society of cardiology/american college of cardiology committee for the redefinition of myocardial infarction. *Eur Heart J* 2000;21:1502-13.
[58] Carroccio A, Giannitrapani L, Soresi M, Not T, Iacono G, Di Rosa C, Panfili E, Notarbartolo A, Montalto G. Guinea pig transglutaminase immunolinked assay does not predict celiac disease in patients with chronic liver disease. *Gut* 2001;49:506-11.
[59] Villalta D, Crovatto M, Stella S, Tonutti E, Tozzoli R, Bizzaro N. False positive reactions for IgA and IgG anti-tissue transglutaminase antibodies in liver cirrhosis are common and method-dependent. *Clin Chim Acta* 2005;356:102-9.
[60] Bizzaro N, Tampoia M, Villalta D, Platzgummer S, Liguori M, Tozzoli R, Tonutti E. Low specificity of anti-tissue transglutaminase antibodies in patients with primary biliary cirrhosis. *J Clin Lab Anal* 2006;20:184-9.
[61] Sárdy M, Csikós M, Geisen C, Preisz K, Kornseé Z, Tomsits E, Töx U, Hunzelmann N, Wieslander J, Kárpáti S, Paulsson M, Smyth N. Tissue transglutaminase ELISA positivity in autoimmune disease independent of gluten-sensitive disease. *Clin Chim Acta* 2007;376:126-35.
[62] Bergamini CM, Griffin M, Pansini FS. Transglutaminase and vascular biology: physiopathologic implications and perspectives for therapeutic interventions. *Curr Med Chem* 2005;12:2357-72.
[63] Kim SY. Transglutaminase 2 in inflammation. *Front Biosci* 2006;11:3026-35.
[64] Sane DC. Antibodies to tissue transglutaminase: an immune link between the gut, the coronaries and the myocardium? *J Intern Med* 2008;263:1-3.

*Chapter VII*

# ELECTROCARDIOGRAPHIC PREDICTORS OF FIBRILLATORY EVENTS IN VENTRICULAR EARLY REPOLARIZATION

*Xingpeng Liu, Ashok J. Shah, Nicolas Derval, Frederic Sacher, Shinsuke Miyazaki, Amir S. Jadidi, Andrei Forclaz, Isabelle Nault, Lena Rivard, Nick Linton, Olivier Xhaet, Daniel Scherr, Pierre Bordachar, Philippe Ritter, Meleze Hocini, Pierre Jais and Michel Haissaguerre.*
Hôpital Cardiologique du Haut-Lévêque and the Université Bordeaux II, Bordeaux, France

## INTRODUCTION

Early repolarization (ER) pattern is a common electrocardiographic (ECG) variant, characterized by J point elevation manifested either as QRS slurring (at the transition from the QRS segment to the ST segment) or notching (a positive deflection inscribed on terminal S wave), ST-segment elevation with upper concavity and prominent T waves in at least two contiguous leads.[1, 2] The prevalence of ER pattern in normal population varies from 1% to 13%, depending on the age (predominant in young adults), the race (highest amongst black population), and the criterion for J point elevation (0.05 mV vs. 0.1 mV).[3-6] Since first described by Tomashewski in 1938,[7] ER pattern has been largely considered as an innocent ECG phenomenon for decades. However, this long-held concept has been getting some new momentum by recently published reports. ER pattern has been associated with ventricular fibrillation (VF) in patients with aborted sudden cardiac arrest. It has also emerged as a marker of increased long-term cardiovascular mortality in the general population. Thus, ER pattern is probably not so benign as traditionally believed. Under such a situation, now, the critical clinical question is how to identify the ER subjects who are potentially at risk of arrhythmia.[8] In this chapter, we review the currently available knowledge on this issue.

# ER Pattern: The Renaissance of an Old ECG Entity

So far, 3 lines of evidence have been advanced suggesting that ER pattern is potentially associated with malignant ventricular arrhythmias: (1) three case-control studies;[3-5] (2) one population-wide long-term follow-up study;[6] and (3) three studies favoring the ER pattern as the key substrate for VF.[3,5,9]

## ERS is More Prevalent in Patients with Idiopathic Ventricular Fibrillation

During the past decade, J wave / ST segment elevation was reported as the only "abnormal" finding in patients diagnosed with idiopathic VF in the literature from around the globe.[10,11] These observations indicated that ER pattern could be potentially associated with malignant ventricular arrhythmias in some patients. However, its relationship with ER was not indicated until recently. In a case-control study reported initially in 2007 and systematically in 2008, we found surprisingly high prevalence of ER pattern in patients with idiopathic VF as compared with well-matched healthy subjects (31% vs 5%, $P<0.001$).[3,12] ER pattern in the inferolateral leads was proposed as a new syndrome associated with sudden cardiac death.[3, 12] Furthermore, based on the data from implantable cardioverter-defibrillators, we found that idiopathic VF survivors with ER pattern experienced higher VF recurrence than idiopathic VF survivors without ER pattern (41% versus 23%; $P = 0.008$). This observation indicates that ER is not only a primary risk factor but also a secondary risk factor. Subsequently, similar results were reported by two other groups. Rosso et al compared the ECGs of 45 idiopathic VF cases with that of 124 age- and gender-matched control subjects and 121 young athletes.[4] In agreement with the previous study, they found that ER pattern was more common among the patients with idiopathic VF than among the control subjects (42% vs. 13%, $p <0.001$). In another study from Korea, baseline ECGs of 11 out of 19 (57.9%) patients with idiopathic VF showed ER pattern in contrast to 3.3% of 1 395 controls representing the general population.[5] Though case-control studies do not establish causation, strong evidence in favour of association between ER pattern and idiopathic VF-related sudden cardiac death has emerged.

## Subjects with ER Pattern Have Higher Incidence of Cardiovascular Mortality

More recently, Tikkanen et al systemically reported the long-term outcome of ER pattern in the general population.[6] The authors assessed the prevalence and prognostic significance of ER pattern on routine ECG performed during a community-based investigational coronary artery disease study involving 10 864 middle-aged subjects. The mean follow-up was 30±11 years with the primary end point of cardiac death and secondary end points of all-cause mortality and arrhythmic death. The prevalence of ER was 5.8% in this cohort. Importantly for the first time ever, ER pattern in the inferior leads was found to be associated with an increased risk of cardiac death (adjusted relative risk, 1.28; 95% confidence interval [CI], 1.04 to 1.59; $P = 0.03$) in the general population. J-point elevation in the lateral leads was of borderline significance in predicting cardiac death and all-cause death. Moreover, the survival curves started to diverge 15 years after first ECG recording which was undertaken in 1980s and continued to diverge at a constant rate throughout the follow-up period. Such a divergent pattern of survival was observed despite continued improvement in the treatment and prognosis of patients with cardiac disease during the past two decades. Although the authors classified cardiac deaths into arrhythmic and non-arrhythmic categories retrospectively, the results strongly challenge the long held benignancy of ER pattern.

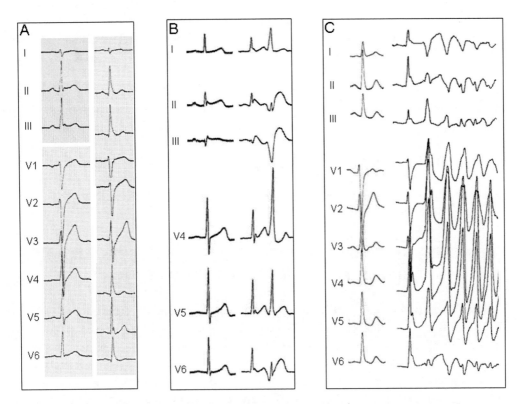

Figure 1. Dynamic nature of J wave magnitude and arrhythmogenesis demonstrated in 3 patients with idiopathic ventricular fibrillation and early repolarization pattern. Each panel shows the QRS complex recorded at baseline (left) and the subsequent complexes recorded just before an arrhythmic event (right). On comparison of the J wave in the two recordings, clear accentuation of early repolarization (arrows) just before the fibrillatory event can be seen. In the patient whose electrocardiogram is shown in Panel A, ventricular fibrillation occurred the following night of the recording shown. Panel B shows a ventricular premature beat (with a left axis); a similar beat triggered ventricular fibrillation a few hours later, as documented on the monitor. Panel C shows the onset of ventricular fibrillation. *This figure needs permission from NEJM*

## Evidence of ER Pattern as the Key Substrate of VF

Because most of the VF episodes cannot be predicted clinically in patients with sporadic episodes of idiopathic VF, it is difficult to get further insights into the role of ER pattern in the mechanism of idiopathic VF. However, some of these patients experience VF storms during hospitalization unraveling the dynamics of ER pattern in VF arrhythmogenesis. We performed serial ECGs during storm (including frequent ventricular ectopy and episodes of ventricular fibrillation) in 18 subjects and all patients showed consistent and marked increase in the amplitude of J wave during the period of storm compared to baseline (from 2.6±1 mm to 4.1±2 mm, P<0.001) (Figure 1).[3] In addition, we found that isoproterenol or quinidine were very effective in preventing arrhythmia recurrence in patients with idiopathic VF and ER pattern; and more importantly, both drugs can significantly reduce the ER pattern or even restore a normal ECG in these patients. Out of 11 patients with idiopathic VF and ER pattern reported by Nam et al., 5 patients experienced VF storm during their stay in the intensive care unit.[5] Interestingly, ECGs recorded within 30 min of the VF storm exhibited global presence of J waves in these patients. These dynamic ECG features of ER pattern appeared spontaneously for a transient period around the VF storm and were not unmasked by sodium channel blockers. These findings are important because they indicate that ER pattern could have been the key substrate for VF in these patients. Moreover, we also provided electrophysiological mapping data in 8 patients with idiopathic VF and ER pattern.[3] Ectopy arising during arrhythmia mapping were found to have originated from the site of repolarization abnormalities in the ventricle. Based on these findings, we consider that the strength of available evidences, even in the absence of prospective validation and exact mechanistic interpretation, is compelling enough to suggest that ER pattern is dynamic and plays a critical role in triggering arrhythmia in some patients with idiopathic VF.

## PREDICTING THE FIBRILLATORY EVENTS IN SUBJECTS WITH ERS USING STANDARD ECG: FACT OR FICTION

Having been convinced that ER pattern could become potentially lethal, more and more cardiologists would like to know how to differentiate the so-called *high risk* ER pattern from the benign ER pattern just from the routine standard ECG. Theoretically, the possible answer of this question could be available through 3 kinds of studies: (1) Prospectively tracking the long term outcome of subjects with ER pattern and finding the characteristic ER patterns related to adverse outcome / events; (2) performing case-control studies to compare the ECG parameters in ER pattern between the patients with and without idiopathic VF; and (3) identifying the internal/external factor(s) capable of amplifying the J wave abnormalities and produce arrhythmia. Keeping these in mind, we explored the possibility of stratifying the ER pattern based on the characteristics of J wave and QRS complex on the routine ECG.

### Magnitude of J Wave

In the study by Tikkanen et al, subjects with J-point elevation of more than 0.2 mV on inferior leads not only had a higher risk of death from cardiac causes (adjusted relative risk, 2.98; 95% CI, 1.85 to 4.92; P<0.001) as compared with J point elevation of more than 0.1 mV, but also had a markedly elevated risk of death from arrhythmia (adjusted relative risk, 2.92; 95% CI, 1.45 to 5.89; P = 0.01).[6] This finding indicates that the magnitude of J-point elevation could be a discriminator of risk. However, this study did not provide the sensitivity and specificity of this measure in predicting the endpoint-events. In accordance with this finding, we also found that the magnitude of J wave elevation in case group was significantly higher than that in the control subjects (2.0±0.8 mV vs 1.2±0.4 mV, P<0.001).[3] It is worthy to note that J point elevation of more than 0.2 mV seems less common in normal population. Of 630 subjects with ER pattern identified in a recently published study, only 68 patients (10.7%) had J wave elevation of more than 0.2 mV.[6] Thus, whether very prominent J wave (>0.2 mV) portends high risk of VF in subjects with ER pattern should be validated in a prospective manner. However, it is necessary to emphasize that the magnitude of J wave elevation can fluctuate in the absence of drug provocation or exercise and therefore it should not be considered as a static entity. Also, the magnitude of J wave can potentially augment.

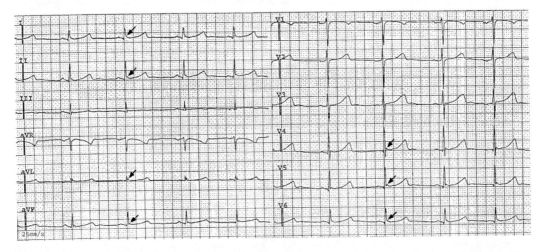

Figure 2. ER pattern is widely distributed in the inferior, lateral, and left precordial leads (marked with arrow) in a patient with idiopathic ventricular fibrillation

## Global J Wave

In normal subjects, ER pattern is confined to inferior leads, lateral leads (I/aVL) or left precordial leads. As reported by Tikkanen et al, only 16 out of 630 subjects with ER (2.5 %) had an ER pattern in both the inferior and lateral leads.[6] In contrast, Haissaguerre et al found that 46.9% of patients in the idiopathic VF group had ER pattern in both the inferior and lateral leads (Figure 2).[3] Similarly, Nam et al found the presence of ER pattern in the left and right precordial and infero-lateral leads (global J wave) in 45.5% of patients with ER and idiopathic VF. On the contrary, none of the 46 subjects having ER pattern without VF from the selected 1395 individuals representing the general population exhibited the global presence of ER pattern.[5] The implications of the wider ECG distribution of ER pattern are unknown, but, theoretically, this feature signifies more diffuse presence of the repolarization abnormality. In a recent *state-of-the-art* review entitled *J wave syndrome*, Antzelevitch et al. proposed division of ER pattern into three subtypes depending on the electrocardiographic distribution of J wave: Type 1, an ER pattern predominantly in the lateral precordial leads, is prevalent among healthy male athletes and rarely seen in the VF survivors; Type 2, an ER pattern predominantly in the inferior or the infero-lateral leads, is associated with a high risk of VF; whereas Type 3, an ER pattern globally in the inferior, lateral and right precordial leads, is associated with the highest level of risk for the development of malignant arrhythmias and is often associated with VF storms.[13] We do believe that global presence of J wave on the ECG represents very high risk of arrhythmic events; however, in our experience, such a pattern seems to be very dynamic and rare in usual clinical practice. Whenever this ER pattern is encountered, it is observed to occur just before an acute attack of VF and fades away after the VF storm.

## Morphology of J Wave

Recently, Merchant et al compared the baseline ECGs of 9 patients with idiopathic VF/VT and ER (so-called malignant ER pattern group) and 61 age- and gender-matched controls with normal ER pattern (so-called benign ER pattern group).[14] The results demonstrated that QRS notching was more prevalent among cases than controls in leads V4 (44% vs 5%, p = 0.001), V5 (44% vs 8%, p = 0.006) and V6 (33% vs 5%, p = 0.013). They concluded that left precordial terminal QRS notching is more prevalent in malignant variants of ER pattern than in benign cases and could be used as a tool for risk stratification of subjects with ER pattern. However, since the study included a small number of cases, the findings should be retested in a larger population. Also, the malignant ER group included 3 patients with idiopathic monomorphic VT without VF.

## Fragmented QRS

Fragmented QRS (fQRS) on the routine ECG is defined as presence of ≥1 additional deflections, notching or slurring within the QRS complex (including top of R wave or nadir of S wave) in at least two contiguous leads.[15] Typical bundle branch block (BBB) pattern (QRS≥120 ms) and incomplete right BBB are excluded from the definition of fQRS. The mechanism of fQRS is not fully known and has been explained by inhomogeneous activation of the ventricles because of myocardial scar and/or ischemia.[16] Published data suggested that fQRS is a new non-invasive maker in risk stratification of mortality and sudden cardiac death in patients with coronary artery disease, cardiomyopathy and Brugada syndrome.[17,18] Recently, QRS complex abnormalities have also been described in some patients with idiopathic VF, in whom the structural heart abnormalities are absent.[19] However, the implications of fQRS in patients with idiopathic VF have not been elucidated. Therefore, we performed a study to investigate the value of fQRS in predicting long-term recurrence of ventricular arrhythmias in patients having idiopathic VF and ER pattern. We reviewed data from 139 patients with idiopathic VF. Only patients satisfying all of the following criteria were included in the analysis, (1) ER pattern on standard ECG; (2) Availability of systematic implantable cardioverter-defibrillator (ICD) follow-up for ≥ 12 months and (3)Availability of signal-averaged ECG. The follow-up data on recurrent VF was made available by serial ICD interrogations. Totally, 44 (31.6%) patients having idiopathic VF and ER were identified. Of them, 16 patients (11 Males, age 37±9 years) met all the inclusion criteria described above. Ventricular late potentials detected by signal-averaged ECG were absent in all but 1 patient. In 7 (43.8%) patients, fQRS was observed in 2-4 (mean: 2.7) leads. fQRS was more frequently present in inferior leads (36.9%) and lateral leads (31.6%) (Figure 3). After a mean follow-up of 67±66 (range 12-264, median 54) months, 5

(71.4%) of 7 patients with fQRS had recurrent VF (ICD shocks ranging from 1-8, mean 3.8), whereas none of the patients lacking fQRS (n=9) experienced appropriate ICD discharges (P<0.01).[20] Therefore, our preliminary data suggest that the presence of fQRS could increase the risk of recurrent ventricular arrhythmias in patients with idiopathic VF and ER. However, this observation should be validated in a larger population. Also, whether fQRS can be used as a maker in stratifying subjects with ER pattern is unknown.

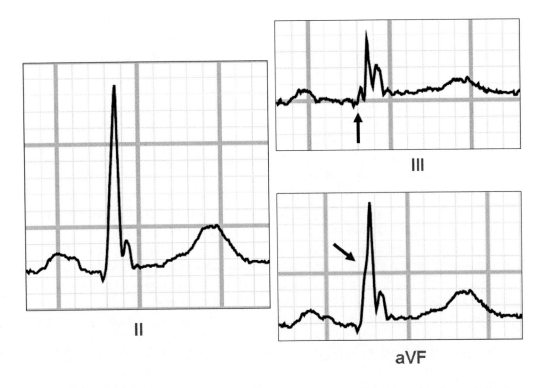

Figure 3. Fragmented QRS in a patient with idiopathic ventricular fibrillation and early repolarization in the inferior leads. Note that the initial part of QRS in the inferior leads presents an additional deflection (lead III) or a slurring on the upstroke of QRS (lead aVF) each of which is marked with an arrow.

# RISK STRATIFICATION OF ERS: INSIGHTS FROM STUDIES USING NOVEL NON-INVASIVE MAPPING SYSTEMS

## Dynamic SA-ECG Mapping

As a marker of ventricular depolarization abnormalities, late potentials (LPs) on the signal-averaged ECG have been widely utilized to detect high-risk individuals among patients with cardiac disorders such as myocardial infarction, arrhythmogenic right ventricular cardiomyopathy and Brugada syndrome.[21,22] More recently, Abe et al investigated the role of LPs in the pathophysiology and risk stratification of ER pattern.[23] This study enrolled 7 patients with idiopathic VF and ER pattern in the infero-lateral leads. The control group comprised of 30 healthy subjects with J wave and another 30 healthy subjects without J wave. The LPs were detected using a newly developed signal-averaging system. This system is capable of analyzing LPs automatically every 30 minutes using data from a digital Holter ECG recorder. The parameters reflecting LPs include the filtered QRS duration, the root mean square voltage of the terminal 40 msec of the filtered QRS complex ($RMS_{40}$), and the duration of low-amplitude signals (<40 µV) in the terminal, filtered QRS complex ($LAS_{40}$), which are same as the conventional signal-averaged ECG analyzing system. The LPs were considered positive when two of three criteria (fQRS >135 msec, $RMS_{40}$<15µV, and $LAS_{40}$ >39 msec) were met. In addition, 2 other markers of repolarization abnormalities viz. T wave alternans (TWA) and QT dispersion were also analyzed in the study population. Of the 7 patients with idiopathic VF and ER pattern, 6 had LPs. In contrast, LPs were detected in only 4 (7%) patients in the 60 control subjects. The incidence of LPs did not differ between subjects with ER pattern and subjects without ER pattern in the latter. Interestingly, in all of the 7 idiopathic VF patients with ER pattern, the values of the parameters of LPs increased during the night and decreased during the day in 6 and *vice versa* in 1. In control subjects with ER pattern, significant circadian variation in LP parameters was not seen. As regards to TWA and QT dispersion, a significant difference was not seen between patients with idiopathic VF and the control subjects. Based on the above findings, the authors concluded that the detection of LP by signal-averaged ECG using 24-hour Holter ECG could be a useful technique to identify the subjects at high risk for arrhythmic events among those with ER pattern. Importantly, although the number of cases is small, the study associates arrhythmogenesis due to high risk ER pattern with abnormalities of depolarization.

## Reconstruction of Epicardial Potentials

This novel noninvasive imaging modality combines 250 body surface ECGs with computed tomography (CT) of the heart-torso geometry to compute potentials, electrograms (typically 600) and activation sequences (isochrones) on the epicardial surface of the heart.[24] In addition, using this system, the local repolarization of the heart can also be depicted by analyzing the local activation-recovery interval (ARI). ARI is the difference between the recovery and activation times and has a good correlation with the local action potential duration (APD).[25] More recently, Ghosh et al. reported the mapping results using ECG imaging in two patients with idiopathic VF and ER pattern in the infero-lateral leads.[26] They found that despite normal ventricular activation, both patients presented with abnormal repolarization characterized by areas with short ARI. The previously reported value of human ARI was 235±21ms;[25] however, the shortest ARI during sinus rhythm in these patients was 140msec and 180 ms, respectively. Also, the electrograms from these short ARI areas showed substantial elevation of the junction of QRS-ST segment while the neighboring electrograms showed flat ST segment. More importantly, abnormally steep localized ARI gradients (107ms/cm and 261msec/cm, respectively) were observed in both the patients. In contrast, the value of ARI gradient in the normal heart computed from previously published data ranged from 4.5ms/cm to 11.3ms/cm.[25] Therefore, the ECG imaging data from both the patients reveal the presence of regions with relatively short action potential durations and abnormally large spatial repolarization gradients, which may be proarrhythmic in high risk ER pattern.

However, whether ECG imaging can be used as a non-invasive modality in differentiating high risk ER pattern from benign ER pattern needs further investigation.

## CONTROVERSIAL ISSUES

Currently, the risk stratification of ER pattern is still an issue of hot debate. Firstly, some investigators do not consider that it is really worth to do such a work. It is well recognized that although ER is common, unexplained sudden cardiac arrest is very rare. Rosso et al calculated the probability of sudden cardiac death in subjects with ER pattern by using the Bayes' law of conditional probabilities.[4] The results suggested that the presence of ER pattern in a young adult would increase the probability of idiopathic VF from 3.4:100 000 to 11:100 000 which is a negligible rise. They, therefore, concluded that the incidental discovery of ER pattern on routine screening should not be interpreted as a marker of "high risk" for sudden death because the odds for this fatal disease would still be approximately 1:10 000. Secondly, there are some investigators who remain suspicious of the possible link between ER pattern and malignant ventricular arrhythmias, and therefore, they do not think that the so-called risk stratification is necessary. For example, rising concerns are expressed on the ER pattern in the athletes in whom it is more prevalent than the general population. As reported by Bianco et al, the ER was observed in up to 89% of top-level endurance-trained athletes.[27] In contrast with the observations made in the general population; most of the ER pattern in the athletes is not consistent and can be reversed after months or years of detraining. Obviously, the meaning of ER in this subgroup of subjects is not the same as that in the general population. Finally, some investigators even consider the term of ER pattern, a misnomer. Since the cardiac repolarization always follows depolarization, the initial repolarization begins as soon as the first ventricular cell is depolarized. In other words, cardiac repolarization normally should be *early*. The data favoring this concept had been published more than 30 years ago.[28,29] Therefore, the propounders consider that so-called ER pattern actually is some kind of normal repolarization. The genesis of the ER pattern on standard ECG is proposed to be the result of distortion of the end of the QRS complex by the augmented voltage and extended duration of ST-T complex which is a normal variant in some individuals, particularly the young adults.[30] Putting the above concerns together, it is obvious that there are many fundamental issues needing clarification on various aspects of ER.

## CONCLUSION

There is a mounting evidence establishing critical association between the ER pattern in the infero-lateral leads and idiopathic VF in some patients. Currently, it is difficult to differentiate the high risk ER from the benign ER on routine ECG due to paucity of information. The role of diffuse distribution of ER pattern and fragmented QRS in characterizing high risk ER patients needs further validation. Novel non-invasive ECG mapping system including dynamic signal-averaged ECG may provide new insights in the mechanisms as well as the risk stratification of ER pattern. In addition, it is also critical to investigate appropriate pharmacological test aiming at stratification of the so-called J wave syndrome in the future.

## REFERENCES

[1] Klatsky AL, Oehm R, Cooper RA, Udalstova N, Armstrong MA. The early repolarization normal variant electrocardiogram: correlates and consequences. *Am J Med* 2003;115: 171-7.
[2] Mehta M, Jain AC, Mehta A. Early repolarization. *Clin Cardiol* 1999; 22: 59-65.
[3] Haïssaguerre M, Derval N, Sacher F, Jesel L, Deisenhofer I, de Roy L, et al. Sudden cardiac arrest associated with early repolarization. *N Engl J Med* 2008; 358: 2016-23
[4] Rosso R, Kogan E, Belhassen B, Rozovski U, Scheinman MM, Zeltser D, et al. J-point elevation in survivors of primary ventricular fibrillation and matched control subjects: incidence and clinical significance. *J Am Coll Cardiol* 2008; 52: 1231-8
[5] Nam GB, Ko KH, Kim J, Park KM, Rhee KS, Choi KJ, et al. Mode of onset of ventricular fibrillation in patients with early repolarization pattern vs Brugada syndrome. *Eur Heart J* 2010; 31: 330-9
[6] Tikkanen JT, Anttonen O, Junttila MJ, Aro AL, Kerola T, Rissanen HA, et al. Long-term outcome associated with early repolarization on electrocardiography. *N Engl J Med* 2009; 361: 2529-37
[7] Tomaszewski W: Changement electrocardiographiques observes chez un homme mort de froid. *Arch Mal Coeur Vaiss* 1938; 31:525-8
[8] Liu X, Shah A, Sacher F, Derval N, Jadidi A, Hocini M, et al. Clinical frontiers in electrocardiographic early repolarization syndrome: does a good guy turn bad now? *Chin Med J* (Engl), 2010: in press
[9] Haïssaguerre M, Sacher F, Nogami A, Komiya N, Bernard A, Probst V, et al. Characteristics of recurrent ventricular fibrillation associated with inferolateral early repolarization: role of drug therapy. *J Am Coll Cardiol* 2009; 53: 612-9
[10] Kalla H, Yan GX, Marinchak R. Ventricular fibrillation in a patient with prominent J (Osborn) waves and ST segment elevation in the inferior electrocardiographic leads: a Brugada syndrome variant? *J Cardiovasc Electrophysiol* 2000;11: 95-8
[11] Tsunoda Y, Taketshi Y, Nozaki N, Kitahara T, Kubota I. Presence of intermittent J waves in multiple leads in relation to episode of atrial and ventricular fibrillation. *J Electrocardiol* 2004; 37: 311-4
[12] Haissaguerre M, Sacher F, Derval N, Jesel L, Deisenhofer I, De Roy L, et al. Early repolarization in the inferolateral leads : a new syndrome associated with sudden cardiac death. *J Interv Cardiac Electrophsiol* 2007; 18: 281
[13] Antzelevitch C, Yan GX. J wave syndrome. *Heart Rhythm 2010*; 7: 549 - 58.
[14] Merchant FM, Noseworthy PA, Weiner RB, Singh SM, Ruskin JN, Reddy VY. Ability of terminal QRS notching to distinguish benign from malignant electrocardiographic forms of early repolarization. *Am J Cardiol* 2009; 104: 1402-6
[15] Das MK, Zipes DP. Fragmented QRS: A predictor of mortality and sudden cardiac death. *Heart Rhythm 2009*;6:S8 –S14

[16] Flowers NC, Horan LG, Thomas JR, et al. The anatomic basis for highfrequency components in the electrocardiogram. *Circulation* 1969;39:531–539.

[17] Das MK, Khan B, Jacob S, et al. Significance of a fragmented QRS complex versus a Q wave in patients with coronary artery disease. *Circulation* 2006;113: 2495–2501.

[18] Morita H, Fukushima K, Miura D, et al. Fragmented QRS as a marker of conduction abnormality and a predictor of prognosis of Brugada syndrome. *Circulation* 2008;118:1697–1704.

[19] Letsas KP, Weber R, Kalusche D, et al. QRS complex abnormalities in subjects with idiopathic ventricular fibrillation. *Int J Cardiol* 2009, doi:10.1016/j.ijcard.2009.12.008

[20] Liu X, Hocini M, Derval N, et al. Fragmented QRS complexes as a predictor of ventricular arrhythmic events in patients with idiopathic ventricular fibrillation and early repolarization. *Heart Rhythm 2010*; 7 (suppl): in press

[21] Gomes JA, Winters SL, Stewart D, et al. A new noninvasive index to predict sustained ventricular tachycardia and sudden death in the first year after myocardial infarction: based on signal-averaged electrocardiogram, radionuclide ejection fraction and Holter monitoring. *J Am Coll Cardiol* 1987; 10: 349-57.

[22] Ikeda T, Sakurada H, Sakabe K, et al.: Assessment of noninvasive markers in identifying patients at risk in the Brugada syndrome: Insight into risk stratification. *J Am Coll Cardiol* 2001; 37: 1628-34

[23] Abe A, Ikeda T, Tsukada T, et al. Circadian variation of late potentials in idiopathic ventricular fibrillation associated with J Waves: insights into pathophysiology and risk stratification. *Heart Rhythm 2010*, doi: 10.1016/j.hrthm.2010.01.023

[24] Rudy Y. Cardiac repolarization: Insights from mathematical modeling and electrocardiographic imaging (ECGI). *Heart Rhythm 2009*;6:S49–S55

[25] Ramanathan C, Jia P, Ghanem R, et al. *Activation and repolarization of the normal human heart under complete physiological conditions.* Proc Natl Acad Sci USA 2006;103: 6309-6314.

[26] Ghosh S, Cooper DH, Vijayakumar D, et al. Early Repolarization associated with Sudden Death: Insights from Noninvasive Electrocardiographic Imaging (ECGI). *Heart Rhythm 2009*, doi: 10.1016/j.hrthm.2009.12.005

[27] Bianco M, Bria S, Gianfelici A, et al. Does early repolarization in the athlete have analogies with the Brugada syndrome? *Eur Heart J* 2001; 22: 504 –10.

[28] Spach MS, Barr RC, Lanning CF, et al. Origin of body surface QRS and T wave potentials from epicardial potential distributions in the intact chimpanzee. *Circulation* 1977; 55: 268.

[29] Spach MS, Barr RC, Benson W, et al. Body surface low level potentials during ventricular repolarization with analysis of the ST segment: variability in normal subjects. *Circulation* 1979; 59: 822.

[30] Liebman J. The early repolarization syndrome is a variation of normal. *J Electrocard* 2007; 40: 391–394

In: Ventricular Fibrillation and Acute Coronary Syndrome
Editor: Joyce E. Mandell

ISBN: 978-1-61728-969-9
© 2011 Nova Science Publishers, Inc.

*Chapter VIII*

# IMPACT OF SODIUM CHANNEL DYSFUNCTION ON ARRHYTHMOGENESIS IN BRUGADA SYNDROME

*Hiroshi Morita[a,b], Douglas P. Zipes[b], Satoshi Nagase[a] and Jiashin Wu[b,c]*

[a]Department of Cardiovascular Medicine, Okayama University Graduate School of Medicine, Dentistry and Pharmaceutical Sciences, Okayama, Japan
[b]Krannert Institute of Cardiology, Indiana University School of Medicine, Indianapolis, IN, USA
[c] Department of Molecular Pharmacology and Physiology, University of South Florida, Tampa, FL, USA

## ABSTRACT

(Background) Patients with Brugada syndrome (BS) have sodium channel (Na-Ch) SCN5A mutations (20%) as well as calcium channel (Ca-Ch) mutations (8%) that reduce the inward current and affect the action potential (AP). We investigated the affects of Na-Ch dysfunction on arrhythmogenesis in patients with BS and in experimental models of BS to understand the mechanisms of arrhythmogenesis and the origins of the ECG characteristics of BS.

(Methods) *Clinical study*: we evaluated 80 BS patients [22 with prior ventricular fibrillation (VF) and implantation of a cardioverter defibrillator], and compared ECG parameters and recurrent VF episodes between the patients with and without SCN5A mutation.

*Experimental study*: We created 2 experimental models of BS in 18 canine right ventricular preparations: 1) Na-Ch dysfunction model (Na-model) by using pilsicainide and pinacidil (n=11); and 2) Ca-Ch dysfunction model (Ca-model) by using verapamil (n=7). We then optically mapped multisite APs on the transmural surface of these tissue models, and analyzed the mechanisms of arrhythmogenesis and origins of characteristic BS ECGs.

(Results) *Clinical Study*: Patients with the SCN5A mutation had longer PQ interval (202 ± 31 ms) than patients without the mutation (182 ± 31 ms, $p<0.05$), but no differences in ST elevation. Patients with mutation experienced earlier recurrence of VF (2.0 ± 0.9 months) than patients without mutation (12.7 ± 19 months, $p<0.05$).

*Experimental study*: Transmural activation time (endocardial stimulation to epicardial breakthrough) took longer in the Na-model than in the Ca-model (50 ± 11, vs. 34 ± 10 ms, p<0.01). The Na-model also had prominent epicardial AP heterogeneity, which promoted frequent ventricular arrhythmias (VA) via phase 2 reentry (incidence of VAs: Na-model 50% vs. Ca-model 0%, p<0.01).

(Conclusion) Conduction disturbances and AP heterogeneity (especially in the epicardium of the right ventricle) were the underlying causes of frequent VAs and ECG characteristics in Brugada syndrome with Na-Ch dysfunction.

# INTRODUCTION

Brugada syndrome (BS) is characterized by ST elevation in the right precordial leads in the electrocardiogram (ECG) and a corresponding repolarization abnormality in the right ventricular outflow tract (RVOT) [1, 2, 3]. The ST elevation in BS can vary on a daily basis or even beat by beat (e.g., T wave alternans) [4] and heightens during ventricular fibrillation (VF) attacks [5].

Brugada syndrome is associated with inherited ion channel abnormalities with $Na^+$ channel gene (SCN5A) mutations [6] in 20%[7] and $Ca^{2+}$ channel gene mutations in 8% of patients [8]. Although the genotypes of BS occur in both sexes, the phenotypes of BS are expressed preferentially in adult male patients. Sodium channel dysfunction reduces the rate the phase 0 depolarization of the action potential (AP) and slows the conduction of excitation in cardiac tissue. A reduced inward $Na^+$ current ($I_{Na}$) combined with heterogeneously distributed transient outward $K^+$ current ($I_{to}$) contribute to a deep phase 1 notch of the AP, especially in the epicardium of the RVOT, and in adult males. Rapid and enhanced early repolarization elevates the ST segment in the ECG. Regional differences in $Na^+$ channel dysfunction and its cascade effects on the other ion currents enhance AP heterogeneity, which is most prominent in the epicardium of the RVOT and can subsequently initiate phase 2 reentry and ventricular tachycardia (VT) [9, 10]. In contrast to the well characterized genotype-phenotype correlations in the long QT syndrome [11], only few reports present the genotype-phenotype correlations in BS[12-14].

In this study, we investigated the electrophysiological mechanisms of BS due to $Na^+$ channelopathy by evaluating patients with and without the SCN5A mutation, as well as experimentally examining the mechanisms of arrhythmogenesis in canine RVOT tissues treated with drugs to replicate the BS.

# CLINICAL STUDY

## Methods

We examined 80 patients with BS (average age 46 ± 12 year-old, male/female = 79/1). All patients had spontaneous type 1 ECG defined by the Second Consensus Reports of Brugada Syndrome [15]. Twenty-two patients were resuscitated from documented VF, 14 had unexplained syncope, and 44 had no symptoms at the registration of this study.

Standard twelve-lead ECGs with 0-150 Hz filter were recorded. ECGs acquired prior to drug therapy were used for analysis. We evaluated the duration of the RR interval, PQ interval, QRS width, QT interval, ST level at J point, and number of spikes within the QRS complex (fragmented QRS) in lead V1-V3 [16, 17].

We determined the presence of late potentials (LPs), and measured the filtered QRS duration, the root mean square voltage of the terminal 40 ms in the filtered QRS complex (RMS40), and the duration of low-amplitude signals <40 μV in the terminal filtered QRS complex (LAS40) using a SAECG (ART 1200EPX). LPs were considered to be positive when two criteria were met (RMS40 <20 μV and LAS40 >38 ms) [15,18].

Electrophysiological study was performed in 73 patients as reported previously [19]. Induction of sustained ventricular tachycardia (VT) or VF was tested with programmed electrical stimulation (PES, from the right ventricular apex, RVOT, or left ventricle, using a maximum of 2 extra stimuli at 2 cycle lengths) prior to antiarrhythmic therapy.

Gene (SCN5A) analysis was performed in compliance with guidelines for human genome studies of the Ethics Committee of Okayama University. Informed consent was obtained from all patients. The presence of SCN5A mutation was tested in all patients as reported previously [20]. SCN5A mutation was detected in 18 patients but not in the other 62 patients. We did not analyze genes of calcium channel, beta-subunits of the sodium channel, transient outward potassium channel, and GPD1-L, all having been reported as causes of Brugada syndrome.

Patients were divided into 2 groups according to the presence or absence of the SCN5A mutation. Data were expressed as mean ± SD values. Comparisons among means were performed with 2-way ANOVA coupled with Scheffe's test. Student's t-test was used to compare unpaired and paired data, as appropriate, between the 2 groups. Fisher's exact test was performed for the comparison of proportions among groups. Significance was defined as $p<0.05$.

## Results

No differences existed between patients with and without SCN5A mutation in age, sex, family history of sudden death, clinical symptoms, presence of late potentials, and the induction of VF by PES (Table).

Both patients with and without SCN5A mutation had ST elevation and negative T waves (Figure 1). Patients with SCN5A mutation had longer PQ and HV intervals than patients without mutations (Figure 2). QRS and QT intervals and ST level were different between the 2 groups.

Using previously published criteria[17] of fragmented QRS complexes (f-QRS) as ≥4 spikes within a single QRS of the leads V1-V3 or the sum the number of spikes in a single QRS complex from each of V1-V3 to be ≥8 spikes, we found no difference in the rate of occurrence of f-QRS between patients with and without mutations, but patients with SCN5A mutation had more spikes in f-QRS than patients without mutation (Table, Figure 3).

## Table 1

| SCN5A | Mutation (−) | Mutation (+) | P value |
|---|---|---|---|
| Total (n) | 62 | 18 | |
| Age (y.o.) | 46 ± 11 | 47 ± 14 | 0.9562 |
| Male (n) | 61 (98%) | 18 (100%) | 0.59 |
| Family History | 20 (32%) | 7 (39%) | 0.6027 |
| Symptom | | | |
|   VF | 18 (29%) | 4 (22%) | 0.5713 |
|   Syncope | 9 (15%) | 5 (28%) | 0.1952 |
|   Asymptomatic | 35 (56%) | 9 (50%) | 0.63 |
| f-QRS | 24 (39%) | 11 (61%) | 0.0937 |
| Late Potential | 44 (71%) | 15 (83%) | 0.2967 |
| PES-induced VF | 30 (52%) | 6 (38%) | 0.288 |

PES: programmed electrical stimulation

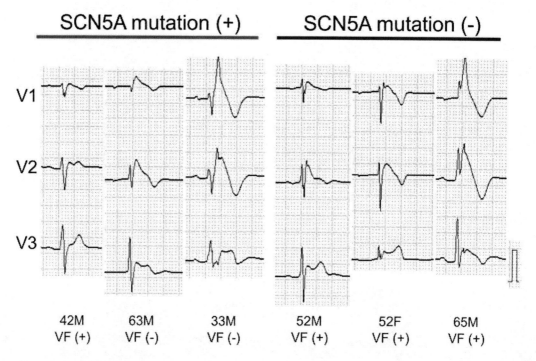

Figure 1. ECGs from patients. Both patients with and without SCN5A mutation had coved-type ST elevation with negative T wave.

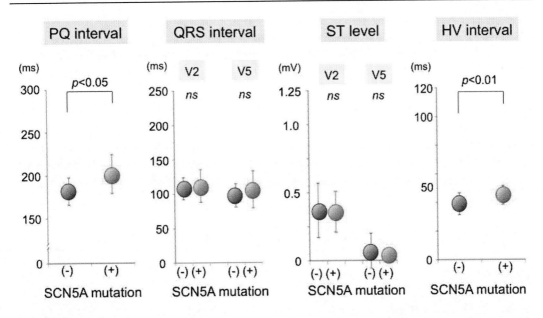

Figure 2. ECG parameters and HV interval in patients with and without SCN5A mutation. Patients with SCN5A mutation had longer PQ and HV intervals than patients without mutation. QRS interval and ST level were not different between the 2 groups.

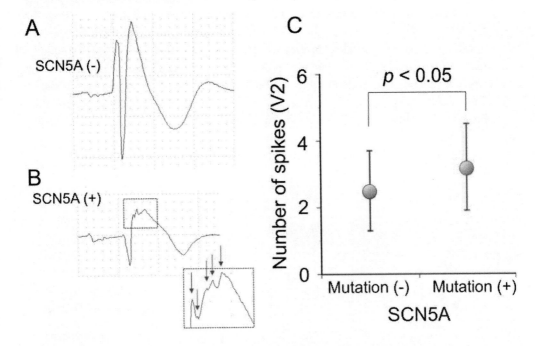

Figure 3. Fragmented QRS. A. ECG from a patient without SCN5A mutation and did not have f-QRS. B. ECG from a patient with mutation and had multiple spikes within QRS complex (arrows). C. Patients with SCN5A mutation had more multiple spikes than patients without mutation.

There were no significant differences in the age of patients at the first VF attack between those with and without SCN5A mutation ( 53 ± 17 vs. 45 ± 11 y.o. p=0.4755). Two asymptomatic patients without mutation experienced new VF events. There was no difference between the 2 groups in the incidence of VF during follow-up. Patients with the SCN5A mutation experienced earlier recurrence of VF than patients without the mutation (the interval between the 1$^{st}$ and 2$^{nd}$ VF episodes: 2.0 ± 0.9 vs. 12.7 ± 19 months, p=0.0157).

## Summary of the Clinical Study

Patients with the SCN5A mutation had prolonged conduction times (longer PQ and HV intervals) and more spikes within the QRS complex, and often experienced earlier recurrence of VF attacks, than patients without the mutation.

## EXPERIMENTAL STUDY

## Methods

### *Arterially Perfused Right Ventricular Tissue Preparations*

The methods for this study were described previously [21] (Figure 4). In brief, we harvested hearts from 18 anesthetized adult male mongrel dogs and immediately perfused the hearts with a cold cardioplegic solution. We isolated one transmural tissue preparation (~0.8x2.5x1.0 cm$^3$) containing a branch of the right coronary artery (diameter: ~1 mm) from the right ventricular free wall of each heart. The tissues were mounted in a warmed chamber with their cut-exposed transmural recording surfaces up, perfused with Tyrode's solution via the coronary artery branch. Two silver electrodes were placed in the bath, 5 mm away from the epicardium (anode) and endocardium (cathode) of the tissue, to register its transmural ECG. The tissues were stained with di-4-ANEPPS (4 mmol/l) and immobilized by cytochalasin D (20-30 μmol/l), shown not to affect the canine AP [22]. An optical mapping system with a 256-element (16x16) photodiode camera collected the fluorescence from a 19.5x19.5 mm2 tissue surface area and converted it into 256 AP channels [23].

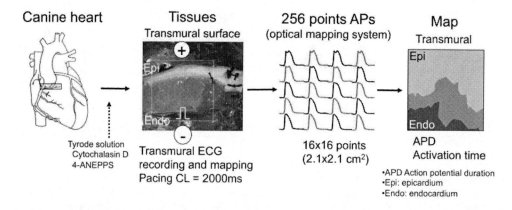

Figure 4. Method of experimental study. Right ventricular free wall tissues from the canine heart were perfused with Tyrode solution. We recorded 256 action potentials (APs) on the transmural surface of the tissue using an optical mapping system and constructed action potential duration (APD) and activation time (AT) maps.

We induced two models of BS[21]: 1) $Na^+$ channelopathy (Na-model, n=11) with pilsicainide, (2.5-12.5 μmol/l), a $Na^+$ channel blocker, and pinacidil (1.25-12.5 μmol/l), a $K_{ATP}$ opener, to produce a characteristic deep phase 1 notch in the AP and 2) $Ca^{2+}$ channelopathy model (Ca-model, n=7) with verapamil (5-10 mol/l). We increased the drug doses progressively until full development of characteristic epicardial AP and ECG of BS at a pacing cycle length (CL) of 2,000 ms [2, 24].

We statistically analyzed AP durations (APDs) at the recording sites along the epicardial and endocardial layers in the preparations. We defined Epi1 and Epi2 as the longest and shortest APDs in the epicardium[2]. Transmural dispersion of APD was calculated as the difference between the endocardial and epicardial APDs. Polymorphic VT was identified using a criterion of ≥ 3 consecutive rapid non-paced activations with changing contours in the ECG [25].

## Results

At control (before the administration of BS-inducing drugs), the epicardial APs had a small phase 1 notch and were homogeneous in the RVOT tissues. Small J wave and positive T wave appeared in the transmural ECG (Figure 5A).

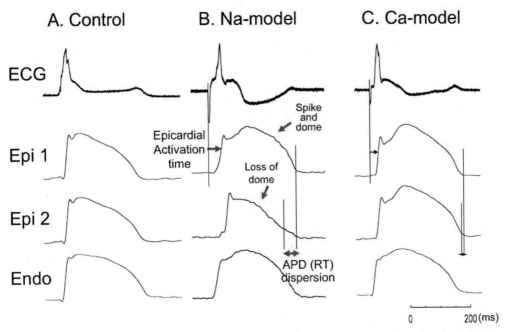

Figure 5. Action potential and ECG before and after induction of Brugada models. A. At control, there was no action potential heterogeneity and transmural ECG had small J wave and positive T wave. After induction of Brugada model, both the Na and Ca-models had ST elevation with negative T wave. The Na-model had longer epicardial activation time (B) than the Ca-model (C). The Na-model had larger action potential heterogeneity within the epicardium than the Ca-model. Modified from reference 21.[21]

After drug administration, both the Na and Ca-models developed a deep phase 1 notch and a large phase 2 dome (spike-and-dome) in the epicardial APs, but not in the endocardial APs. Transmural activation time (measured from endocardial stimulation to epicardial breakthrough) took longer in the Na-model than the Ca-model (Figure 5B, 5C, 6A). Although the phase 2 dome was prominent initially, continued deepening of the phase 1 notch of the AP eliminated the phase 2 dome. Heterogeneity in the response of the phase 2 dome to the BS-induction drugs caused simultaneous presence of epicardial regions with and without a phase 2 dome, resulting in large APD dispersion and voltage gradient within the epicardium in the Na-model (Figure 5B, 6B). Compared to the Na-model, the Ca-model had less AP heterogeneity in the epicardium, although both models had spike-and-dome type APs.

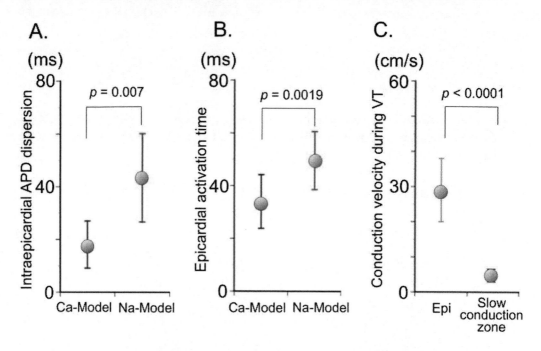

Figure 6. Electrophysiological parameters in the Brugada models. The Na-models had longer activation time (A) and larger APD dispersion (B) than the Ca-models. C. Slow conduction zone was observed at the initiation of VT and facilitated the maintenance of reentrant circuit in the epicardium of the Na-model.

Increased dispersion of repolarization induced premature ventricular activations (PVAs), which conducted in the form of phase 2 reentry following the recovery of tissue excitability in the RVOT tissue. Sustained reentry produced polymorphic VT in the transmural ECG. This mechanism of arrhythmogenesis occurred frequently in the Na-model but not in the Ca-model, which had less AP heterogeneity (Figure 7).

Figure 8 demonstrates the initiation of polymorphic VT in the $Na^+$ channel dysfunction model. Increased epicardial AP heterogeneity caused reentrant conduction of the phase 2 dome that initiated VT. Slow conduction between the short APD (Epi2) and long APD areas (Epi1 and mid-endocardium) facilitated the maintenance of functional reentry.

# Impact of Sodium Channel Dysfunction on Arrhythmogenesis in Brugada Syndrome

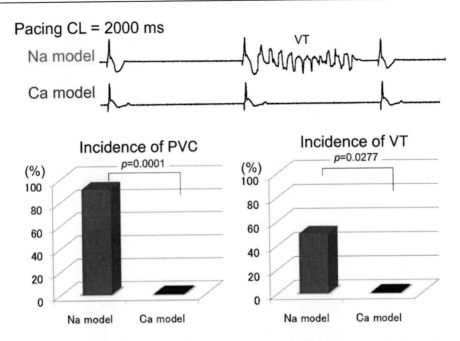

Figure 7. Occurrence of ventricular arrhythmias. Action potential heterogeneity often promoted ventricular arrhythmias in the Na-model but not in the Ca-model (A). Incidences of PVC and VT were more frequent in the Na-model than in the Ca-model (B, C). Modified from reference 21.[21]

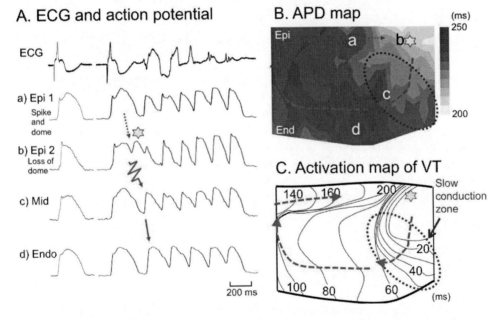

Figure 8. Initiation of the ventricular tachycardia in a Na-model. A. Transmural ECG and action potentials (APs). Epicardium had both spike-and-dome and loss-of-dome type APs simultaneously. AP heterogeneity initiated VT at the Epi2 (star), which then propagated within the transmural tissue. B. Transmural distribution of APD. Extensive AP heterogeneity existed in the epicardium. C. Activation sequence of the initial beat during a VT sequence. Initial activation (star) in the epicardium propagated within the transmural tissue (phase 2 reentry). Slow conduction zone (the dotted circle in B and C) between the short and long APD areas facilitated the maintenance of reentry. Dotted arrows represent activation direction of the VT.

## Summary of the Experimental Study

Compared with the $Ca^{2+}$ channel dysfunction model, the $Na^+$ channel dysfunction model had extensive epicardial AP heterogeneity leading to frequent premature ventricular activations. That, along with conduction slowing, facilitated the maintenance of the reentrant circuit causing frequent episodes of polymorphic VT.

## DISCUSSION

Activation of cardiac myocytes triggers the $I_{Na}$ that produces the phase 0 rise of the AP. Subsequent activation of the $I_{to}$ induces a phase 1 notch in the AP. A balance of the inward depolarizing $Ca^{2+}$ current ($I_{Ca-L}$) and outward rectifier $K^+$ currents gives rise to a plateau (phase 2 dome), which is followed by phase 3 repolarization and finally restoration of the resting potential (phase 4) [26]. Cardiac $Na^+$ current is the main driving current for the propagation of excitation. In addition to causing Brugada syndrome[6], inherited $Na^+$ channel dysfunction can also cause progressive cardiac conduction disease [27], sick sinus syndrome (loss of function of $Na^+$ channel) [28-30], and long QT syndrome (type 3) (gain of function) [31]. Although $Ca^{2+}$ [8] and $K^+$ [32] channelopathies have also been reported in the patients with Brugada syndrome, their occurrences are rare and their detailed clinical phenotypes are still unknown.

## CONDUCTION DELAY IN PATIENTS WITH SCN5A MUTATION

Although Brugada type ECG occurs in patients with and without SCN5A mutation, patients with SCN5A mutation usually have conduction disturbances. Smits et al. [12-14] reported that patients with SCN5A mutation had longer PQ and HV intervals than patients without mutation. Administration of sodium channel blocker, flecainide, aggravated conduction slowing and resulted in prominent PQ and QRS prolongation in patients with SCN5A mutation[12]. Aging also aggravated conduction disturbances and prolonged PQ and QRS more in patients with, than without, SCN5A mutation[13]. Although SCN5A mutation has been associated with conduction slowing, its impact on the prognosis of BS is still unknown.

## OBSERVATIONS FROM THE PRESENT STUDY

We found that, compared to the patients without SCN5A mutation, patients with mutation have longer PQ and HV intervals, a higher occurrence of fragmented QRS[17] but similar ST elevation. Patients with SCN5A mutation had abnormalities in both the repolarization (ST elevation and T wave inversion) and depolarization (prolongation of PQ and QRS intervals, and fragmented QRS), whereas patients without SCN5A mutation had abnormalities frequently in repolarization but less frequently in depolarization. Although the incidence of new onset of VF in both groups was low, recurrent VF occurred earlier in patients with, than without, SCN5A mutation. The depolarization abnormality appears to be a predisposing factor in the recurrence of VF in patients with BS[33, 34].

Our experimental tissue models demonstrated the mechanisms of arrhythmogenesis in BS: premature activations and phase 2 reentry, leading to VT/VF, similar to the mechanisms reported by Antzelevitch et al[10, 35, 36]. Zones of slow conduction facilitated the maintenance of the reentrant circuit in these tissue models. Both delayed repolarization in the long APD area (usually observed in the epicardium with spike-and-dome type AP rather than the mid and endocardium) and $Na^+$ channel dysfunction contributed to the regional slow conduction. Thus, the repolarization heterogeneity initiated premature activation and the depolarization abnormality contributed to the maintenance of functional reentry in the Na-model.

## CONCLUSION

Conduction disturbances and AP heterogeneity were associated with more frequent occurrences of ventricular arrhythmias in both the BS patients and in the experimental model of BS caused by $Na^+$ channel dysfunction than by the Ca channelopathy.

## REFERENCES

[1] Shimizu W, Antzelevitch C, Suyama K, et al. Effect of sodium channel blockers on ST segment, QRS duration, and corrected QT interval in patients with Brugada syndrome. *J Cardiovasc Electrophysiol* 2000;11:1320-9.

[2] Morita H, Zipes DP, Morita ST, Wu J. Differences in arrhythmogenicity between the canine right ventricular outflow tract and anteroinferior right ventricle in a model of Brugada syndrome. *Heart Rhythm* 2007;4:66-74.

[3] Morita H, Zipes DP, Fukushima-Kusano K, et al. Repolarization heterogeneity in the right ventricular outflow tract: correlation with ventricular arrhythmias in Brugada patients and in an in vitro canine Brugada model. *Heart Rhythm* 2008;5:725-33.

[4] Morita H, Zipes DP, Lopshire J, Morita ST, Wu J. T wave alternans in an in vitro canine tissue model of Brugada syndrome. *Am J Physiol Heart Circ Physiol* 2006;291:H421-8.

[5] Matsuo K, Shimizu W, Kurita T, Inagaki M, Aihara N, Kamakura S. Dynamic changes of 12-lead electrocardiograms in a patient with Brugada syndrome. *J Cardiovasc Electrophysiol* 1998;9:508-12.

[6] Chen Q, Kirsch GE, Zhang D, et al. Genetic basis and molecular mechanism for idiopathic ventricular fibrillation. *Nature* 1998;392:293-6.

[7] Priori SG, Napolitano C, Gasparini M, et al. Natural history of Brugada syndrome: insights for risk stratification and management. *Circulation* 2002;105:1342-7.

[8] Antzelevitch C, Pollevick GD, Cordeiro JM, et al. Loss-of-function mutations in the cardiac calcium channel underlie a new clinical entity characterized by ST-segment elevation, short QT intervals, and sudden cardiac death. *Circulation* 2007;115:442-9.

[9] Morita H, Zipes DP, Wu J. Brugada syndrome: insights of ST elevation, arrhythmogenicity, and risk stratification from experimental observations. *Heart Rhythm* 2009;6:S34-43.

[10] Yan GX, Antzelevitch C. Cellular basis for the Brugada syndrome and other mechanisms of arrhythmogenesis associated with ST-segment elevation. *Circulation* 1999;100:1660-6.

[11] Schwartz PJ, Priori SG, Spazzolini C, et al. Genotype-phenotype correlation in the long-QT syndrome: gene-specific triggers for life-threatening arrhythmias. *Circulation* 2001;103:89-95.

[12] Smits JP, Eckardt L, Probst V, et al. Genotype-phenotype relationship in Brugada syndrome: electrocardiographic features differentiate SCN5A-related patients from non-SCN5A-related patients. *J Am Coll Cardiol* 2002;40:350-6.

[13] Yokokawa M, Noda T, Okamura H, et al. Comparison of long-term follow-up of electrocardiographic features in Brugada syndrome between the SCN5A-positive probands and the SCN5A-negative probands. *Am J Cardiol* 2007;100:649-55.

[14] Morita H, Nagase S, Miura D, et al. Differential effects of cardiac sodium channel mutations on initiation of ventricular arrhythmias in patients with Brugada syndrome. *Heart Rhythm* 2009;6:487-92.

[15] Antzelevitch C, Brugada P, Borggrefe M, et al. Brugada syndrome: report of the second consensus conference: endorsed by the Heart Rhythm Society and the European Heart Rhythm Association. *Circulation* 2005;111:659-70.

[16] Takenaka S, Kusano KF, Hisamatsu K, et al. Relatively benign clinical course in asymptomatic patients with brugada-type electrocardiogram without family history of sudden death. *J Cardiovasc Electrophysiol* 2001;12:2-6.

[17] Morita H, Kusano KF, Miura D, et al. Fragmented QRS as a marker of conduction abnormality and a predictor of prognosis of Brugada syndrome. *Circulation* 2008;118:1697-704.

[18] Morita H, Morita ST, Nagase S, et al. Ventricular arrhythmia induced by sodium channel blocker in patients with Brugada syndrome. *J Am Coll Cardiol* 2003;42:1624-31.

[19] Morita H, Fukushima-Kusano K, Nagase S, et al. Site-specific arrhythmogenesis in patients with Brugada syndrome. *J Cardiovasc Electrophysiol* 2003;14:373-9.

[20] Tada T, Kusano KF, Nagase S, et al. Clinical significance of macroscopic T-wave alternans after sodium channel blocker administration in patients with Brugada syndrome. *J Cardiovasc Electrophysiol* 2008;19:56-61.

[21] Morita H, Zipes DP, Morita ST, Wu J. Genotype-phenotype correlation in tissue models of Brugada syndrome simulating patients with sodium and calcium channelopathies. *Heart Rhythm* 2010.

[22] Wu J, Biermann M, Rubart M, Zipes DP. Cytochalasin D as excitation-contraction uncoupler for optically mapping action potentials in wedges of ventricular myocardium. *J Cardiovasc Electrophysiol* 1998;9:1336-47.

[23] Wu J, Zipes DP. Transmural reentry during acute global ischemia and reperfusion in canine ventricular muscle. *Am J Physiol Heart Circ Physiol* 2001;280:H2717-25.

[24] Morita H, Zipes DP, Morita ST, Lopshire JC, Wu J. Epicardial ablation eliminates ventricular arrhythmias in an experimental model of Brugada syndrome. *Heart Rhythm* 2009;6:665-71.

[25] Morita H, Zipes DP, Morita ST, Wu J. Temperature modulation of ventricular arrhythmogenicity in a canine tissue model of Brugada syndrome. *Heart Rhythm* 2007;4:188-97.

[26] Morita H, Wu J, Zipes DP. The QT syndromes: long and short. *Lancet* 2008;372:750-63.

[27] Kyndt F, Probst V, Potet F, et al. Novel SCN5A mutation leading either to isolated cardiac conduction defect or Brugada syndrome in a large French family. *Circulation* 2001;104:3081-6.

[28] Grant AO, Carboni MP, Neplioueva V, et al. Long QT syndrome, Brugada syndrome, and conduction system disease are linked to a single sodium channel mutation. *J Clin Invest* 2002;110:1201-9.

[29] Wang DW, Viswanathan PC, Balser JR, George AL, Jr., Benson DW. Clinical, genetic, and biophysical characterization of SCN5A mutations associated with atrioventricular conduction block. *Circulation* 2002;105:341-6.

[30] Lei M, Huang CL, Zhang Y. Genetic Na+ channelopathies and sinus node dysfunction. *Prog Biophys Mol Biol* 2008;98:171-8.

[31] Wang Q, Shen J, Li Z, et al. Cardiac sodium channel mutations in patients with long QT syndrome, an inherited cardiac arrhythmia. *Hum Mol Genet* 1995;4:1603-7.

[32] Delpon E, Cordeiro JM, Nunez L, et al. Functional effects of KCNE3 mutation and its role in the development of Brugada syndrome. *Circ Arrhythm Electrophysiol* 2008;1:209-18.

[33] Takagi M, Yokoyama Y, Aonuma K, Aihara N, Hiraoka M. Clinical characteristics and risk stratification in symptomatic and asymptomatic patients with brugada syndrome: multicenter study in Japan. *J Cardiovasc Electrophysiol* 2007;18:1244-51.

[34] Aiba T, Shimizu W, Hidaka I, et al. Cellular basis for trigger and maintenance of ventricular fibrillation in the Brugada syndrome model: high-resolution optical mapping study. *J Am Coll Cardiol* 2006;47:2074-85.

[35] Di Diego JM, Cordeiro JM, Goodrow RJ, et al. Ionic and cellular basis for the predominance of the Brugada syndrome phenotype in males. *Circulation* 2002;106:2004-11.

[36] Fish JM, Welchons DR, Kim YS, Lee SH, Ho WK, Antzelevitch C. Dimethyl lithospermate B, an extract of Danshen, suppresses arrhythmogenesis associated with the Brugada syndrome. *Circulation* 2006;113:1393-400.

*Chapter IX*

# VENTRICULAR FIBRILLATION: CAUSES, SYMPTOMS AND TREATMENT

## *Pasquale Notarstefano, Aureliano Fraticelli, Raffaele Guida and Leonardo Bolognese*
Cardiovascular Departmentm S. Donato Hospital, Arezzo (IT)

Ventricular fibrillation (VF) is a disorganised series of very rapid, ineffective contractions of the ventricular muscle caused by several chaotic electrical wavefronts. Its electrocardiographic hallmark is a rapid and grossly irregular ventricular rhythm with marked variability in QRS cycle length, morphology and amplitude (1, 2) (figure). As consequence of poorly synchronized and inadequate myocardial contractions, the heart immediately loses its pump function, with subsequent tissue hypoperfusion and global tissue ischemia. VF very rarely terminates spontaneously. Loss of consciousness occurs in seconds and few minutes are sufficient to cause irreversible brain damage due to cerebral anoxya, followed by death (1, 2).

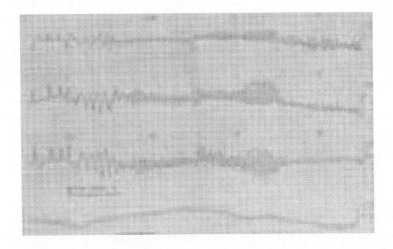

Figure 1. Ventricular Fibrillation

**Table 1**

| Etiologies of ventricular fibrillation |
|---|
| **Structural heart disease** |
| Coronary artery disease |
| -during acute Myocardial infarction or ischemia |
| -in absence of acute Myocardial Infarction or ischemia |
| Cardiomyopathy |
| -Dilated |
| -Hypertrophic |
| -Arrhythmogenic right ventricular cardiomyopathy or dysplasia |
| Valvular Heart disease |
| Myocarditis |
| Congenital heart disease |
| **Cardiac, apparently no structural heart disease** |
| Channelopathies |
| -Catecholaminergic polymorphic ventricular tachycardia |
| -Long QT syndrome |
| -Short QT syndrome |
| -Brugada syndrome |
| Mechanical (commotio cordis) or electrical accidents |
| After supraventricular tachycardia in Wolff-Parkinson-White syndrome |
| Heart block |
| Idiopathic Ventricular Fibrillation |
| **Non cardiac** |
| Drug-induced QT prolongation with torsades de pointes |
| Aortic dissection |
| Bronchospasm |
| Sleep apnea |
| Primary pulmonary hypertension |
| Pulmonary embolism |
| Tension pneumothorax |
| Metabolic or toxic |
| Electrolyte disturbances and acidosis |
| Medications or drug ingestion |
| Environmental poisoning |
| Sepsis |
| Neurologic |
| Cerebrovascular accident |
| Drowning |

# CAUSES

Principal causes of VF are listed in table. VF can be viewed as a continuum of electromechanical states leading to sudden cardiac death. Ventricular tachycardia degenerating first to ventricular fibrillation and later to asystole appears to be the most common pathophysiological cascade involved in out of hospital cardiac arrest (3). Coronary artery disease represents the most common substrate associated to cardiac arrest (2, 3). Two common patterns in the initiation of fatal arrhythmias have been recognized in patients with ischemic heart disease (4, 5, 6): ventricular tachyarrhythmia triggered by acute myocardial ischemia in patients with or without previous myocardial infarction, and ventricular tachyarrhythmia related to an anatomical substrate, such as scarring from a previous infarction without clinically evident myocardial ischemia (2). The boundaries zones between fibrosis and ventricular muscle are zone of slow conduction where muscle fibers are separated an disoriented by connective tissue and provide the substrate for reentrant circuites that give rise to ventricular tachycardia and subsequently ventricular fibrillation (2).

In Dilated non-ischemic cardiomyopathy, patchy areas of interstitial fibrosis represent a substrate for the development of VF. The degree of left ventricular impairment is correlated with the risk of sudden death. (3, 4, 7).

In patients with hypertrophic cardiomypathy (HCM), sudden death events are caused by rapid ventricular tachycardia and/or VF. Myocardial disarray and fibrosis as consequence of silent microvascular ischemia represent the most probable electrophysiological substrate for malignant arrhythmias. High risk factors for sudden death are massive left ventricular hypertrophy, syncope, sustained ventricular tachycardia, family hystory of sudden death, abnormal blood pressure response to exercise (8).

Other cardiac diseases predisposing to SCD include arrhythmogenic right ventricular cardiomyopaty (ARVD) (9), in which some areas of right ventricular myocardium are replaced by fibrous and fatty tissue, congenital abnormalities (i.e. coronary artery anomalies), and rarely myocarditis (3, 7, 10).

In patients with Wolff-Parkinson-White (WPW) syndrome VF can occur when atrial fibrillation or flutter waves pass rapidly through a bypass tract to the ventricular muscolature.(11, 12)

Among valvulopathies, aortic stenosis is associated with a risk of sudden cardiac death ranging from 5% to 20%. In these patients death can be the result not only of ventricular arrhythmias, but also of bradycardia, out-flow obstruction and ischemia (13)

In 5% to 10% of cases, SCD occurs in the absence of structural heart disease. Channellopathies such as Long QT syndrome (LQTS), Short QT Syndrome (SQTS), Brugada Syndrome and Catecholaminergic Ventricular Tachycardia are a group of inherited abnormalities associated to increased risk of fatal arhhythmias in the absence of evident structural cardiac abonormalities (14, 15, 16, 17, 18, 19).

Bradycardia, especially if associated to electrolyte imbalance and drugs effect, can lead to prolongation and dispersion of the QT interval, torsades de pointes and VF (2).

The toxic potential of drugs for VF is an important trigger of VF. Antiarrhythmic drug themselves may be a cause of fatal arrhythmias (20), especially in patients with coronary artery disease and left ventricular dysfunction, as highlighted in the Cardiac Arrhythmia Suppression Trial (CAST) and the Survival with d-Sotalol (SWORD) Trial (21, 22).

Hypokalemia is another well recognised triggering factor for the occurrence of VF (23). Several other triggers have been reported (7, 24, 25). The interaction between triggering elements and predisposing conditions like ischemia, cardiac structural abnormalities, or primary electrophysiological abnormalities, results in a complex of factors that can induce VF and sudden death (3).

The term of Idiopatic VF is reserved for those patients resuscitated from VF and in which it is not possible to identify triggers factors or a predisposing substrate. Within this limited category of patients, recent evidences suggest an higher prevalence then expected of early repolarization in inferolateral leads, an ECG aspect hystorically considered benign (26). The reasons for this association are under investigation. Experimental findings indicate the presence of transmural electrical heterogeneity, which can be amplified under certain conditions, favoring the occurrence of fatal arrhythmias (26, 27).

## SYMPTOMS

VF often occurs without forewarning. The absence of organised ventricular contractions rapidly causes loss of consciousness and death. Depending on the underlyng disease, symptoms such as chest pain, dyspnea, palpitations or syncope can immediatly preceede the occurence of VF. The patient becomes cyanotic, there is no pulse or respiration, heart tones are absent. The electrocardiogram shows wide and disorganised complexes, then a fine, irregular pattern, and finally isoelectric asystolic line if VF is not interrupted (1,2).

## TREATMENT

Even if spontaneous restoring of sinus rhythm is rarely noted during ECG monitoring, the management of VF generally requires the immediate delivery of electrical defibrillation (ED) (1, 2). Unsynchronised direct electrical current is delivered to the heart to uniformly and simultaneously depolarize myocardial muscle, with the objective to interfere with all reentrant circuits that determine the arrhythmia. The percentage of success and the energy required are strictly dependent on the time between the onset of VF and the delivery of the shock. The loss of pump function during VF rapidly causes energy reserve depletion and consequent impaired active ion transport. Cardio Pulmonary Resuscitation (CPR) slows the progression of these events, determining a minimal cardiac perfusion, improving metabolic state of myocardium and making it more sensible to the ED (28). It is demonstrated that both early CPR (before arrival of Emergency Medical System- EMS) and early defibrillation improve survival (28). After ED temporary asystole or pulseless electrical activity (PEA) may occour. In this case immediate CPR is recommended after ED, because CPR can be able to convert PEA or asystole in perfusing rhythm (29, 30).

The patients survived an episode of VF are by definition at high risk of recurrence, unless a clear and completely reversible cause or predisposing factor has been identified and eliminated (i.e. revascularization of ischemic myocardium, catheter ablation of atrioventricular bypass tract). There is no evidence that drug treatment prevent the recurrence of life threatening arrhythmic event. The only evidence-based therapeutic strategy for these patients is the implantation of a cardioverter-defibrillator (ICD). (31, 32, 33).

In terms of primary prevention of sudden death due to malignant arrhythmia, largest observational studies of risk factors and interventional trials of therapy have been conducted in patients with ischemic heart disease or dilated cardiomyopathy. For those patients with previous Myocardial infarction and low ejection fraction, implantation of defibrillator is associated to improved survival, even in absence of arrhythmic markers (34). The SCD-HeFT Trial compared amiodarone and ICD in addition to best medical therapy in patients with coronary heart disease or non ischemic cardiomyopathy who were in NYHA class II or III and with ejection fraction less than 35%. The total mortality was 7,2% per year in the medical group, with a risk reduction of 23% in ICD group versus placebo. There was no mortality difference between placebo an amiodarone groups (35).

Among other categories of patients, the implantable defibrillator is indicated in subgroup patients with specific high risk markers for SD. However it must be keep in mind that most of SD, in terms of absolute number of events, occur in the general population and in patients with non specific and intermediate risk profiles (3, 7). As a consequence most of cardiac arrest happen out of hospital. Identify time saving strategies is a crucial an challenging objective in this setting. The most successful one include the distribution in the territory of automatic or semi automatic external defibrillator, able to make diagnosis and therapy of VF.

## PUBLIC ACCESS DEFIBRILLATION

In Out-of Hospital cardiac arrest (OHCA) conventional emergency medical system response times are rarely sufficiently rapid to allow survival; as a consequence, OHCA survival rates are usually lower than 8 %(36). The last two decades have witnessed the spreading of "public access defibrillation" (PAD) programmes, which are based on the deployment of early defibrillation by individuals who do not belong to health professional categories ("lay persons") but who can rapidly assist OHCA victims. Technological, cultural and legislative progress have allowed this unique treatment strategy. The development of semi-automatic and automatic external defibrillators (AED) have been a crucial first step. The principle of the AED operation is reliable, automatic recognition of shockable rhythms (i.e. VF or VT) through adhesive paddles applied to the thorax of a patient with definite or suspected cardiac arrest; in a fully-automatic device, a shock is readily delivered; in semiautomatic defibrillators a vocal message prompts the rescuer to release a shock, which can be done simply by pressing a button. Several types of AEDs have been produced in the last decade, and after approval by the FDA and other regulatory agencies, they have been widely distributed, some models being sold even to private customers "over the counter" and through the internet. AEDs models may differ in waveform (biphasic vs monophasic), energy level (150 to 360 Joules), type of instructions (vocal vs visual), modality for paediatric defibrillation activation and so on. Automatic diagnosis by sensitive and specific algorithms and ease of operation are the key for deployment of AEDs by lay persons with minimal training.

Effective AEDs training, alone (36) or within a basic life support programme (BLS-D) have been demonstrated in several settings, which include professional categories (policeman, fire fighters ) (37, 38), the general public, and experimentally even primary school children (39, 40, 41).

The legal implications of a medical act, i.e. defibrillation, performed by lay rescuers to patients at a high risk of death, have been an obstacle to the diffusion of PAD programmes, especially in an early phase. Several countries have passed laws such as the U.S. "Good Samaritan" legislation, (36) that allows lay defibrillation and affords legal protection to lay rescuers, even though some issues remain uncertain in many circumstances, including the case of totally untrained rescuers.

A series of observational studies have given support to the notion that PAD programmes may effectively increase OHCA survival. Impressive results have been reported in settings where high density of potential witnesses, availability of AEDs and trained personnel, and limited distance to reach an OHCA victim favour early intervention, such as airplanes and casinos (42, 43, 44, 45) with survival rates as high as 53%.

The PAD (Public Access Defibrillation) trial (39) is the first randomized study giving strong scientific evidence to the benefits of early defibrillation by lay persons. The study involved over 19,000 volunteers in almost 1000, mostly (84%) public community locations, such as shopping centres, recreational facilities, large hotels or office buildings, randomized to two types of volunteer-based emergency response to cardiac arrest: a CPR only, and an AED plus CPR system. The latter granted a significantly higher number of cardiac arrest survivors (30 out of 127 cardiac arrests, vs 15 out of 107 in the control group, p = 0.03). Following the publication of the PAD trial, the American Heart Association issued a statement (46) in support of the development of lay rescuers AED programmes.

The high proportion of cardiac arrests occurring at home has generated the hypothesis that home dissemination of AEDs in categories of patients at risk may be an effective primary prevention strategy.

The HAT study (47) is a randomized trial involving 7000 survivors of anterior myocardial infarction who were not candidate for ICD implant. Patients were randomly assigned to two treatments, to be applied in case of home cardiac arrest: home AED operated by family members, followed by calling the emergency medical system and CPR, or conventional emergency call and CPR. The primary end-point of total mortality was not improved in the AED arm. Reasons advocated for this negative results include the low event rate and the fact that the AED was deployed in only one quarter of total home cardiac arrests, (and in half of the witnessed ones). This latter observation indicates that AED training for family members of patients with myocardial infarction is a limiting factor even within a randomized clinical trial.

In conclusion, the use of AEDs by trained lay personnel in the setting of cardiac arrest occuring in public venues has been supported by respected scientific boards since the midnineties. Guidelines stress the importance of several keys issues in order to assure effective operation of public access defibrillation projects, which include thorough planning, strict interplay with the emergency medical system, proper maintenance and quality programmes.

# REFERENCES

[1] American Heart Association. 2005 American Heart Association Guidelines for Cardiopulmonary Resuscitation and Emergency Cardiovascular Care. *Circulation*. Dec 13 2005;112(24 Suppl):IV1-203.

[2] Zipes DP, Jalife J. *Cardiac Electrophysiology: from Cell to Bedside*, 4rd ed. Saunders, 2004.

[3] Huikuri HV, Castellanos A, Myerburg RJ: Sudden death due to cardiac arrhythmias. *N Engl J Med* 345:1473, 2001

[4] Zipes DP, Wellens HJJ. Sudden cardiac death. *Circulation* 1998;98: 2334-51.

[5] Wit AL, Janse MJ. Experimental models of ventricular tachycardia and fibrillation caused by ischemia and infarction. *Circulation* 1992;85:Suppl I: I-32–I-42.

[6] Mehta D, Curwin J, Gomes JA, Fuster V. Sudden death in coronary artery disease: acute ischemia versus myocardial substrate. *Circulation* 1997;96:3215-23.

[7] Myerburg RJ, Kessler KM, Castellanos A. Sudden cardiac death. Structure, function and time-dependence of risk. *Circulation* 1992; 85:I2-10.

[8] Maron BJ: Contemporary Insights and Strategies for Risk Stratification and Prevention of Sudden Death in Hypertrophic Cardiomyopathy *Circulation* 2010;121;445-456

[9] Basso C, Corrado D, Marcus F, et al. Arrhythmogenic right ventricular cardiomyopathy. *Lancet* 2009; 373:1289-1300.

[10] Blauwet LA, Cooper LT. Myocarditis. Progr Cardiovasc Dis 2010; 52:274-288.

[11] Timmermans C, Smeets JL, Rodriguez LM et al. Aborted Sudden death in the Wolff-Parkinson-White Syndrome. *Am J Cardiol* 1995; 76:492-4.

[12] Munger TM, Packer DL, Hammil SC et al. A population study of the natural hystory of Wolff-Parkinson-White Syndrome in Olmsted Country, Minnesota, 1953-1989. *Circulation*1993; 87:866-73.

[13] Schwartz L, GoldfischerJ, SpragueGJ, et al. Syncope and sudden death in aortic stenosis. *Am J Cardiol* 23:647, 1969.

[14] Moss AJ, Robinson J. Clinical features of the idiopathic long QT syndrome. *Circulation* 1992;85:140 –144.

[15] Priori SG, Schwartz PJ, Napolitano C et al. Risk stratification in the long QT Syndrome. *N Engl J Med* 2003;348:1866-74.

[16] Gaita F, Giustetto C, Bianchi F, et al. Short QT syndrome: a familial cause of sudden death. *Circulation* 2003;108:965–970.

[17] Brugada J, Brugada R, Brugada P. Determinants of sudden cardiac death in individuals with the electrocardiographic pattern of Brugada syndrome and no previous cardiac arrest. *Circulation* 2003;108:3092–3096.

[18] Priori SG, Napolitano C, Gasparini M et al. Natural hystory of Brugada Syndrome: insights for risk stratification an management. *Circulation* 2002; 105:1342-1347.

[19] Priori SG, Napolitano C, Memmi M, et al. Clinical and molecular characterization of patients with cathecolaminergic polymorphyc ventricular tachycardia. *Circulation* 2002;106:69-74.

[20] Ruskin JN, McGovern B, Garan H, et al: Antiarrhythmic drugs: A possible cause of out of hospital cardiac arrest. *N Engl J Med* 309:1302, 1983.

[21] Echt DS, Liesbon PR, Mitchell LB, et al: Mortality an morbidity in patients receiving encainide, flecainide, or placebo: The Cardiac Arrhythmia Suppression Trial. *N Engl J Med* 1991;324:781-788.

[22] Waldo AL, Camm AJ, DeRuyter H et al: Effect of d-sotalol on mortality in patients with left ventricular dysfunction after recent and remote myocardial infarction.The SWORD Investigators. Survival With Oral d-Sotalol. *Lancet* 1996; 348:7-12.

[23] Podrid PJ. Potassium and ventricular arrhythmias *Am J Cardiol*. 1990 Mar 6;65(10):33E-44E.

[24] Myerburg RJ, Kessler KM, Castellanos A. Sudden cardiac death: epidemiology, transient risk, and intervention assessment. Ann Intern Med 1993;119:1187-97.

[25] Myerburg RJ, Interian A Jr, Mitrani RM, Kessler KM, Castellanos A. Frequency of sudden cardiac death and profiles of risk. *Am J Cardiol* 1997; 80:10F-19F.

[26] Haissaguerre, M, Derval N, Sacher F, et al. Sudden cardiac arrest associated with early Repolarization. *N Engl J Med* 2008;358:2016-23.
[27] Gussak I, Antzelevich C. Early repolarization syndrome: clinical characteristics and possible cellular and ionic mechanisms. *J Electrocardiol* 2000;33:299-309.
[28] Achleitner U, Wenzel V, StrohmengerHU et al The beneficial of basic life support on ventricular fibrilation mean frequency and coronary perfusion. *Resuscitation* 2001;51:151-158.
[29] Cummins RO, Ornato JP, Thies WH et al Improving survival from sudden cardiac arrest.. *Circulation* 1991; 83: 1832-1847 .
[30] International Liaison Committee on Resuscitation. 2005 International Consensus on Cardiopulmonary Resuscitation and Emergency Cardiovascular Care Science with Treatment Recommendations. Part 3: defibrillation. *Resuscitation*. 2005 Nov-Dec;67(2-3):203-11.
[31] The Antiarrhythmics versus Implantable Defibrillators (AVID) Investigators. A comparison of antiarrhythmic-drug therapy with implantable de- fibrillators in patients resuscitated from near-fatal ventricular arrhythmias. *N Engl J Med* 1997;337:1576-83.
[32] Kuck KH, Cappato R, Siebels J, Ruppel R. Randomized comparison of antiarrhythmic drug therapy with implantable defibrillators in patients resuscitated from cardiac arrest: the Cardiac Arrest Study Hamburg (CASH). *Circulation* 2000;102:748-54.
[33] Connolly SJ, Gent M, Roberts RS, et al. Canadian Implantable Defibrillator Study (CIDS): a randomized trial of the implantable cardioverter defibrillator against amiodarone. *Circulation* 2000;101:1287-302.
[34] Moss AJ. Madit II and its implications. *Eur Heart J* 2003;24:8-16.
[35] Bardy GH, Lee KL, Mark DB, et al. Amiodarone or an Impiantable Cardioverter-defibrillator for congestive Heart Failure.*N Eng J Med* 2005; 352:225-37.
[36] Nichol G, Stiell IG, Laupacis A, et al. A cumulative meta-analysis of the effectiveness of defibrillator-capable emergency medical services for victims of out-of-hospital cardiac arrest. *Ann Emerg Med*. 1999;34:517-25.
[37] Capucci A, Aschieri D, Piepoli MF, et al Tripling survival from sudden cardiac arrest via early defibrillation without traditional education in cardiopulmonary resuscitation. *Circulation*. 2002 Aug 27;106:1065-70.
[38] White RD, Bunch TJ, Hankins DG. Evolution of a community-wide early defibrillation programme experience over 13 years using police/fire personnel and paramedics as responders. *Resuscitation*. 2005 Jun;65:279-83.
[39] Hallstrom AP, Ornato JP, Weisfeldt M, et al. Public Access Defibrillation Trial Investigators. Public-access defibrillation and survival after out-of-hospital cardiac arrest. *N Engl J Med*. 2004 Aug 12;35:637-46.
[40] Uray T, Lunzer A, Ochsenhofer A, et al. Feasibility of life-supporting first-aid (LSFA) training as a mandatory subject in primary schools. *Resuscitation*. 2003 Nov;59:211-20.
[41] Toner P, Connolly M, Laverty L, et al. Teaching basic life support to school children using medical students and teachers in a 'peer-training' model--results of the 'ABC for life' programme. *Resuscitation*. 2007 Oct;75:169-75.
[42] Caffrey SL, Willoughby PJ, Pepe PE, Becker LB. Public use of automated external defibrillators. *N Engl J Med*. 2002 Oct 17;347:1242-7

[43] Aufderheide T, Hazinski MF, Nichol G, et al. American Heart Association Emergency Cardiovascular Care Committee; Council on Clinical Cardiology; Office of State Advocacy. Community lay rescuer automated external defibrillation programs: key state legislative components and implementation strategies: a summary of a decade of experience for healthcare providers, policymakers, legislators, employers, and community leaders from the American Heart Association Emergency Cardiovascular Care Committee, Council on Clinical Cardiology, and Office of State Advocacy. *Circulation*. 2006 Mar 7;113:1260-70.

[44] Page RL, Joglar JA, Kowal RC, et al. Use of automated external defibrillators by a U.S. airline. *N Engl J Med*. 2000 Oct 26;343(17):1210-6.

[45] Valenzuela TD, Roe DJ, Nichol G, et al. Outcomes of rapid defibrillation by security officers after cardiac arrest in casinos. *N Engl J Med*. 2000 Oct 26;343(17):1206-9.

[46] Hazinski MF, Idris AH, Kerber RE, et al. American Heart Association Emergency Cardiovascular Committee; Council on Cardiopulmonary, Perioperative, and Critical Care; Council on Clinical Cardiology. Lay rescuer automated external defibrillator ("public access defibrillation") programs: lessons learned from an international multicenter trial: advisory statement from the American Heart Association Emergency Cardiovascular Committee; the Council on Cardiopulmonary, Perioperative, and Critical Care; and the Council on Clinical Cardiology. *Circulation*. 2005 Jun 21;111(24):3336-40.

[47] Bardy GH, Lee KL, Mark DB, et al. HAT Investigators. Home use of automated external defibrillators for sudden cardiac arrest. *N Engl J Med*. 2008 Apr 24;358(17):1793-804.

*Chapter X*

# PRIMARY VENTRICULAR FIBRILLATION IN "TAKO-TSUBO" SYNDROME

## *J. Villegas del Ojo[a], E. Moreno Millán[b], A.M. García Fernandez[b], F. Bocanegra Martin[c], and P. Martinez Romero[d]*

[a]Servicio de Medicina Intensiva Hospital Virgen del Camino, Sanlúcar de Barrameda. Spain
[b]Servicio de Medicina Intensiva Hospital Santa Bárbara. Puertollano. Spain
[c]Unidad de Gestión Clínica Barrio Bajo. Sanlúcar de Barrameda. Spain
[d]Servicio de Cardiología. Hospital Universitario de Puerto Real. Spain

## ABSTRACT

Introduction: The "tako-tsubo" syndrome is a recently described process that clinically mimics an acute coronary disease, understanding the association of chest pain with ST-T elevation without coronary artery occlusion, and with a typical and reversible deformation of left ventricle as a result of anteroapical diskinesia with basal hyperkinesia.

Case report: a 64-year-old woman without cardiovascular risk factors, featuring presyncope and chest pain and showing in the hospital ST segment elevation in inferiorposterolateral area, proceeding to fibrinolysis with tenecteplase, showing 15 minutes after an episode of ventricular fibrillation (VF) that is treated with shock of 360 joules, recovering effective spontaneous circulation. The electrocardiographic ST segment elevation persistence 90 minutes postfibrinolisis, by that an emergency angiography was made showing no signs of coronary arteries occlusion, and finding on ventriculography anteroapical dyskinesia with basal hyperkinesia.

Discussion and Conclusion: Today, there are new diseases, probably undiagnosed, as the "tako-tsubo" syndrome, predominantly female and generated by stress, which simulates an acute coronary syndrome with ST segment elevation and may be responsible for sudden death by primary VF. It is very important to recognize this syndrome, as its management and prognosis are different from the acute myocardial infarction resulting from coronary thrombotic occlusion.

## INTRODUCTION

The main mechanism of sudden cardiac death (SCD) is the ventricular fibrillation (VF), and it is defined as idiopathic ventricular fibrillation (IVF) when it occurs in the absence of structural heart disease, cardiotoxicity, electrolyte abnormalities or predisposing or hereditary condition (1). The etiology of VF remains incompletely understood, being presented in the setting of acute cardiac ischemia or infarction. Acute myocardial infarction (AMI) is diagnosed in up to half of SCD survivors, occurring in 5–10% of survivors of extrahospitalary SCD (2). The incidence of SCD is also relatively high in the postinfarction period. In addition, abnormal rapid stimulation of the ventricles can lead to VF; this can be present during ventricular tachycardia (VT) and other settings (Wolff-Parkinson-White syndrome, atrial fibrillation or flutter, severe left ventricular dysfunction, cardiomyopathies, acquired or idiopathic long QT syndrome and Brugrada syndrome). VF is more common in young males showing a circadian pattern appearing more frequently midnight and mid-morning (3). It is also prevalent worldwide, with a reported predominance in the northern hemisphere. The incidence of SCD in the United States is approximately 300,000 cases per year. Among some European populations, the annual incidence of cardiac arrests exceeds 6 cases per 10,000 people. The distribution of rhythms found in patients with SCD depends largely on the average duration of the arrest state and, thus, the emergency medical system (EMS) response time, but where average response times are less than 5 minutes, the initial rhythm is VF in approximately 70% of patients. Improved outcomes occur in patients who have a witnessed arrest, receiving bystander cardiopulmonary resuscitation (CPR) and obtaining defibrillation and advanced cardiac life support from EMS personnel within 10 minutes of onset, and present with an initial rhythm of VF (4,5,6). The rate of survival from VF in the community varies from 4–33%. The survival rate of all SCD victims regardless of presenting rhythm has been reported between 2–18% in various EMS systems. These low rates of survival have been attributed to low rate of bystander CPR, longer response intervals, and that few patients present VF as initial rhythm. VF begins as a quasiperiodic reentrant pattern of excitation in the ventricles, resulting in poorly synchronized and inadequate myocardial contractions (7). Consequently the heart loses immediately its ability to function as a pump, with subsequent tissue hypoperfusion that creates global tissue ischemia.

The tako-tsubo syndrome (TTS), or transient left ventricular dysfunction, was described in Japan by Sato et al. (8,9). The clinic is indistinguishable from an acute coronary syndrome (ACS), including their complications. Coronary angiography shows no significant coronary lesions and in ventriculography the apical hypokinesia gives a typical image, which resembles a narrow-necked globular and wide vessel as those used in Japan to trap octopus, called tako-tsubo, giving its name to this syndrome. Characteristically, TTS is accompanied by a recovery within two weeks of abnormal segmental contractility. It usually affects women around the 60–80 years without relevant cardiovascular risk factors, often associated with emotional and/or physical exertion, showing a benign course. The etiology is unknown, but several causes have been postulated like viral myocarditis, direct toxic effect of catecholamines, coronary spasm, coronary thrombosis, transient and anatomical variations of the anterior descending artery, and even could be a spontaneous mechanical abortion of the myocardial infarct.

## CASE REPORT

We report the case of a 57-year-old woman that comes to the emergency department (ED) of our hospital translated by EMS. She presented acute sweating, discomfort and chest pain, Being attended by primary care physician, showing on the first examination profuse sweating, and hypotension with a blood pressure (BP) 50/30 mmHg, with spontaneous resolution (BP 110/70 mmHg). An electrocardiogram was made showing ST-segment elevation in inferoposterolateral area. The patient did not have familiar medical history, and in her personal medical history included: no cardiovascular risk factors, osteoporosis, and her regular treatment was calcium, vitamin D, biphosphonates and glicofosfopeptical. She had been in an excellent health until the day prior the admission. When she arrived to the ED, on examination she was conscience, breath rate was 15 per minute, saturation 100% with oxygen, pulse rate was 89 beats per minute, and BP was 150/90 mmHg, she was sweaty and presented discomfort without others interest sings at the examination time. Then we decided to admit her into ICU. The regular blood tests were within normal limits. Electrocardiogram (ECG) showed sinus tachycardia, ST-segment descent in V4, V5, V6 and ST-segment elevation in II, III, AVF. In the Rx chest posterior-anterior showed no signs of abnormality. With the diagnostic of acute coronary syndrom ST-segment elevation (STEMI), we started antisiquemic treatment with A.A.S. 300 mg, clopidogrel 300 mg, endovenous nitroglycerine, enoxaparin 30 mg and fibrinolysis with 6500 UI of tenecteplase without electrocardiographics signs of reperfusion. Twenty-five minutes later, she suffered VF recovering spontaneous circulation after one 360 J defibrillation shock. After 90 minutes postfibrinolysis, the patient showed in the ECG persistent ST-segment elevation. Therefore, we contacted with reference Hemodynamics Unit and traslated her to do a rescue coronariography, showing no significant coronary stenosis and with global normal contractility in left ventricle with ejection fraction of 59%, with anterior, apical and inferior hypokinesia in the ventriculography (Figure 1).

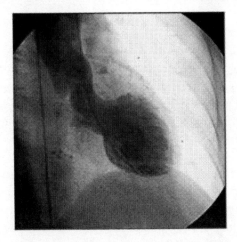

Figure 1. Catheterization with ventriculography. Abalone left apical characteristic of the syndrome Tako-Tsubo at the beginning and end of systole.

A transthoracic echocardiography was made 48 hours later presenting normal global contractility and no dilated left ventricle, with apical and inferior hypokinesia left atrial and aortic root not dilated; normal diastolic function; mitral, trycuspide and pulmonar valves without alterations and sclerotic aortic valve. Therefore, she was moved to the Cardiology Unit and she was discharged from hospital in 10 days. Finally, after analyzed all complementary tests and considering the absence of obstruction in angiography and the apical hypokinesia, we conclude that the patient presents a TTS. Presently, a year after the event, she continues with the double antiaggregant treatment, beta-blockers and statins and she is asymptomatic and without recurrence.

## DISCUSSION

Some authors doubt if TTS could also represent a spontaneous myocardial infarct abortion. Could it be that in this population the balance between coronary thrombosis and endogenous fibrinolysis, falls on the fibrinolysis side and, therefore, no thrombus is seen on angiography? This AMI abortion could also induce wall motion abnormalities that may recover some days later, because of auto-thrombolysis (10). Therefore, in the early phase, these patients present the same complications the ACS, as ventricular arrhithmyas. TTS patients present on angiography no coronary artery stenosis, usually maked in the subacute phase and under the state-of-the-art antithrombotic–anticoagulant therapy. Could we diagnose an aborted AMI when the thrombus responsible for the event has been completely lysed? This hypothesis becomes more plausible when it has been reported in TTS patients a disrupted eccentric atherosclerotic plaques in anterior descending artery, these findings have been visualized by intravascular ultrasound (IVUS), but were not visible by contrast angiography (11). Could the transient akinesia seen in these patients be secondary to stunned myocardium because of multiple episodes of occlusion–reperfusion? After relief of ischaemia, the post-ischaemic but viable myocardium requires hours to days before the function is fully restored. The length of time for the ventricular function to return is dependent on the number and duration of the ischaemic episodes and we know that after a 15 minute of coronary artery occlusion, 48 h of reperfusion was needed for full recovery of systolic function (12). Therefore, we believe that the TTS patients could represent the paradigm of AMI abortion secondary to spontaneous auto-thrombolysis.

There is always a trigger event which is usually an episode of physical stress, unusual physical exertion, surgery, or severe emotional stress. Although its exact etiology is unknown, microvascular abnormalities and/or excessive sympathetic stimulation and catecholamine release, viral infections, microvascular spasm, have been postulated as probable etiology of this syndrome, which produces vasoconstriction of the microvasculature heart and coronary spasms (although only 21% of patients present vasospasm with acetylcholine), dynamic medioventricular obstruction and some times it can be seen the existence of a large recurrent descending anterior coronary segment (13). In studies performed by PET and contrast perfusion –echocardiography has shown decreased distal blood flow in apical region of the septum, while middle and lateral areas blood perfusion is preserved (14). The incidence is unclear and is not known how many of the AMI with normal coronary arteries (6%) could be TTS. The clinical presentation is similar to an ACS. The onset symptoms are chest pain (53-71%), dyspnea (7-20%) and more rarely cardiogenic shock (5%). The initial ECG may be similar to ACS (show ST elevation in precordial leads (90%) and/or negative T wave in precordial leads (44%), Q-wave (15-27%), and rarely mirrored in the inferior face). ECG changes may last for days or weeks and evolved into disappearance of the Q wave (90-100%), normalization of the ST and the presence of negative and deep T waves (84-97%). These changes are explained by the difference between repolarization of apical dyskinetic and basal hyperkinetic area. In the ultrasound performed at baseline, there is a dyskinesia or akinesia of the left ventricular apex, with normo or basal hyperkinesia.(15). Cardiac enzymes may be elevated slightly (56% CPK, troponin almost 100%) but present a curve that is moving rapidly toward normalization, not following the typical curve of AMI. Histological findings on endomyocardial biopsy include focal myocytolysis, mononuclear infiltrates, and necrosis contraction band without evidence of myocarditis. The possible complications are ventricular arrhythmias (9%) like in our case, severe bradycardia (10%), heart failure (22%) and cardiogenic shock (15%). The clinical recovery and hemodynamic improvement, usually starts in 2-3 ° day, the ECG changes may last for days or weeks and ultrasonographic changes are normalized within days or weeks (16). The evolution is usually benign, with a 1% of mortality and recurrence is rare. Being the TTS a recently described entity, long-term implications are unknown and its optimal treatment (acute and long-term) is not clear. In the acute phase of the TTS, the hypovolemia, inotropes and an intraaortic balloon worsen dynamic intraventricular obstruction and thereby decrease output cardiac, and should therefore be avoided, but betablockers can be used to decrease the ventricular gradient. However, it seems that there is an ischemic microvascular base in this disease; therefore, it seems advisable to maintain the treatment of the AMI for a long period, with the exception of the renin angiotensin aldosterone inhibitors because ventricular dysfunction is temporary.

## CONCLUSION

Distinguishing in the ED, with clinical and ECG findings, a TTS of ACS is difficult, both syndromes are very similar; thereby, we find high complexity to make a differential diagnosis in the acute phase, but it is important, since the ventricular dysfunction is the main important prognostic factor. It is resolved in TTS over the following weeks, which suggests its lower severity, once the acute phase finished.

Presently, there are new diseases, probably undiagnosed, as TTS, that may be responsible for SCD by VF. Our patient suffered this complication, that is a typical complication of the ACS. It is very important to recognize this syndrome, as its management, because its prognosis is different from the ACS, being the quick defibrillation the priority. The way we described it, TTS has many and different clinical presentation and complications; therefore, this etiology is to be considered in patients without cardiovascular risk factors and SCD.

The early management until the completion of angiography with ventriculography, the choice diagnostic test, must be the same treatment for an ACS.

In addition, we would highly suggest the use of a technique that visualizes the entire vessel wall such as IVUS, to explore the presence of disrupted plaques in patients with ACS and without obstruction in the angiography.

In relation with the treatment, new studies are required to assess what treatment is appropriate, the need for secondary prophylaxis and subsequent implications, to clear up questions not answered in the current literature.

## REFERENCES

[1] Lown B. Sudden cardiac death: biobehavioral perspective. *Circulation* 1987; 76: I 186-196.

[2] Kasanuki H, Ohnishi S, Ohtuka M, Matsuda N, Nirei T, Isogai R et al. . Idiopathic ventricular fibrillation induced with vagal activity in patients without obvious heart disease. *Circulation* 1997; 95: 2277- 2285.

[3] Markus FI. Idiopathic ventricular Fibrillation. *J Cardiovasc Electrophysiol* 1997; 8: 1075-1083.

[4] Mewis C, Kuhlkamp V, Spyridopoulos I, Bosch Rf, Seipel L. Late outcome of idiopathic ventricular fibrillation. *Am J Cardiol* 1998; 81: 999-1003.

[5] Haissaguerre M, Shoda M, Jais P, Nogami A, Shah Dc, Kautzner J et al. Mapping and ablation of idiopathic ventricular fibrillation. *Circulation* 2002; 106: 962-967.

[6] Consensus Statement of the Joint Steering committees of the unexplained Cardiac Arrest Registry of Europe (UCARE) and of the Idiopathic Ventricular Fibrillation Registry of the United States (IVF-USNeed for definition and Standardized clinical evaluation. *Circulation* 1997; 95: 265-272.

[7] Priori Sg, Crotti L. Idiopathic ventricular fibrillation. *Cardiac Electrophysiol Rev* 1999; 3: 198-201.

[8] Kurisu S, Sato H, Kawagoe T, Ishihara M, Shimatani Y, Nishioka K, et al. Tako-Tsubo-like left ventricular dysfunction with ST-segment elevation: a novel cardiac syndrome mimicking acute myocardial infarction. *Am Heart J* 2002; 143:448-55.

[9] Gaspar J, Gomez Cruz RA. Tako-Tsubo syndrome (transient antero-apical dyskinesia): first case reported in Latin America and review of the literature. *Arch Cardiol Mex* 2004; 74:205-14.

[10] Verheugt FW, Gersh BJ, Armstrong PW. Aborted myocardial infarction: a new target for reperfusion therapy. *Eur Heart J* 2006; 27:901–904.

[11] Ibanez B, Navarro F, Cordoba M, Alberca P, Farre J. Tako-tsubo transient left ventricular apical ballooning: is intravascular ultrasound the key to resolve the enigma? *Heart* 2005; 91:102–104.

[12] Charlat ML, O'Neill PG, Hartley CJ, Roberts R, Bolli R. Prolonged abnormalities of left ventricular diastolic wall thinning in the 'stunned' myocardium in conscious dogs: time course and relation to systolic function. *J Am Coll Cardiol* 1989;13:185–194.

[13] Ibanez B, Navarro F, Farre J, Marcos-Alberca P, Orejas M, Rabago R, Rey M, Romero J, Iniguez A, Cordoba M. Tako-tsubo syndrome associated with a long course of the left anterior descending coronary artery along the apical diaphragmatic surface of the left ventricle. *Rev Esp Cardiol* 2004;57:209–216.

[14] Upadya SP, Hoq SM, Pannala R, Alsous F, Tuohy E, Zarich S. Tako–Tsubo Cardiomyopathy (Transient Left Ventricular Apical Ballooning): a case report Myocardial Perfusion Echocardiogram Study. *J Am Soc Echocardiogr* 2005; 18:883.

[15] Kurisu S, Inoue I, Kawagoe T, Ishihara M, Shimatani Y, Nakamura S, et al. Time course of electrocardiographic changes in patients with tako-tsubo syndrome: comparison with acute myocardial infarction with minimal enzymatic release. *Circ J* 2004; 68:77-81.

[16] 16.Nyui N, Yamanaka O, Nakayama R, Sawano M, Kawai S. 'Tako-Tsubo' transient ventricular dysfunction: a case report. *Jpn Circ J* 2000; 64: 715-9.

In: Ventricular Fibrillation and Acute Coronary Syndrome
Editor: Joyce E. Mandell

ISBN: 978-1-61728-969-9
© 2011 Nova Science Publishers, Inc.

*Chapter XI*

# VENTRICULAR FIBRILLATION IN THE ABSENCE OF APPARENT STRUCTURAL HEART DISEASE: ELECTROPHYSIOLOGICAL MECHANISMS, CLINICAL PROGNOSIS AND THERAPEUTIC MANAGEMENT.

### *Osmar Antonio Centurión*[*]

Division of Electrophysiology and Arrhythmia Cardiovascular Institute. Sanatorio Migone-Battilana. Asunción, Paraguay. Departamento de Cardiología. Primera Cátedra de Clínica Médica. Hospital de Clínicas. Universidad Nacional de Asunción

### ABSTRACT

Up to a third of all cases of unexplained sudden cardiac arrest may be primarily due to cardiac arrhythmias, with ventricular fibrillation (VF) being the culprit arrhythmia in the majority of patients. Sudden cardiac death in the truly normal heart is an uncommon occurrence. The majority of patients without apparent structural heart disease who died suddenly do not actually have "normal" hearts. Idiopathic ventricular fibrillation (IVF) is an uncommon disease of unknown etiology that manifests as syncope, cardiac arrest or seizures caused by rapid polymorphic ventricular tachycardia (VT) or VF in the absence of structural heart disease or identifiable channelopathy. Usually during an arrhythmic storm, it is relatively easy to diagnose IVF in a cardiac arrest survivor when the onset of spontaneous polymorphic VT/VF can be recorded, and this shows initiation of polymorphic VT/VF by very short coupled ventricular ectopy. Conduction block was found responsible for wave front fractionation and reentry, an important mechanism in proliferation of wave fronts and rotors during VF. IVF is essentially a diagnosis by exclusion. However, typical clinical and electrophysiological characteristics present in some patients often allows for a positive diagnosis. Since the rate of recurrence of malignant ventricular arrhythmias in IVF is unacceptably high in the absence of therapy, once a diagnosis of IVF is made, some form of therapy is mandatory. Therapy may include ICD implantation, drug therapy, radiofrequency catheter ablation of the triggering

---

[*] Address for correspondence: Prof. Dr. Osmar A. Centurión, MD, PhD, FACC., Associate Professor of Medicine, Faculty of Medical Sciences, Asunción National University, Trejo y Sanabria 1657, Sajonia, Asunción, Paraguay, E-mail: osmarcenturion@hotmail.com, Tel-fax: 595-21-421423

focus or combinations of the above. In this chapter, it will be discussed the electrophysiological mechanisms, clinical prognosis and therapeutic management of VF in the absence of apparent structural heart disease.

## INTRODUCTION

During the last two decades, important advances have been made in the understanding of the genesis, the electrophysiological mechanism, clinical prognosis and the therapeutic management of idiopathic ventricular fibrillation (IVF) patients. IVF is a rare disorder encountered in only 3% to 9% of cases of out-of-hospital VF not related to an acute coronary syndrome. The majority of patients without apparent structural heart disease who died suddenly do not actually have "normal" hearts. Sudden cardiac death (SCD) in the truly normal heart is an uncommon occurrence. Most individuals suffering from SCD become unconscious within seconds to minutes as a result of insufficient cerebral blood flow. There are usually no premonitory symptoms or signs. Symptoms, if present, are nonspecific and include chest discomfort, palpitations, shortness of breath, and weakness. The actual auxiliary diagnostic methods preclude identification of structural or functional derangement. Although the risks of SCD are higher in patients with structural heart disease, and the underlying pathophysiology for the majority of these deaths is due to coronary artery disease, SCD events also occur in individuals with apparently normal hearts (1-5).

In a small number of cases of survivors of SCD, despite extensive clinical evaluation, no underlying structural heart disease can be found. In the past decade, increasing attention has focused on this group of survivors of out-of-hospital cardiac arrest, which is also known as IVF (1-3). The etiology of many of these deaths was unknown and deemed "idiopathic." However, subsequent discoveries have identified the cause of death in many of these patients. In 1929, Dock described the case of a 36-year-old male with clusters of syncope caused by documented VF that terminated spontaneously (1). Organic heart disease was appropriately excluded with the technologies then available. Similar case reports followed and in 1987 Belhassen published the first series of IVF (2), emphasizing the importance of electrophysiological evaluation with programmed ventricular stimulation and the high efficacy of quinidine for preventing inducible and spontaneous VF (2). The first systematic review on IVF was published in 1990 (3). The typical clinical characteristics of IVF were summarized and are stated in Table 1. The mode of onset of spontaneous arrhythmias in IVF, namely, the triggering of rapid polymorphic VT/VF by premature ventricular contractions (PVCs) with very short (R-on-T) coupling intervals is shown in Figure 1. Haissaguerre et al demonstrated that the short-coupled PVCs triggering VF in this disease are very-early PVCs originating from Purkinje fibers (6). The differential diagnosis of IVF included the following arrhythmia-disorders: the long QT syndrome (7-9), the catecholamine sensitive polymorphic VT (CPVT) (10), and the syndrome of nocturnal sudden death of South East Asia (11). However, in 1992, the Brugada brothers described patients with otherwise IVF who had a peculiar electrocardiogram showing right bundle branch block with persistent ST-segment elevation in the right precordial leads (12). It soon became evident that more than 20% of patients thought until then to have IVF had the Brugada syndrome (13). Moreover, in 1997 it became clear that the syndrome of unexplained nocturnal sudden death in South East Asia was in fact, an endemic manifestation of Brugada syndrome in Asia (14). More recently, patients with the congenital short QT syndrome (15, 16) proved to have inducible (15), and spontaneous (17, 18) ventricular arrhythmias indistinguishable from those of IVF patients. Therefore, considering the light shed lately by interesting studies, it will be discussed in this chapter the electrophysiological mechanisms, clinical prognosis and therapeutic management of VF in the absence of apparent structural heart disease.

**Table 1. Typical clinical characteristics of Idiopathic Ventricular Fibrillation**

| | |
|---|---|
| 1. | The onset of symptoms during early adulthood in both genders. |
| 2. | The relatively high incidence of arrhythmic storms with clusters of VF episodes. |
| 3. | The high inducibility rate of VF with programmed ventricular stimulation. |
| 4. | The excellent response to quinidine therapy. |

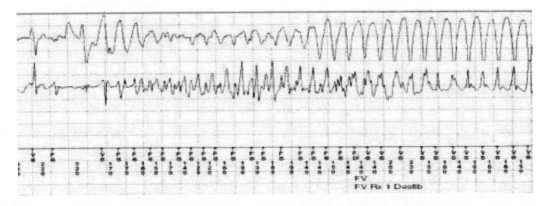

Figure 1. Recorded strip from an ICD placed in a young adult with idiopathic VF and recurrent syncope. It shows the beginning of an episode of IVF.

# ELECTROPHYSIOLOGICAL DATA AND MECHANISMS IN IVF

Electrophysiological studies in animals and humans have determined the existence of a vulnerable period in the cardiac cycle, during which a single premature stimulus of appropriate strength can reproducibly induce VF. The most vulnerable phase, as judged from the stimulus strength needed to induce VF, is the upslope of the T wave, but the peak and early phases of the T wave down-slope are also within this vulnerable phase. Stimulation during this vulnerable period, at a time when there is maximal dispersion of refractoriness in the ventricle, leads to functional unidirectional block and multiple reentrant waves of VF even in a normal ventricle. Some investigators have reported the presence of fractionated right ventricular potentials during ventricular extra-stimulation in patients with IVF. Conduction block was found responsible for wave front fractionation and reentry, an important mechanism in proliferation of wave fronts and rotors during VF. Induction of polymorphic VT by programmed ventricular stimulation is often viewed as an artifact or a non-clinical arrhythmia in patients without organic heart disease. In addition, the odds of inducing polymorphic VT or VF are inversely related to the coupling intervals used during ventricular extra-stimulation. Therefore, induction of sustained polymorphic VT and VF in patients with a history of cardiac arrest may be clinically relevant. Moreover, the spontaneous arrhythmias leading to cardiac arrest in IVF are indeed polymorphic and are precipitated by PVCs with a short coupling interval. Thus, whenever IVF is suspected following an episode of cardiac arrest, protocols of programmed extra-stimulation using short coupling intervals should be considered.

There are some interesting findings lately that shed some light into the understanding of the mechanism and etiology of IVF. Almost 8 decades after the original description of IVF (1), the etiology of this disorder remains a mystery. There are some clinical and electrophysiological data which suggest that IVF is a channelopathy. The spontaneous and inducible ventricular arrhythmias of IVF are remarkably similar to those observed in two well-described channelopathies involving hereditary malfunction of sodium channels (Brugada syndrome) (19) or potassium channels (short QT syndromes) (20-22). Moreover, patients with the Brugada syndrome may have the typical diagnostic electrocardiogram with ST segment elevation in the right precordial leads at some times, but may have normal or near-normal electrocardiograms at other times, making distinction of patients with IVF and Brugada syndrome challenging. In fact, a diagnosis of IVF is not considered definite until the Brugada syndrome with near normal electrocardiogram is excluded by performing a drug-challenge with a sodium-channel blocker, namely, ajmaline (23-25), flecainide (25-27), disopyramide (28) or procainamide (29). These drugs will worsen any inborn malfunction of sodium channels, augmenting the ST segment elevation in up to 40% of patients with Brugada syndrome who have a normal electrocardiogram (19, 25, 30). On the other hand, the fact that only a minority of patients with IVF report a familial history of sudden death (3, 31-36) is a strong argument against the role of genetic channelopathies in this disease.

The electrocardiogram of patients with IVF is normal during sinus rhythm. Japanese investigators reported that patients with IVF often have J-point elevation in the inferior leads (37). Male patients with IVF have a disproportionally high prevalence of relatively short QT (18). The Tpeak-Tend interval, that is the interval from the summit to the end of the T wave, which is a marker of the ventricular dispersion of repolarization and arrhythmic risk in the long QT syndromes (38, 39) and Brugada syndrome (40), is normal in IVF (18). PVCs only rarely occur in patients with IVF, but when they do, they have varying coupling intervals with some PVCs closely coupled to the preceding complex. The mean coupling interval was 297±41 ms in the series of Haissaguerre (32), and 300±35 in the series of Champagne (34). Because of the short coupling interval, the PVCs fall on the summit or the descending limb of the T wave. There appears to be an inverse relationship between the coupling interval of the PVCs and the risk for malignant arrhythmias with longer bursts of polymorphic VT triggered by PVCs with shorter coupling intervals (32). In contrast to the polymorphic ventricular arrhythmias recorded in the long QT syndrome (41, 42), the QT (357±41 ms) and QTc (397±56 ms) of the sinus complexes immediately before the onset of arrhythmias are normal (5, 34) and arrhythmias are as a rule not pause dependent (3, 31-34). In early reports showing the onset of IVF (1, 3, 43), a similar ECG pattern of the first short-coupled PVC was observed, namely left bundle branch block pattern and left axis deviation. However, later reports (32, 33), showed that PVCs with other patterns do exist, suggesting various possible origin sites. Interestingly, when multiple episodes of polymorphic VT are recorded with 12-leads recordings, the morphology of the initiating beats of all these episodes is similar. This applies not only to the first complex, but to the second and third complexes of the polymorphic arrhythmias as well. The last observation supports the notion that IVF has a focal origin. In this regard, Haissaguerre et al recently proposed that IVF represents a "focal VF" triggered by ectopic beats originating from Purkinje fibers (33). These Purkinje PVCs are so premature that fall on the vulnerable period of the surrounding ventricular tissue, initiating reentrant VF. Radiofrequency ablation directed to this very early VPC with a recorded Purkinje potential terminated IVF in selected patients. Figure 2 shows a recorded Purkinje potential with the ablation catheter prior to radiofrequency ablation. The very-early Purkinje ectopic beats have been demonstrated by intracardiac recordings (33) but the reason for this very-premature focal activity remains to be determined.

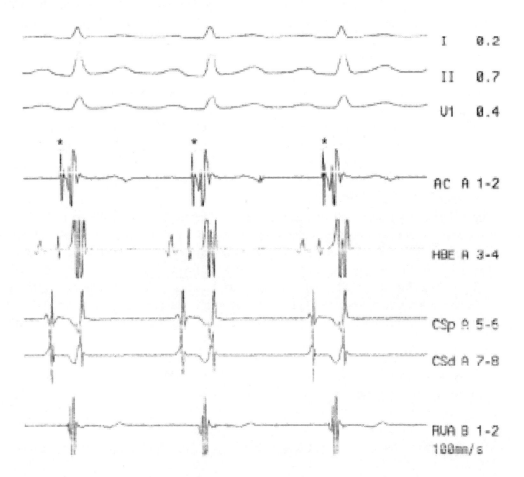

Figure 2. Endocardial mapping during the electrophysiological study that demonstrates a Purkinje potential (shown with asterisks), at the ablation catheter site, prior to radiofrequency ablation. The Purkinje potential preceded the local myocardial activation by 14 ms during sinus rhythm.

Electrophysiological studies performed in patients with IVF demonstrate normal A-H and H-V intervals, and their ventricular refractory periods are within normal limits (2, 44). This is in contrast to patients with Brugada syndrome, who often have prolonged H-V interval (12) and patients with short QT syndrome, who invariably have short refractory periods in the atrium and the ventricle (15, 45, 46). The ventricular arrhythmias induced by programmed ventricular stimulation are invariably of polymorphic morphology, namely polymorphic VT or VF. Induction of monomorphic VT excludes the diagnosis of IVF. This is different in patients with Brugada syndrome who also have primarily VF (47), but rarely have monomorphic VT (48-53). The inducibility rate is a function of the protocol used during programmed ventricular stimulation. In earlier small studies, 9% of healthy individuals without documented or suspected spontaneous ventricular arrhythmias had inducible VF when the coupling intervals were limited only by ventricular refractoriness. Moreover, an additional 40% had inducible non-sustained polymorphic VT and this lead to premature discontinuation of the pacing protocol. Therefore, one must recognize that at least 9% of healthy individuals will have inducible VF if aggressive protocols of extra-stimulation are utilized (54-56). On the other hand, as many as 80% of patients with IVF have inducible VF with aggressive protocols of extra-stimulation consisting of double and triple ventricular extra-stimuli at two right ventricular pacing sites and using repetition of extra-stimulation at the shortest coupling interval that captures the ventricle (44, 57). This very high-inducibility rate suggests that the induction of VF, with aggressive protocols of extra-stimulation, is a valid endpoint of programmed ventricular stimulation that then may be used for guiding anti-arrhythmic therapy in patients with IVF.

Recently, using endocardial recordings in patients with IVF at a time when they had frequent spontaneous PVCs and/or bursts of polymorphic VT, the investigators were able to locate the site of origin of these ventricular arrhythmias in 27 patients (32, 33). Successful localization of the site of origin of the ventricular arrhythmias was guided by recording of very early endocardial electrograms and confirmed by abolition of ventricular arrhythmias following radiofrequency ablation of the firing focus (Figure 2). Purkinje potentials were recorded at the site of origin of ventricular arrhythmias in 23 (85%) out these 27 patients (in the left ventricular septum in 10 patients, the anterior right ventricle in 9 patients and in both locations in 4). The Purkinje potentials preceded the local myocardial activation by 11±5 ms during sinus rhythm and by 10±15 ms during spontaneous PVC (32). Based on these endocardial recordings, it seems that the arrhythmias in IVF have a focal origin and that the triggering focus is within the Purkinje fibers in the majority of patients. Of note, the firing focus was not within the Purkinje network in only 4 (15%) patients and in all these patients the arrhythmias originated in the right ventricular outflow tract (RVOT). Other sites were also described in detail, Noda and Shimizu recently reported a large series of patients with polymorphic VT/VF originating in the RVOT (41, 58).

## CLINICAL MANIFESTATIONS AND DIFFERENTIAL DIAGNOSIS IN IVF

There are some clinical characteristics in IVF patients that need consideration. Patients with IVF present with either syncope or cardiac arrest in early adulthood. It is not clear why some events of polymorphic VT terminate spontaneously causing syncope, while others deteriorate to fine ventricular fibrillation causing cardiac arrest. In Figure 3 there is an example of IVF that terminates spontaneously causing sometimes dizziness or syncope. The mean age at presentation in several series has been 35-45 years and the vast majority is older than 20 years and younger than 65 years old at the time of presentation (31, 34). Two thirds of the patients are males. The arrhythmias provoking syncope and those causing cardiac arrest are similar in terms of mode of onset, ventricular rate and polymorphic morphology. The proportion of patients presenting with cardiac arrest, as opposed to syncope, is much higher in

IVF than in other channelopathies causing polymorphic ventricular tachyarrhythmias like the long QT syndrome or CPVT (35). In other words, arrhythmias in IVF occur rarely, but once they occur they are generally sustained. As a rule, syncope and cardiac arrest in IVF are not related to effort or emotional stress (3, 31, 32). Sleep-related arrhythmias, which are common in sodium channelopathies, are rare in IVF (13, 32). Finally, about 25% of patients with IVF present with arrhythmic storms, that is, with clusters of VF episodes recurring within 24-48 hours (3, 31). Some of these VF clusters have been triggered by fever (36).

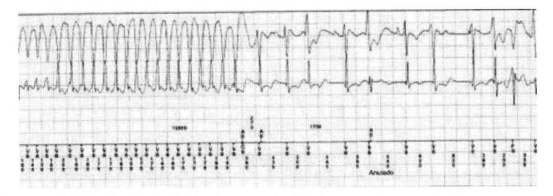

Figure 3. Recorded strip from an ICD placed in a young adult with idiopathic VF and recurrent syncope. It demonstrates the spontaneous termination of the arrhythmia.

IVF is a diagnosis by exclusion. Several times the patients are admitted after resuscitation from cardiac arrest and have documented ventricular fibrillation, but recordings of the initiation of the arrhythmia are not available. In such cases, the diagnosis of IVF is established by excluding all identifiable causes and further supported by the inducibility of VF with programmed ventricular stimulation. However, several etiologies for VF may be difficult to exclude even with invasive studies. For example, genotyping of families with a congenital long QT syndrome has demonstrated considerable overlapping in the duration of the QT interval between patients affected with a long QT gene and unaffected controls. However, during an arrhythmic storm, diagnosing IVF in a cardiac arrest survivor is relatively easy when the onset of spontaneous polymorphic VT/VF is recorded, showing initiation of polymorphic VT/VF by very short coupled PVCs (3, 31, 42). Other conditions that lead to such characteristic mode of VF initiation, namely myocardial ischemia (59-60), Brugada syndrome (61), and short QT syndrome (17) can be identified with appropriate testing.

The diagnosis of IVF must be considered in patients presenting with syncope without documented arrhythmias. In the majority of patients presenting with syncope in the absence of heart disease a diagnosis of vasovagal syncope, rather than arrhythmic syncope, will be evident already from the clinical history. Also, the vast majority of patients with syncope who does not appear to be of vasovagal origin have electrocardiographic or echocardiographic abnormalities that will suggest an underlying diagnosis. Non-invasive studies including drug challenges to exclude Brugada syndrome (25, 30), long QT syndrome (62-65) and Wolff Parkinson White (66) should be performed. Moreover, electrophysiologic evaluation can be performed to exclude intra-His block as the cause of syncope.

## Minimal Organic Heart Disease

Although not easy to be done, excluding all forms of organic heart disease is essential before the diagnosis of IVF is considered. However, it should be noted that some forms of organic heart disease, namely hypertrophic cardiomyopathy, and right ventricular dysplasia, may cause malignant ventricular arrhythmias at a time when the anatomic abnormalities are minimal and difficult to detect by imaging modalities. For example, patients with hypertrophic cardiomyopathy due to Troponin-T mutations may be at risk for arrhythmic death at a time when left ventricular hypertrophy is still mild (67, 68). Arrithmogenic right ventricular dysplasia is sometimes identified as the underlying cause of sudden death only during forensic examination and despite negative extensive diagnostic workup (69). Other subtle anatomic abnormalities, like mitral valve prolapse without hemodynamic significance, should not necessarily be accepted as the cause of cardiac arrest. On the other hand, signs of severe left ventricular dysfunction after resuscitation should not necessarily be used to exclude the diagnosis of IVF because prolonged resuscitation may result in transient electrocardiographic and echocardiographic abnormalities that are indistinguishable from those seen in patients with dilated cardiomyopathy (70). If such abnormalities resolved during the follow-up period, the diagnosis of IVF should obviously be considered.

## Wolff-Parkinson-White (WPW) Syndrome

Different electrophysiological properties in WPW patients may preclude the diagnosis of pre-excitation during sinus rhythm. Patients with atrioventricular accessory pathways may have minimal or no ventricular preexcitation. Patients may have narrow QRS complexes if they also have fast conduction along the AV node or if their accessory pathway is located on the left lateral wall far away from the sinus node. Patients with accessory pathways that have short refractory periods may develop atrial fibrillation with rapid ventricular rates that may deteriorate to VF (71). If the preexcited atrial fibrillation is not recorded and the patient is found in VF, the near-normal electrocardiogram during sinus rhythm may lead to a wrong diagnosis of "IVF" because all imaging tests will be normal. The wrong diagnosis of IVF may gain further support from electrophysiologic studies if atrial stimulation is not performed prior to ventricular pacing because programmed ventricular stimulation is likely to induce VF in patients with WPW (71). Therefore, excluding accessory pathways, either with adenosine injection as a bedside test or with atrial pacing during electrophysiologic studies, is a mandatory step in the work-up of VF survivors even when the electrocardiogram is judged to be normal. Of note, rare cases of cardiac arrest caused by very rapid supraventricular tachyarrhythmias in patients without Wolff-Parkinson-White have also been described (72).

## Catecholamine Sensitive Polymorphic VT (CPVT)

Exercise stress test should be performed in survivors of cardiac arrest events. Physicians may not perform an exercise test in cardiac arrest survivors reasoning that coronary angiography will eventually reveal any significant coronary lesion. However, there are patients with CPVT who were erroneously diagnosed as IVF only because exercise stress testing was not performed. Since all other tests, including electrophysiologic studies, are invariably normal in this disease, exercise stress test is a mandatory test in cardiac arrest survivors. The majority of patients with CPVT have a pathognomonic response to exercise, namely, exercise-induced atrial fibrillation followed my multifocal PVCs, bidirectional VT and polymorphic VT. However, it was recently recognized that some patients with genetically proven CPVT have only single PVCs that look like typical benign right ventricular outflow tract (RVOT) extrasystoles during maximal exercise (73). Such patients may be wrongly diagnosed as having IVF.

## Long QT Syndrome (LQTS)

The QTc intervals of the healthy population, as well as the QTc of patients with LQTS have a normal distribution and there is considerable overlapping between the QTc of both populations. Importantly, 12% of patients with genetically proven LQTS have a normal QT when the latter is defined as QTc <440 msec (74). Identifying patients with LQTS who have borderline QT interval is especially challenging in the LQT1 genotype because the T-wave morphology, which is frequently abnormal in LQT2 and LQT3, is most often normal in LQT1. Fortunately, the epinephrine challenge test is especially effective for unraveling abnormal QT responses in LQT1 (62-64, 75).

## Short QT Syndrome (SQTS)

Distinguishing IVF from SQTS is not easy. The newly described SQTS (15, 16) is caused by genetic mutations involving the same potassium channels that cause the LQTS but with an opposite effect (20, 22, 30, 76-78). In the SQTS there is excessive outflow of potassium currents, shortening the action potential duration and the effective ventricular refractory period. Although the original cases of SQTS had extremely short QT intervals (QTc shorter than 300 ms) (15, 16), more recently described cases of genetically proven SQTS have QTc intervals of 320 ms (22). It was also described that relatively short QT intervals (QTc <360 ms) are frequently observed in healthy males but are statistically more common in males with IVF (18). Moreover, patients with IVF have normal QT intervals at normal heart rates, but their QT fails to lengthen as their heart rate slows down, leading to abnormally short QTc values during bradycardia (79-81). Finally, patients with SQTS and patients with IVF share the following clinically characteristics: 1) Both patient groups have similar spontaneous (5, 17) and inducible (3, 46) ventricular arrhythmias; 2) both patient groups appear to respond especially well to quinidine therapy (2, 44, 45, 82); 3) both patient groups are at risk for inappropriate ICD-shocks because of intracardiac T-wave oversensing (83, 84). Patients with SQTS may be misdiagnosed as "IVF" if the QT interval is measured only during relatively rapid heart rates. This is because the main problem in the SQTS is failure of appropriate QT lengthening during bradycardia (46). This familial syndrome of an abnormally shortened QT interval and arrhythmias is characterized by the features stated in Table 2.

**Table 2. Characteristics and features of the Short QT interval syndrome**

| | |
|---|---|
| 1) | An autosomal dominant pattern of inheritance. |
| 2) | A corrected QT interval (QTc) equal to or more than 340 ms. |
| 3) | An increased risk of sudden cardiac death due to ventricular fibrillation. |
| 4) | Atrial fibrillation, which often occurs at a young age. |
| 5) | Short atrial and ventricular refractory periods at electrophysiological study. |

## Brugada Syndrome

The Brugada syndrome is a genetically transmitted arrhythmogenic disease that is associated with an increased risk of SCD. The Brugada brothers described patients with otherwise IVF who had a peculiar electrocardiogram showing right bundle branch block with persistent ST-segment elevation in the right precordial leads (12). It is estimated that 20% of patients originally diagnosed as IVF have in fact Brugada syndrome (13) and very similar incidences were reported by others (85). Moreover, if all patients with IVF undergo systematic testing with repeated electrocardiograms, placing the right precordial electrodes in places at higher positions (86), and with pharmacological challenge test using sodium-channel blockers to unravel subtle sodium-channel malfunction, as many as 40% with IVF could be diagnosed as Brugada syndrome (19).

## Short-Coupled Variant of Right Ventricular Outflow Tachycardia

The right ventricular outflow tract (RVOT) is the site of origin of the most common type of VT occurring in patients without organic heart disease (31). This RVOT-VT has a distinctive morphology, QRS complexes with left bundle branch block pattern and tall R waves in the inferior leads. RVOT-VT is generally considered a benign arrhythmia that does not produce hemodynamic alteration (31). However, it was recently described (58, 87) certain patients with otherwise typical benign RVOT PVCs who went on to develop spontaneous VF or polymorphic VT (88). It is not clear if patients with IVF and patients with this newly described form of polymorphic VT from the RVOT (58, 87, 89) represent different aspects of one disease or two distinct disorders (88). However, several characteristics differ among both groups: 1) otherwise typical monomorphic RVOT-VT is also seen in patients with malignant polymorphic RVOT-VT (58, 87) but is never seen in IVF (3, 31, 32). 2) Only 5% of patients with malignant polymorphic VT have inducible VF by programmed ventricular stimulation, whereas the majority of patients with IVF have inducible VF (44). 3) the coupling interval of the PVCs initiating the malignant ventricular arrhythmias is invariably very short in IVF (5, 32) but is longer, varying from relatively short (87) to normal (58) in the polymorphic RVOT-VT. The last observation is consistent with the results of intracardiac mapping performed by Haissaguerre et al (32). In that series, IVF originated from Purkinje fibers in 86% of the patients and from the RVOT in the remaining 14%. Again, the coupling interval of the PVCs initiating VF was longer for arrhythmias originating in the RVOT than for arrhythmias triggered by Purkinje fibers ($355\pm30$ ms vs. $280\pm26$ ms, $p<0.01$).

## PROGNOSIS AND THERAPEUTIC MANAGEMENT IN IVF

Among survivors of SCD due to IVF, the reported rate of recurrent VF ranges between 22 and 37 percent at two to four years. Because they have no structural heart disease, these patients have an excellent prognosis for long-term survival if VF is prevented. As a result, such patients are best treated with an ICD. At a mean follow-up of 6 years, more than 40% of patients have recurrent VF and the risk is higher for those with normal electrocardiograms, that is, after excluding those with possible Brugada syndrome (90). In a recent series of IVF patients with exclusion not only those with Brugada-type electrocardiogram at baseline but also those who developed ST-segment elevation when challenged with sodium channel blockers, the risk for recurrent VF was 39% at 3 years (34). Therefore, once a diagnosis of IVF is made, some form of therapy is mandatory. Therapy may include ICD implantation, drug therapy, radiofrequency catheter ablation of the triggering focus or combinations of the above.

## Pharmacological Therapy

The very first patients with IVF were treated with quinidine after multiple episodes of spontaneous polymorphic VT and VF were clearly documented. Both patients had an excellent response (1, 91-93). In 1987, Belhassen pioneered the therapy of IVF with EPS-guided quinidine after observing that VF is easily inducible at the baseline state but no longer inducible after quinidine therapy (2). Of note, one of the patients included in that original report (43), recently completed 25 uneventful years of electrophysiologic-guided therapy with amiodarone and quinidine after experiencing arrhythmic storms of VF in the absence of therapy and recurrent arrhythmic syncope on amiodarone alone (93).

It was found that the recurrence rate of cardiac arrest was high during therapy with other antiarrhythmic drugs, including amiodarone, beta-blockers or verapamil (3). The high-rate of arrhythmia recurrence with verapamil is worth noting because that drug was empirically proposed by Leenhardt and Coumel to treat the short-coupled variant of torsade de pointes (4), an entity that probably represents IVF. In contrast, there was no recurrence reported with quinidine (3). The criteria for quinidine therapy in IVF survivors are stated in Table 3, and may be summarized as follows: Of 34 patients with IVF with aborted sudden cardiac arrest, 26 (80%) had inducible VF at baseline electrophysiologic study and all but one of them were rendered non-inducible with quinidine. Side effects from quinidine led to discontinuation of quinidine therapy in 14% of our patients. Nevertheless, 23 patients remained on quinidine therapy without ICD back-up, and all are alive and completely free of arrhythmic symptoms that now exceeds 10 years. It is very important to consider the risks of most anti-arrhythmic drugs with regard to the potential for loss of efficacy or pro-arrhythmia under a number of clinical conditions including hypokalemia, hypomagnesemia, bradycardia, therapy with other agents that alter repolarization, metabolic inhibitors, and changes in myocardial substrate. Nevertheless, it is no longer recommend empiric use of quinidine for non-inducible patients, a subgroup of patients for whom ICD implantation is mandatory. The excellent response of VF storms in IVF with Brugada syndrome has also been repeatedly reported (95-97).

### Table 3. Criteria for quinidine therapy in IVF survivors

| | |
|---|---|
| 1) | Diagnosis of IVF with or without Brugada syndrome. |
| 2) | Inducible VF in the absence of drugs with programmed ventricular stimulation. |
| 3) | No-inducible arrhythmias during oral quinidine therapy despite a very aggressive protocol of ventricular stimulation. |
| 4) | Informed consent by a patient who is well informed of the risk and benefits of ICD and quinidine therapy for this disease. |
| 5) | Repeated assertion of drug compliance during long-term follow-up (compliance is assessed with quinidine serum levels and quinidine-effect on the QT interval). |

## Radiofrequency Catheter Ablation

The optimal timing for the electrophysiologic mapping and ablation procedure is when the patient has frequent PVCs. The origin of the PVCs is localized by mapping the earliest site of electrical activity and/or pace mapping. Purkinje origin is identified by the Purkinje potential, a sharp spike of less than 10 ms duration, occurring before the PVC. Catheter-based radiofrequency ablation of the triggering focus is now an accepted mode of therapy for IVF. This form of therapy has been used primarily to treat patients with implanted ICDs who are receiving multiple ICD shocks because of arrhythmic storms (32, 98, 99). The first successful ablation was reported by Aizawa in 1992 (98) whereas relatively large series have been reported by others (32, 33, 58). The series of Haissaguerre (32, 33) and Noda and Shimizu (58) differ in the site of origin of the targeted arrhythmias: Noda and Shimizu targeted polymorphic VT originating from the RVOT (58). In contrast, 85% of the polymorphic ventricular arrhythmias ablated by Haissaguerre et al. were mapped to the Purkinje system in the right or left ventricle while the site of origin of the VF was in the RVOT in only 4 (15%) patients (32). An acute successful ablation was achieved in all cases while 24 patients (89%) had no recurrence of VF without drug during follow-up. Such favorable results do certainly stimulate adopting such a curative option for treating patients with IVF. However, since the etiology of IVF is unknown, at this moment it is hard to understand that this is a focal disease.

## Implantable Cardioverter-Defibrillator

An implantable cardioverter-defibrillator (ICD) is the preferred therapeutic modality in most survivors of SCD. An ICD shock does certainly terminate an episode of spontaneous or induced IVF (Figure 4). This change in practice is based upon improvements in device technology, clinical trials demonstrating improved outcomes with an ICD compared to pharmacological therapy, and concerns about the toxicity associated with antiarrhythmic drugs. No doubt that ICD offers the most effective therapy for preventing arrhythmic death in IVF. Indeed, ICD implantation is considered the only effective therapy for IVF by most authors. However, the complication rate of the implantation procedure has also to be considered. In the AVID trial, a large multicenter study of ICD implantation for malignant ventricular arrhythmias in patients with organic heart disease (100), the risk of adverse events serious enough to warrant re-intervention, was 12% (101). Considering that an ICD terminates episodes of IVF (Figure 4) but does not prevent arrhythmias, patients who have frequent symptoms or device discharges from recurrent arrhythmias may benefit from adjunctive anti-arrhythmic drug therapy, usually beginning with empiric amiodarone. Such drug therapy, by reducing the frequency of appropriate shocks, can improve the patient's quality of life. Anti-arrhythmic drugs, again beginning with empiric amiodarone, are also indicated in SCD survivors who are not candidates for or refuse an ICD.

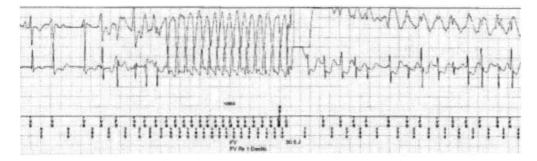

Figure 4. Recorded strip from an ICD placed in a young adult with idiopathic VF and recurrent syncope. It demonstrates termination of the arrhythmia with a 30 joules ICD shock.

## CONCLUSION

VF is a challenging arrhythmia for physicians, with only a limited number of treatment options available. ICD therapy is the treatment of choice for patients with both primary and secondary prevention with the role of antiarrhythmic therapy aimed at reducing the number of recurrences. Implantable devices do not prevent arrhythmias, thus, patients who have frequent symptoms or device discharges from recurrent arrhythmias may benefit from adjunctive anti-arrhythmic drug therapy. Drug therapy usually begins with empiric amiodarone, or quinidine therapy for appropriately selected patients with IVF. Such therapy, by reducing the frequency of appropriate shocks, can improve the patient's quality of life. In some patients, antiarrhythmic drug treatment is still an efficient approach, but predicting which patients will respond positively to drug treatment is often hampered by the absence of a reliable parameter to predict a favourable outcome.

Secondary and primary prevention trials have demonstrated the superiority of ICD compared with antiarrhythmic medication in preventing death. Although, ICD therapy represents the gold standard treatment for this condition the underlying substrate for the arrhythmia is unchanged. Considering that the trigger for VF is ventricular ectopy in the majority of patients, ablation of this trigger lead to abolition of VF in many cases. Therefore, catheter ablation is an accepted treatment for a number of patients with IVF. The Purkinje network is critical in the triggering and maintenance of VF, thus, catheter ablation targeting the PVCs or Purkinje potentials responsible for triggering VF was shown to be both possible and efficacious in IVF. Although the long-term results are awaited, the short-term results are very encouraging, and the procedure appears robust as it is being repeated by a number of different groups around the world. Long-term follow-up studies are required to demonstrate whether ablation of the trigger results in a definitive cure for these patients.

# REFERENCES

[1] Dock W. Transitory ventricular fibrillation as a cause of syncope and its prevention by quinidine sulfate. *Am Heart J* 1929;4:709-14.
[2] Belhassen B, Shapira I, Shoshani D, Paredes A, Miller H, Laniado S. Idiopathic ventricular fibrillation: inducibility and beneficial effects of class I antiarrhythmic agents. *Circulation* 1987;75:809-16.
[3] Viskin S, Belhassen B. Idiopathic ventricular fibrillation. *Am Heart J* 1990;120:661-71.
[4] Leenhardt A, Glaser E, Burguera M, Nurnberg M, Maison-Blanche P, Coumel P. Short-coupled variant of torsade de pointes. A new electrocardiographic entity in the spectrum of idiopathic ventricular tachyarrhythmias. *Circulation* 1994;89:206-15.
[5] Viskin S, Lesh M, Eldar M, et al. Mode of onset of malignant ventricular arrhythmias in idiopathic ventricular fibrillation. *J Cardiovasc Electrophysiol* 1997;8:1115-20.
[6] Haissaguerre M, Extramiana F, Hocini M, et al. Mapping and ablation of ventricular fibrillation associated with long-QT and Brugada syndromes. *Circulation* 2003;108:925-8.
[7] Jervell A, Lange-Nielsen F. Congenital deaf-mutism, functional heart disease with prolongation of the Q-T interval and sudden death. *Am Heart J* 1957;54:59-68.
[8] Romano C, Gemme G, Pongiglione R. Aritmie cardiache rare dell'eta pediatrica. *Clin Pediat* 1963;45:656-83.
[9] Ward OC. A new familial cardiac syndrome in children. *J Irish Med Assoc* 1964;54:103-6.
[10] Leenhardt A, Lucet V, Denjoy I, Grau F, Ngoc D, Coumel P. Catecholaminergic polymorphic ventricular tachycardia in children. A 7-year follow-up of 21 patients. *Circulation* 1995;91:1512-9.
[11] Aponte G. The enigma of "Bangungut". *Ann Intern Med* 1960;52:1258-63.
[12] Brugada P, Brugada J. Right bundle branch block, persistent ST segment elevation and sudden cardiac death: a distinct clinical and electrocardiographic syndrome. A multicenter report. *J Am Coll Cardiol* 1992;20:1391-6.
[13] Viskin S, Fish R, Eldar M, et al. Prevalence of the Brugada sign in idiopathic ventricular fibrillation and healthy controls. *Heart* 2000;84:31-6.
[14] Nademanee K, Veerakul G, Nimmannit S, et al. Arrhythmogenic marker for the sudden unexpected death syndrome in Thai men. *Circulation* 1997;96:2595-600.
[15] Gaita F, Giustetto C, Bianchi F, et al. Short QT Syndrome: a familial cause of sudden death. *Circulation* 2003;108:965-70.
[16] Gussak I, Brugada P, Brugada J, et al. Idiopathic short QT interval: a new clinical syndrome? *Cardiology* 2000;94:99-102.
[17] Schimpf R, Bauersfeld U, Gaita F, Wolpert C. Short QT syndrome: successful prevention of sudden cardiac death in an adolescent by implantable cardioverter-defibrillator treatment for primary prophylaxis. *Heart Rhythm* 2005;2:416-7.
[18] Viskin S, Zeltser D, Ish-Shalom M, et al. Is idiopathic ventricular fibrillation a short QT syndrome? Comparison of QT intervals of patients with idiopathic ventricular fibrillation and healthy controls. *Heart Rhythm* 2004;1:587-91.
[19] Chen Q, Kirsch GE, Zhang D, et al. Genetic basis and molecular mechanism for idiopathic ventricular fibrillation. *Nature* 1998;392:293-6.

[20] Bellocq C, van Ginneken AC, Bezzina CR, et al. Mutation in the KCNQ1 gene leading to the short QT-interval syndrome. *Circulation* 2004;109:2394-7.

[21] Brugada R, Hong K, Dumaine R, et al. Sudden death associated with short-QT syndrome linked to mutations in HERG. *Circulation* 2004;109:30-5.

[22] Priori SG, Pandit SV, Rivolta I, et al. A novel form of short QT syndrome (SQT3) is caused by a mutation in the KCNJ2 gene. *Circ Res* 2005;96:800-7.

[23] Hong K, Brugada J, Oliva A, et al. Value of electrocardiographic parameters and ajmaline test in the diagnosis of Brugada syndrome caused by SCN5A mutations. *Circulation* 2004;110:3023-7.

[24] Rolf S, Bruns HJ, Wichter T, et al. The ajmaline challenge in Brugada syndrome: diagnostic impact, safety, and recommended protocol. *Eur Heart J* 2003;24:1104-12.

[25] Wolpert C, Echternach C, Veltmann C, et al. Intravenous drug challenge using flecainide and ajmaline in patients with Brugada syndrome. *Heart Rhythm* 2005;2:254-60.

[26] Meregalli PG, Ruijter JM, Hofman N, Bezzina CR, Wilde AA, Tan HL. Diagnostic value of flecainide testing in unmasking SCN5A-related Brugada syndrome. *J Cardiovasc Electrophysiol* 2006 (in press).

[27] Priori SG, Napolitano C, Schwartz PJ, Bloise R, Crotti L, Ronchetti E. The elusive link between LQT3 and Brugada syndrome: the role of flecainide challenge. *Circulation* 2000;102:945-7.

[28] Chinushi M, Aizawa Y, Ogawa Y, Shiba M, Takahashi K. Discrepant drug action of disopyramide on ECG abnormalities and induction of ventricular arrhythmias in a patient with Brugada syndrome. *J Electrocardiol* 1997;30:133-6.

[29] Sangwatanaroj S, Prechawat S, Sunsaneewitayakul B, Sitthisook S, Tosukhowong P, Tungsanga K. New electrocardiographic leads and the procainamide test for the detection of the Brugada sign in sudden unexplained death syndrome survivors and their relatives. *Eur Heart J* 2001;22:2290-6.

[30] Hong K, Bjerregaard P, Gussak I, Brugada R. Short QT syndrome and atrial fibrillation caused by mutation in KCNH2. *J Cardiovasc Electrophysiol* 2005;16:394-6.

[31] Belhassen B, Viskin S. Idiopathic ventricular tachycardia and fibrillation. *J Cardiovasc Electrophysiol* 1993;4:356-68.

[32] Haissaguerre M, Shoda M, Jais P, et al. Mapping and ablation of idiopathic ventricular fibrillation. *Circulation* 2002;106:962-7.

[33] Haissaguerre M, Shah DC, Jais P, et al. Role of Purkinje conducting system in triggering of idiopathic ventricular fibrillation. *Lancet* 2002;359:677-8.

[34] Champagne J, Geelen P, Philippon F, Brugada P. Recurrent cardiac events in patients with idiopathic ventricular fibrillation, excluding patients with the Brugada syndrome. *BMC Med* 2005;3:1-6.

[35] Viskin S, Belhassen B. Polymorphic ventricular tachyarrhythmias in the absence of organic heart disease. Classification, differential diagnosis and implications for therapy. *Prog Cardiovasc Dis* 1998;41:17-34.

[36] Pasquie JL, Sanders P, Hocini M, et al. Fever as a precipitant of idiopathic ventricular fibrillation in patients with normal hearts. J Cardiovasc Electrophysiol 2004;15:1271-6.

[37] Takagi M, Aihara N, Takaki H, et al. Clinical characteristics of patients with spontaneous or inducible ventricular fibrillation without apparent heart disease

presenting with J wave and ST segment elevation in inferior leads. *J Cardiovasc Electrophysiol* 2000;11:844-8.

[38] Shimizu W, Horie M, Ohno S, et al. Mutation site-specific differences in arrhythmic risk and sensitivity to sympathetic stimulation in the LQT1 form of congenital long QT syndrome: multicenter study in Japan. *J Am Coll Cardiol* 2004;44:117-25.

[39] Yan GX, Antzelevitch C. Cellular basis for the normal T wave and the electrocardiographic manifestations of the long-QT syndrome. *Circulation* 1998;98:1928-36.

[40] Castro Hevia J, Antzelevitch C, Tornes Barzaga F, et al. Tpeak-Tend and Tpeak-Tend dispersion as risk factors for ventricular tachycardia/ventricular fibrillation in patients with the Brugada syndrome. *J Am Coll Cardiol* 2006;47:1828-34.

[41] Noda T, Shimizu W, Satomi K, et al. Classification and mechanism of Torsade de Pointes initiation in patients with congenital long QT syndrome. *Eur Heart J* 2004;25:2149-54.

[42] Viskin S, Alla SR, Barron HV, et al. Mode of onset of torsade de pointes in congenital long QT syndrome. *J Am Coll Cardiol* 1996;28:1262-8.

[43] Belhassen B, Pelleg A, Miller HI, Laniado S. Serial electrophysiological studies in a young patient with recurrent ventricular fibrillation. *PACE* 1981;4:92-9.

[44] Belhassen B, Viskin S, Fish R, Glick A, Setbon I, Eldar M. Effects of electrophysiologic-guided therapy with Class IA antiarrhythmic drugs on the long-term outcome of patients with idiopathic ventricular fibrillation with or without the Brugada syndrome. *J Cardiovasc Electrophysiol* 1999;10:1301-12.

[45] Gaita F, Giustetto C, Bianchi F, et al. Short QT syndrome: pharmacological treatment. *J Am Coll Cardiol* 2004;43:1494-9.

[46] Gussak I, Bjerregaard P. Short QT syndrome--5 years of progress. *J Electrocardiol* 2005;38:375-7.

[47] Brugada P, Geelen P, Brugada R, Mont L, Brugada J. Prognostic value of electrophysiologic investigations in Brugada syndrome. *J Cardiovasc Electrophysiol* 2001;12:1004-7.

[48] Boersma LV, Jaarsma W, Jessurun ER, Van Hemel NH, Wever EF. Brugada syndrome: a case report of monomorphic ventricular tachycardia. *Pacing Clin Electrophysiol* 2001;24:112-5.

[49] Dinckal MH, Davutoglu V, Akdemir I, Soydinc S, Kirilmaz A, Aksoy M. Incessant monomorphic ventricular tachycardia during febrile illness in a patient with Brugada syndrome: fatal electrical storm. *Europace* 2003;5:257-61.

[50] Mok NS, Chan NY. Brugada syndrome presenting with sustained monomorphic ventricular tachycardia. *Int J Cardiol* 2004;97:307-9.

[51] Sastry BK, Narasimhan C, Soma Raju B. Brugada syndrome with monomorphic ventricular tachycardia in a one-year-old child. *Indian Heart J* 2001;53:203-5.

[52] Shimada M, Miyazaki T, Miyoshi S, et al. Sustained monomorphic ventricular tachycardia in a patient with Brugada syndrome. *Jpn Circ J* 1996;60:364-70.

[53] Viskin S, Belhassen B. Clinical problem solving: When you only live twice. *N Engl J Med* 1995;332:1221-5.

[54] Brugada P, Green M, Abdollah H, Wellens HJ. Significance of ventricular arrhythmias initiated by programmed ventricular stimulation: the importance of the type of

ventricular arrhythmia induced and the number of premature stimuli required. *Circulation* 1984;69:87-92.

[55] Morady F, DiCarlo L, Baerman J, de Buitleir M. Comparison of coupling intervals that induce clinical and nonclinical forms of ventricular tachycardia during programmed stimulation. *Am J Cardiol* 1986;57:1269-73.

[56] Stevenson WG, Brugada P, Waldecker B, Zehender M, Wellens HJ. Can potentially significant polymorphic ventricular arrhythmias initiated by programmed stimulation be distinguished from those that are nonspecific? *Am Heart J* 1986;111:1073-80.

[57] Belhassen B, Shapira I, Sheps D, Laniado S. Programmed ventricular stimulation using up to two extrastimuli and repetition of double extrastimulation for induction of ventricular tachycardia: a new highly sensitive and specific protocol. *Am J Cardiol* 1990;65:615-22.

[58] Noda T, Shimizu W, Taguchi A, et al. Malignant entity of idiopathic ventricular fibrillation and polymorphic ventricular tachycardia initiated by premature extrasystoles originating from the right ventricular outflow tract. *J Am Coll Cardiol* 2005;46:1288-94.

[59] Myerburg R, Kessler K, Mallon S, et al. Life-threatening ventricular arrhythmias in patients with silent myocardial ischemia due to coronary-artery spasm. *N Engl J Med* 1992;326:1451-5.

[60] Wolfe CL, Nibley C, Bhandari A, Chatterjee K, Scheinman M. Polymorphous ventricular tachycardia associated with acute myocardial infarction. *Circulation* 1991;84:1543-51.

[61] Kakishita M, Kurita T, Matsuo K, et al. Mode of onset of ventricular fibrillation in patients with Brugada syndrome detected by implantable cardioverter defibrillator therapy. *J Am Coll Cardiol* 2000;36:1646-53.

[62] Ackerman MJ, Khositseth A, Tester DJ, Hejlik JB, Shen WK, Porter CB. Epinephrine-induced QT interval prolongation: a gene-specific paradoxical response in congenital long QT syndrome. *Mayo Clin Proc* 2002;77:413-21.

[63] Shimizu W, Noda T, Takaki H, et al. Epinephrine unmasks latent mutation carriers with LQT1 form of congenital long-QT syndrome. *J Am Coll Cardiol* 2003;41:633-42.

[64] Viskin S. Drug challenge with epinephrine or isoproterenol for diagnosing a long QT syndrome: Should we try this at home? *J Cardiovasc Electrophysiol* 2005;16:285-7.

[65] Viskin S, Rosso R, Rogowski O, et al. Provocation of sudden heart rate oscillation with adenosine exposes abnormal QT responses in patients with long QT syndrome: a bedside test for diagnosing long QT syndrome. *Eur Heart J* 2006;27:469-75.

[66] Garratt CJ, Antoniou A, Griffith MJ, Ward DE, Camm AJ. Use of intravenous adenosine in sinus rhythm as a diagnostic test for latent preexcitation. *Am J Cardiol* 1990;65:868-73.

[67] Varnava A, Baboonian C, Davison F, et al. A new mutation of the cardiac troponin T gene causing familial hypertrophic cardiomyopathy without left ventricular hypertrophy. *Heart* 1999;82:621-4.

[68] Varnava AM, Elliott PM, Baboonian C, Davison F, Davies MJ, McKenna WJ. Hypertrophic cardiomyopathy: histopathological features of sudden death in cardiac troponin T disease. *Circulation* 2001;104:1380-4.

[69] Fontaine G, Fornes P, Hebert JL. Ventricular tachycardia in arrhythmogenic right ventricular cardiomyopathies. In: Zipes DP, Jalife J, eds. *Cardiac Electrophysiology: From Cell to Bedside*. 3rd ed. Philadelphia: W.B Saunders; 2003.

[70] Deantonio HJ, Kaul S, Lerman BB. Reversible myocardial depression in survivors of cardiac arrest. *Pacing Clin Electrophysiol* 1990;13:982-5.

[71] Centurión OA, Shimizu A, Isomoto S, Konoe A. Mechanisms for the genesis of paroxysmal atrial fibrillation in the Wolff-Parkinson-White syndrome: Intrinsic atrial muscle vulnerability vs. electrophysiological properties of the accessory pathway. *Europace* 2008;10:294-302.

[72] Wang Y, Griffin J, Lesh M, Cohen T, Chien W, Scheinman M. Patients with supraventricular tachycardia presenting with aborted sudden death: incidence, mechanism and long-term follow-up. *J Am Coll Cardiol* 1991;18:1720-1.

[73] Tester DJ, Kopplin LJ, Will ML, Ackerman MJ. Spectrum and prevalence of cardiac ryanodine receptor (RyR2) mutations in a cohort of unrelated patients referred explicitly for long QT syndrome genetic testing. *Heart Rhythm* 2005;2:1099-105.

[74] Vincent GM, Timothy KW, Leppert M, Keating M. The spectrum of symptoms and QT intervals in carriers of the gene for the long QT syndrome. *N Engl J Med* 1992;327:846-52.

[75] Shimizu W, Noda T, Takaki H, et al. Diagnostic value of epinephrine test for genotyping LQT1, LQT2, and LQT3 forms of congenital long QT syndrome. *Heart Rhythm* 2004;3:273-86.

[76] Borggrefe M, Wolpert C, Antzelevitch C, et al. Short QT syndrome. Genotype-phenotype correlations. *J Electrocardiol* 2005;38:75-80.

[77] Hong K, Piper DR, Diaz-Valdecantos A, et al. De novo KCNQ1 mutation responsible for atrial fibrillation and short QT syndrome in utero. *Cardiovasc Res* 2005;68:433-40.

[78] McPate MJ, Duncan RS, Milnes JT, Witchel HJ, Hancox JC. The N588K-HERG K+ channel mutation in the 'short QT syndrome': mechanism of gain-in-function determined at 37 degrees C. *Biochem Biophys Res Commun* 2005;334:441-9.

[79] Fujiki A, Sugao M, Nishida K, et al. Repolarization abnormality in idiopathic ventricular fibrillation: assessment using 24-hour QT-RR and QaT-RR relationships. *J Cardiovasc Electrophysiol* 2004;15:59-63.

[80] Sugao M, Fujiki A, Nishida K, et al. Repolarization dynamics in patients with idiopathic ventricular fibrillation: pharmacological therapy with bepridil and disopyramide. *J Cardiovasc Pharmacol* 2005;45:545-9.

[81] Sugao M, Fujiki A, Sakabe M, et al. New quantitative methods for evaluation of dynamic changes in QT interval on 24 hour Holter ECG recordings: QT interval in idiopathic ventricular fibrillation and long QT syndrome. *Heart* 2006;92:201-7.

[82] Wolpert C, Schimpf R, Giustetto C, et al. Further insights into the effect of quinidine in short QT syndrome caused by a mutation in HERG. *J Cardiovasc Electrophysiol* 2005;16:54-8.

[83] Schimpf R, Wolpert C, Bianchi F, et al. Congenital short QT syndrome and implantable cardioverter defibrillator treatment: inherent risk for inappropriate shock delivery. *J Cardiovasc Electrophysiol* 2003;14:1273-7.

[84] Strohmer B, Schernthaner C, Pichler M. T-wave oversensing by an implantable cardioverter defibrillator after successful ablation of idiopathic ventricular fibrillation. *Pacing Clin Electrophysiol* 2006;29:431-5.

[85] Remme CA, Wever EF, Wilde AA, Derksen R, Hauer RN. Diagnosis and long-term follow-up of the Brugada syndrome in patients with idiopathic ventricular fibrillation. *Eur Heart J* 2001;22:400-9.

[86] Shimizu W, Matsuo K, Takagi M, et al. Body surface distribution and response to drugs of ST segment elevation in Brugada syndrome: clinical implication of eighty-seven-lead body surface potential mapping and its application to twelve-lead electrocardiograms. *J Cardiovasc Electrophysiol* 2000;11:396-404.

[87] Viskin S, Rosso R, Rogowski O, Belhassen B. The short-coupled variant of right ventricular outflow ventricular tachycardia. A not-so-benign form of benign ventricular tachycardia. *J Cardiovasc Electrophysiol* 2005;16:912-6.

[88] Viskin S, Antzelevitch C. The cardiologists' worst nightmare sudden death from "benign" ventricular arrhythmias. *J Am Coll Cardiol* 2005;46:1295-7.

[89] Ashida K, Kaji Y, Sasaki Y. Abolition of Torsade de Pointes after radiofrequency catheter ablation at right ventricular outflow tract. *Int J Cardiol* 1997;59:171-5.

[90] Wever EF, Robles de Medina EO. Sudden death in patients without structural heart disease. *J Am Coll Cardiol* 2004;43:1137-44.

[91] Moe T. Morgagni-Adams-Stokes attacks caused by transient recurrent ventricular fibrillation in a patient without apparent heart disease. *Am Heart J* 1949;37:811-8.

[92] Konty F, Dale J. Self-terminating idiopathic ventricular fibrillation presenting as syncope: a 40-year follow-up report. *J Intern Med* 1990;227:211-3.

[93] Belhassen B. A 25-year control of idiopathic ventricular fibrillation with electrophysiologic-guided antiarrhythmic drug therapy. *Heart Rhythm* 2004;1:352-4.

[94] Belhassen B, Viskin S. Management of idiopathic ventricular fibrillation: implantable defibrillators? antiarrhythmic drugs? *Ann Noninvasive Electrocardiol* 1998;3:125-8.

[95] Haghjoo M, Arya A, Heidari A, Sadr-Ameli MA. Suppression of electrical storm by oral quinidine in a patient with Brugada syndrome. *J Cardiovasc Electrophysiol* 2005;16:674.

[96] Marquez MF, Rivera J, Hermosillo AG, et al. Arrhythmic storm responsive to quinidine in a patient with Brugada syndrome and vasovagal syncope. *Pacing Clin Electrophysiol* 2005;28:870-3.

[97] Mok NS, Chan NY, Chiu AC. Successful use of quinidine in treatment of electrical storm in Brugada syndrome. *Pacing Clin Electrophysiol* 2004;27:821-3.

[98] Aizawa Y, Tamura M, Chinushi M, et al. An attempt at electrical catheter ablation of the arrhythmogenic area in idiopathic ventricular fibrillation. *Am Heart J* 1992;123:257-60.

[99] Kusano KF, Yamamoto M, Emori T, Morita H, Ohe T. Successful catheter ablation in a patient with polymorphic ventricular tachycardia. *J Cardiovasc Electrophysiol* 2000;11:682-5.

[100] The Antiarrhythmic Versus Implantable Defibrillators (AVID) Investigators. A comparison of antiarrhythmic-drug therapy with implantable defibrillators in patients resuscitated from near-fatal ventricular arrhythmias. *N Engl J Med* 1997;337:1576-83.

[101] Kron J, Herre J, Renfroe EG, et al. Lead- and device-related complications in the antiarrhythmics versus implantable defibrillators trial. *Am Heart J* 2001;141:92-8.

# INDEX

## A

abolition, 133, 208, 215
Abraham, 23, 58
acetylcholine, 101, 198
acid, 57, 100, 102, 103, 106, 107, 142, 145, 148
acidosis, 186
acquired immunity, 132
action potential, x, 166, 171, 172, 176, 177, 179, 182, 211
active site, 141, 143
adenine, 55
adenosine, 2, 27, 75, 78, 90, 95, 96, 97, 104, 110, 111, 210, 219
adenosine triphosphate, 75, 78, 95, 96, 104
adhesion, ix, 34, 38, 76, 90, 102, 106, 112, 119, 121, 124, 128, 129, 139, 144, 145, 146, 149, 152
adiponectin, 36, 50
adipose, 31, 57
adipose tissue, 57
adjunctive therapy, 95, 98, 127, 136
adjustment, 76, 77, 79, 120
ADP, viii, 2, 5, 8, 10, 12, 14, 15, 18, 19, 26, 78, 89, 90, 91, 93, 96, 98, 100, 102, 103, 104, 105, 106, 108, 109, 110, 111
adulthood, 205, 208
adventitia, 42, 43
adverse event, 3, 4, 7, 10, 11, 21, 99, 100, 103, 214
agencies, 189
agglutination, 8
aggregation, 3, 4, 5, 10, 12, 18, 62, 73, 90, 93, 95, 100, 102, 104
agonist, 4, 5, 102
akinesia, 198, 199
albumin, 42
allergic reaction, viii, 89, 91
alteplase, 110

American Heart Association, 17, 22, 25, 26, 28, 79, 105, 190, 193
amines, 148
amino acids, 45
ammonia, 141, 144
amplitude, xi, 162, 166, 173, 185
amylase, 31
androgen, 156
anemia, 75, 76, 79, 149
aneurysm, 34, 41, 54, 78
angina, 62, 63, 68, 77, 92, 106, 121, 132, 151
angiogenesis, ix, 40, 52, 53, 139, 142, 144, 145, 146, 151, 152, 154
angiogram, 98
angiography, xi, 10, 14, 19, 92, 98, 103, 195, 196, 198, 199, 210
angioplasty, 10, 92, 118, 119, 130, 132, 136
ankylosing spondylitis, 145
ANOVA, 173
antagonism, 105, 111, 146
antibody, ix, 102, 127, 136, 139, 150, 152, 153, 154, 155
anti-cancer, 146
anticoagulant, 66, 76, 198
anticoagulation, viii, 61
antigen, x, 31, 33, 35, 39, 120, 122, 123, 128, 129, 130, 131, 132, 140, 150, 151, 154
antigen-presenting cell, 122, 131
antihypertensive drugs, 38
anti-inflammatory agents, 126
aorta, 33, 34, 40, 42, 46, 47, 55
aortic stenosis, 187, 191
aortic valve, 39, 53, 198
apnea, 186
apoptosis, ix, 35, 48, 50, 120, 121, 122, 124, 126, 127, 129, 131, 135, 137, 139, 145, 152, 157
ARC, 95, 103
arrest, xi, 186, 189, 190, 196, 203, 206, 208, 209, 210, 213

# Index

arrests, 190
arrhythmia, vii, x, xi, 159, 162, 182, 188, 203, 204, 205, 209, 212, 213, 215, 219
arteries, vii, viii, ix, 29, 37, 40, 42, 43, 46, 55, 90, 139, 152
artery, xi, 18, 23, 25, 40, 42, 43, 46, 50, 62, 92, 93, 102, 109, 121, 130, 143, 176, 186, 187, 195, 196, 198, 200, 219
arthritis, 128
Asia, 204
aspartate, 141
assessment, vii, 1, 3, 4, 8, 28, 50, 65, 66, 68, 103, 134, 191, 220
asthma, 126
astrocytes, 144
asymptomatic, 35, 175, 182, 183, 198
ataxia, 148, 149, 150, 157
atherosclerosis, viii, ix, 27, 29, 31, 33, 35, 36, 40, 42, 46, 48, 50, 54, 55, 56, 58, 59, 74, 105, 110, 111, 115, 116, 121, 123, 125, 132, 133, 134, 135, 136, 137, 138, 139, 142, 152
atherosclerotic plaque, viii, ix, 35, 36, 46, 50, 51, 56, 58, 62, 89, 90, 101, 121, 124, 125, 131, 132, 140, 143, 151, 153, 198
atherosclerotic vascular disease, 90, 103, 105, 131
athletes, 160, 163, 167
ATP, 14, 18, 104
atrial fibrillation, 187, 196, 210, 211, 217, 220
authors, 18, 65, 93, 98, 102, 105, 151, 158, 160, 166, 198, 214
autoantibodies, 156, 157, 158
autoimmune diseases, 126
autoimmunity, 130, 137, 143, 145, 147, 148, 150, 158
autopsy, 55
autosomal dominant, 212
autosomal recessive, 143, 147, 155

## B

Bacillus subtilis, 56
background, 65
bacteria, 141, 150
basic research, 40
BBB, 164
behaviors, 42
beneficial effect, 124, 126, 127, 129, 216
benign, x, 147, 157, 159, 162, 164, 167, 168, 182, 188, 196, 199, 211, 212, 221
bioavailability, 5, 100
biochemistry, 156
bioinformatics, 47
biological activity, 98
biological processes, 130

biomarkers, 30, 31, 32, 34, 35, 36, 40, 44, 46, 47, 48, 49, 50, 56, 58, 113, 133
biopsy, 40, 54, 155, 199
biotin, 43
bleeding, vii, viii, 2, 6, 7, 11, 12, 13, 15, 16, 17, 18, 61, 62, 63, 64, 65, 66, 67, 68, 69, 71, 72, 73, 74, 75, 76, 77, 78, 79, 90, 92, 93, 94, 95, 96, 97, 98, 99, 100, 101, 102, 103, 104, 105, 142
bleeding time, 95, 98, 101, 102
blood clot, 142
blood flow, 8, 9, 134, 146, 198
blood monocytes, 51
blood particles, 37
blood pressure, 142, 187, 197
blood transfusion, 64, 75, 76, 77, 79
blood transfusions, 75, 76, 77
blood vessels, 43, 128, 143
bloodstream, 143
BMI, 70
body fluid, 36, 44
body mass index, 5
body weight, 74
bonds, 141, 142
bone, 37, 39, 53, 74, 143
bone marrow, 37, 39, 53, 74, 143
bone marrow transplant, 53
bradyarrhythmia, 97
bradycardia, 187, 199, 211, 213
brain, xi, 42, 55, 143, 146, 147, 149, 185
brain damage, xi, 185
breast cancer, 45, 57
brothers, 204, 212
budding, 143
bundle branch block, 164, 204, 206, 212, 216

## C

$Ca^{2+}$, 143, 144, 145, 147, 148, 172, 177, 180
calcification, 42
calcium, x, 6, 42, 142, 144, 171, 173, 181, 182, 197
calcium channel blocker, 6
cancer, 31, 44, 55, 56, 57, 117, 146, 147, 149, 157
cancerous cells, 147
candidates, 31, 32, 34, 105, 215
capillary, 44, 56, 118
capsule, 37
cardiac arrest, vii, x, xi, 159, 167, 168, 186, 189, 190, 191, 192, 193, 196, 203, 204, 205, 208, 209, 210, 213, 220
cardiac arrhythmia, xi, 183, 190, 203
cardiac catheterization, 16, 20, 94
cardiogenic shock, 76, 134, 198
cardiomyopathy, 164, 165, 186, 187, 188, 191, 210, 219

cardiovascular disease, 3, 31, 32, 34, 36, 39, 47, 48, 49, 50, 56, 62, 91, 106, 126
cardiovascular function, 32
cardiovascular risk, xi, 3, 105, 106, 134, 195, 196, 197, 199
cardiovascular system, 140, 141, 146, 152, 154
carotid arteries, 55, 131
carotid endarterectomy, 46
casinos, 190, 193
catalysis, 141
catalytic activity, 141, 142
catecholamines, 196
catheter, xii, 78, 188, 203, 207, 213, 215, 221
catheterizations, 74
causation, 119, 160
CEC, 39, 48
cell culture, 44, 45, 46
cell cycle, 145
cell death, 45, 51, 144, 145, 146, 147, 157
cell line, 44, 45, 57, 100
cell lines, 44, 57, 100
cell organelles, 42
cell signaling, 58
cell surface, 39, 130, 144, 145
Central Europe, 62
central nervous system, 144, 147, 149
cerebral blood flow, 204
cerebrospinal fluid, 148
cerebrovascular disease, 39, 91
challenges, 129, 209
changing environment, 150
channel blocker, 7, 23, 162, 177, 180, 181, 182, 206, 212, 213
chemokine receptor, 128
chemokines, 44, 129, 137, 145
cholesterol, 39, 129, 131
chromatography, 38, 43
chromosome, 157
chronic obstructive pulmonary disease, 18
cimetidine, 78
circulation, vii, viii, xi, 29, 31, 47, 101, 195, 197
classification, 17, 65
cleavage, 142
clinical presentation, 31, 198, 199
clinical symptoms, 173
clinical syndrome, 216
clinical trials, viii, 2, 4, 5, 8, 10, 11, 14, 18, 32, 40, 61, 62, 64, 66, 67, 68, 73, 74, 79, 99, 103, 126, 127, 131, 132, 214
close relationships, 147
closure, 8, 78
clustering, 106
clusters, 204, 205, 209
CNS, 147, 149, 156
collagen, viii, 5, 8, 10, 29, 36, 90, 100, 101, 102, 103, 104, 119, 123, 126
collateral, 54, 152
color, iv
combination therapy, 92
combined effect, 142
community, 135, 151, 160, 190, 192, 193, 196
complement, 35, 124, 127, 129, 135, 136
complexity, 32, 42, 44, 121, 199
compliance, 5, 12, 173, 214
complications, viii, 2, 6, 12, 29, 63, 64, 66, 74, 75, 76, 77, 93, 105, 107, 196, 198, 199, 221
compounds, 46, 76, 100, 146
computed tomography, 166
condensation, 145
conditioning, 43
conduction, 169, 172, 176, 178, 179, 180, 181, 182, 183, 187, 210
conference, 182
congestive heart failure, 76
conjugation, 47
connective tissue, 187
consciousness, xi, 185
consensus, 23, 158, 182
consent, 173, 214
contamination, 42, 130
contradiction, 131
control group, 121, 165, 190
coronary angioplasty, 135
coronary arteries, xi, 40, 63, 68, 195, 198
coronary artery bypass graft, 17, 97
coronary artery disease, viii, 17, 21, 26, 27, 28, 35, 36, 38, 39, 50, 52, 53, 89, 91, 93, 96, 99, 101, 105, 108, 112, 113, 132, 133, 134, 137, 160, 164, 169, 187, 191, 204
coronary heart disease, 188
coronary thrombosis, 106, 121, 125, 196, 198
correlation, 4, 39, 58, 116, 153, 166, 181, 182
correlations, 172, 220
corticosteroids, 124, 126, 136
cost, 75, 94, 95, 97, 101
cough, 97
creatinine, 17, 97
CRP, 36, 48, 116, 119
culture, 39, 40, 43, 45, 145, 155, 156
culture conditions, 45
culture media, 45
CVD, 30, 31, 35, 36, 47, 62
cyanotic, 188
cyclooxygenase, 104
cytochrome, 5, 7, 93, 98

cytokines, ix, 38, 44, 90, 115, 119, 120, 121, 122, 125, 128, 131, 145
cytometry, 8, 9, 23, 39
cytoskeleton, 38

# D

death rate, 62, 66
deaths, vii, 61, 117, 161, 204
defects, 143
defibrillation, 188, 189, 190, 192, 193, 196, 199
defibrillator, x, 164, 171, 188, 189, 192, 193, 214, 216, 219, 220
deficiency, 122, 142, 143, 154, 155
deformability, 75
deformation, xi, 195
degradation, 36, 42, 43, 143
dehydration, 143
dendritic cell, 122, 132
Denmark, 88
deoxyribose, 40
dephosphorylation, 18
depolarization, 165, 167, 172, 180, 181
deposition, 100, 126, 146
deposits, 147
depression, 220
deprivation, 45
deregulation, ix, 115, 120, 121, 124, 125
dermatitis, 147, 150, 156
dermatitis herpetiformis, 147, 150, 156
detection, 19, 34, 44, 47, 52, 107, 155, 166, 217
detention, 47
developed countries, viii, 31, 89, 90
deviant behaviour, 134
deviation, 206
diabetes, 5, 15, 26, 27, 34, 39, 50, 94, 109, 125, 146
diabetic patients, 13, 35
diet, 46, 129, 131, 148
differential diagnosis, 151, 199, 204, 217
diffusion, 189
dilated cardiomyopathy, ix, 139, 146, 151, 153, 188, 210
discharges, 62, 165, 215
discomfort, 151, 197, 204
disease progression, 38, 151
disorder, ix, 37, 140, 145, 148, 152, 154, 157, 204, 206
dispersion, 166, 177, 178, 187, 205, 206, 218
disturbances, xi, 153, 172, 180, 181, 186
dizziness, 208
DNA, 133, 144
dogs, 102, 126, 176, 200
Doha, 61
donors, 144

dosage, 4, 12
dosing, 5, 15, 20, 77, 98
double-blind trial, 78
down-regulation, 122, 132
drawing, 8, 18
drug action, 217
drug interaction, 5, 6, 22
drug resistance, 20, 146
drug therapy, xii, 46, 168, 173, 192, 203, 213, 215, 221
drug treatment, 188, 215
drugs, vii, 1, 2, 3, 4, 6, 14, 18, 19, 27, 31, 68, 73, 74, 76, 106, 107, 113, 129, 132, 146, 162, 172, 177, 178, 187, 191, 206, 213, 214, 218, 221
dynamics, 161, 220
dysplasia, 186, 210
dyspnea, 17, 151, 188, 198

# E

East Asia, 204
ECM, viii, 29, 47, 141, 144, 145, 146, 147, 150, 152
economic status, 71
edema, 152
effluent, 41
elafin, 146, 152
election, 42
electrocardiogram, 161, 168, 169, 172, 182, 188, 197, 204, 206, 210, 212, 213
electrodes, 176, 212
electrolyte, 187, 196
electrolyte imbalance, 187
electrophoresis, 36, 52, 54, 55, 142
electroporation, 138
ELISA, 34, 35, 158
embolism, 186
emergency response, 190
encoding, 133, 147, 156, 157
endocardium, 176, 178, 181
endocrine, 31
endothelial cells, 31, 39, 43, 52, 53, 57, 121, 129, 132, 157
endothelial dysfunction, 36
endothelium, viii, 38, 39, 89, 90, 118, 125, 127, 128, 147
endurance, 167
England, 62, 89
enrollment, 19, 96
enzymatic activity, ix, 40, 140, 141, 146, 148, 152, 153, 154
enzyme-linked immunosorbent assay, 151
enzymes, 5, 14, 128, 141, 145, 154, 199
EPC, 39, 40, 48
epicardium, xi, 172, 176, 177, 178, 179, 181

epidemiology, 191
epidermis, 147, 149, 155, 157
epinephrine, 5, 8, 211, 219, 220
epithelial cells, 147, 157
epithelium, 143, 149
equipment, 8
erosion, 2, 51
erythrocytes, 9, 143
erythropoietin, 79
ESI, 33
etiology, xi, 196, 198, 199, 203, 204, 206, 214
exaggeration, 76
excitability, 178
excitation, 172, 180, 182, 196, 210
exclusion, xi, 203, 209, 213
exercise, 163, 187, 210
exertion, 196, 198
experimental condition, 41
extracellular matrix, viii, 29, 37, 128, 129, 141, 152
extraction, 34, 42, 55

## F

family history, 173, 182
family members, 141, 190
fat, 131
fatal arrhythmia, 187, 188
FDA, 15, 16, 32, 49, 189
FDA approval, 32
ferritin, 33, 56
fever, 209
fibers, 187, 204, 207, 208, 212
fibrillation, vii, xi, 161, 168, 185, 187, 191, 196, 203, 210, 212, 216, 217
fibrin, 142, 154
fibrinogen, 8, 33, 90, 100, 134, 142
fibrinolysis, xi, 142, 195, 197, 198
fibroblast proliferation, 119
fibroblasts, 143
fibrogenesis, ix, 139, 144, 145
fibrosis, 126, 131, 146, 152, 187
fibrous cap, viii, 29, 121, 124, 125, 146
fibrous tissue, viii, 29
fluid, 36, 40, 145, 149
fluorescence, 176
fragments, 36, 37, 136
France, 8, 159
frequencies, 131
fusion, 129, 130, 137

## G

gastrointestinal bleeding, 78, 96
gel, 43, 45, 51, 52, 55

gene promoter, 145
gene therapy, ix, 115, 131, 133, 138
gene transfer, 138
genes, 6, 45, 142, 157, 173
genetic factors, 4
genetic mutations, 211
genetic testing, 6, 220
genome, 44, 56
genomics, 50, 51
genotype, 15, 111, 133, 172, 211
Georgia, 16
Germany, 8
germline mutations, 143
gland, 156
glucocorticoid receptor, 126
glucose, 35, 156
glucose tolerance, 35, 156
glutamic acid, 144
glutathione, 33
glycoproteins, 39
Gori, 24, 25, 26, 53
granules, 104
graph, 140
Great Britain, 62
growth factor, 39, 40, 44, 104
guidance, 13
guidelines, vii, 1, 4, 6, 12, 13, 14, 22, 173
guilt, 157
Guinea, 158

## H

haemostasis, 8
hair, 147, 149
hair follicle, 147
half-life, 16, 18, 73, 96
haptoglobin, 33, 34
harmful effects, 126
heart attack, 62, 106
heart disease, xi, 31, 58, 61, 95, 120, 132, 133, 186, 187, 188, 196, 200, 203, 204, 205, 209, 210, 212, 213, 214, 216, 217, 221
heart failure, ix, 5, 36, 72, 75, 133, 135, 137, 139, 146, 151, 152, 156, 199
heart rate, 211, 219
heat shock protein, 58
hematemesis, 63
hematocrit, 63, 64
hematoma, 63, 64, 78
hematomas, 78
hematopoietic stem cells, 39
hematuria, 63
hemisphere, 196
hemoglobin, 34, 42, 49, 54, 63, 64, 66, 75, 79

hemolytic anemia, 142
hemorrhage, 42, 63, 64, 79
hemostasis, 63, 68, 142, 143
hepatitis, 131
hepatocytes, 143
hereditary spherocytosis, 142
heterogeneity, x, xi, 51, 172, 177, 178, 179, 180, 181, 188
histidine, 141
histone, 145
HLA, 148, 150
homeostasis, 38, 125, 129
homocysteine, 134
hospitalization, 36, 62, 161
human experience, 110
human genome, 173
human subjects, 93
hydrogen, 51
hydrogen peroxide, 51
hydrolysis, 141
hyperkinesia, xi, 195, 199
hyperplasia, viii, 29, 147, 148, 149, 157
hypersensitivity, 126
hypertension, 39, 46, 58, 74, 112, 146, 149
hypertrophic cardiomyopathy, 210, 219
hypertrophy, 146, 152, 187, 210, 219
hyperuricemia, 18
hypokalemia, 213
hypokinesia, 117, 196
hypomagnesemia, 213
hypotension, 64, 75, 76, 197
hypothesis, ix, 56, 124, 140, 152, 154, 190, 198
hypovolemia, 199
hypoxemia, 75, 76

# I

IBD, 146, 149, 154
ICAM, 124, 129
ideal, 40, 47
idiopathic, 160, 161, 162, 163, 164, 165, 166, 167, 169, 181, 191, 196, 200, 204, 205, 209, 215, 216, 217, 218, 219, 220, 221
IFN, 145
IL-13, 121
imaging modalities, 210
immune reaction, 75, 122
immune response, ix, 36, 38, 44, 115, 120, 122, 125, 128, 130, 132, 133, 135, 148, 150
immune system, ix, 115, 116, 120, 121, 122, 124, 129, 133, 148
immunity, 123, 131, 132, 133, 134, 148, 155
immunodeficiency, 121
immunoglobulin, 122, 128, 129, 151
immunohistochemistry, 35
immunomodulation, 123, 132, 133, 136
immunomodulatory, 131, 132
immunosuppression, 120, 154
immunotherapy, 137
impurities, 151
in utero, 220
in vivo, 7, 41, 44, 53, 56, 96, 97, 106, 108, 124, 130, 132, 133
incidence, xi, 2, 10, 13, 14, 16, 17, 18, 20, 24, 25, 26, 36, 62, 65, 66, 67, 71, 72, 73, 74, 75, 76, 77, 79, 93, 120, 132, 166, 168, 172, 176, 180, 196, 198, 205, 220
inclusion, 4, 164
incubation period, 45
inducer, 35, 50, 145
induction, ix, 123, 129, 131, 132, 139, 150, 152, 173, 177, 178, 205, 208, 217, 219
infarction, x, 12, 20, 35, 39, 49, 72, 76, 77, 91, 94, 99, 103, 127, 130, 131, 134, 135, 136, 138, 140, 154, 158, 186, 187, 188, 190, 191, 196
inflammation, ix, 37, 39, 75, 90, 116, 119, 120, 123, 126, 130, 132, 133, 134, 135, 137, 138, 139, 144, 145, 152, 157, 158
inflammatory bowel disease, 131, 146, 149, 155, 156
inflammatory cells, viii, 29, 116, 118
inflammatory disease, viii, 29, 117, 128, 130, 131, 132, 133
inflammatory mediators, 90, 133
inflammatory responses, 130, 131
ingestion, 14, 186
inheritance, 212
inherited disorder, 142, 154
inhibition, vii, ix, 1, 2, 3, 4, 5, 7, 8, 9, 10, 11, 12, 13, 15, 16, 17, 18, 19, 20, 21, 22, 23, 27, 28, 78, 91, 93, 95, 96, 98, 99, 100, 102, 106, 108, 109, 110, 111, 115, 123, 126, 127, 128, 130, 131, 132, 133, 135, 136, 137, 138, 154
inhibitor, 16, 18, 19, 23, 54, 55, 68, 77, 93, 95, 97, 102, 108, 110, 112, 142
initiation, xi, 126, 178, 182, 187, 203, 209, 218
innate immunity, 51, 116
insight, ix, 115
insulin, 15, 35, 47, 50, 57, 146
insulin resistance, 47
insulin signaling, 146
integrin, 106, 127, 129, 136, 138, 144, 145
intensive care unit, 64, 162
intercellular adhesion molecule, 121, 124, 129
interference, 45
interferon, 51, 121, 122
interferon-γ, 121, 122
interrogations, 164

intervention, 19, 20, 21, 22, 23, 24, 25, 27, 28, 35, 38, 63, 64, 71, 99, 103, 107, 108, 109, 111, 113, 127, 134, 136, 190, 191, 214
intestine, ix, 139, 143, 150, 151
intima, viii, 29, 34, 35, 36, 42, 43, 55, 56
intracellular cytokines, 132
intraocular, 63, 64
intravenously, 95, 96, 97
ions, 142, 144
ischaemic heart disease, vii, 109
ischemia, xi, 19, 54, 55, 62, 72, 75, 76, 77, 95, 96, 104, 127, 130, 136, 137, 164, 182, 185, 186, 187, 191, 196
ischemia reperfusion injury, 54
isotope, 31, 45, 49, 57
issues, viii, 39, 61, 62, 167, 189, 190
Italy, 139

## J

Japan, 171, 183, 196, 218

## K

$K^+$, 172, 180, 220
keratin, 143, 146
keratinocyte, 143, 147, 149
keratinocytes, 143
kidney, 31
kidneys, 144
Korea, 160

## L

labeling, 43, 45, 57, 58
laboratory tests, 3
landscape, 122
Latin America, 200
LDL, 129, 131
leakage, 40, 45, 145
left ventricle, xi, 131, 173, 195, 197, 200, 214
legal protection, 189
legislation, 189
lesions, viii, 2, 29, 31, 38, 46, 51, 52, 53, 129, 196
leucocyte, 135
leukocyte function antigen, 132, 138
leukocytosis, 116, 134
LFA, 132
ligand, 35, 48, 119, 129, 132
light transmission, 8
light transmittance, 10
lipids, 42
lipoproteins, viii, 29
liquid chromatography, 47, 56, 59
liver, 31, 91, 119, 143, 146, 149, 158

liver cirrhosis, 158
liver disease, 146, 149, 158
localization, ix, 52, 139, 148, 150, 208
loss of consciousness, 188
lovastatin, 6
low molecular weight heparins, 73
low-density lipoprotein, 123, 124, 129, 136
LTA, 98
lumen, 38, 39, 42, 152
lymph, 130, 131
lymph node, 130, 131
lymphocytes, viii, ix, 29, 31, 38, 115, 116, 118, 120, 128, 129, 143, 150
lymphocytosis, 148
lysine, 141, 148
lysis, 45
lysozyme, 35, 50

## M

macrophage inflammatory protein, 129
macrophages, viii, 29, 31, 37, 46, 50, 51, 119, 121, 123, 130, 143, 145, 149
magnetic resonance, 19, 116, 117, 134
magnetic resonance imaging, 19, 117, 134
majority, viii, xi, 36, 61, 62, 128, 203, 204, 208, 209, 211, 212, 215
malabsorption, 74
management, vii, viii, xi, xii, 1, 2, 3, 12, 14, 17, 22, 61, 62, 74, 76, 77, 78, 79, 91, 105, 125, 154, 181, 188, 191, 195, 199, 204, 205
mapping, 8, 162, 166, 167, 176, 182, 183, 207, 212, 214, 221
Marfan syndrome, 54
marrow, 39, 52, 53, 143
masking, 47
mass spectrometry, 49, 52, 54, 55, 56, 57, 59
mast cells, 131
matrix, 37, 51, 52, 90, 101
MCP, 129
MCP-1, 129
mechanical ventilation, 76
media, 35, 42, 43, 45, 46, 55, 56, 57, 58, 62, 156
median, 65, 68, 70, 117, 120, 164
medication, 64, 215
megakaryocyte, 143
messenger ribonucleic acid, 90
meta-analysis, 4, 11, 77, 79, 91, 106, 192
metabolic pathways, 47
metabolism, 5, 34, 36, 37, 44, 47, 122
metabolites, 46, 91
metalloproteinase, 138, 146
methodology, 3, 43, 44
methylprednisolone, 138

MHC, 132
mice, 34, 43, 44, 47, 58, 98, 110, 112, 121, 123, 128, 129, 131, 136, 137, 142, 146, 156
Middle East, 82
migration, ix, 40, 119, 124, 139, 144, 145, 149
MIP, 129
miscarriage, 142, 149
mitochondria, 54, 55, 144, 145
mitral valve, 210
mitral valve prolapse, 210
MMP, 47
MMPs, viii, 29, 128, 132
molecular mass, 146
molecular weight, 77, 95
molecules, 37, 44, 47, 100, 101, 119, 121, 124, 128, 129, 130, 132, 145, 152
momentum, x, 159
monoclonal antibody, 102, 112, 129, 136
monocyte chemoattractant protein, 129
monomers, 142
Moon, 84
morbidity, viii, 61, 62, 75, 76, 79, 90, 191
morphology, xi, 51, 185, 206, 207, 208, 211, 212
mortality rate, 67
Moses, 24, 85
motif, 129
mRNA, 38, 131
mucosa, 150, 155
multiple sclerosis, 129, 131, 137
mutation, x, 147, 156, 157, 171, 172, 173, 174, 175, 176, 180, 183, 217, 219, 220
myeloid cells, 57
myocardial ischemia, vii, ix, 47, 58, 62, 101, 127, 135, 136, 139, 151, 152, 187, 209, 219
myocardial necrosis, 126, 127, 151, 153
myocarditis, x, 133, 138, 140, 152, 154, 187, 199
myocardium, x, 41, 46, 54, 76, 126, 127, 129, 131, 132, 133, 136, 140, 146, 154, 158, 182, 187, 188, 198, 200
myocyte, 127
myoglobin, 134, 151, 153
myosin, 35, 42, 55

## N

Na$^+$, 172, 177, 178, 180, 181, 183
natural killer cell, 131
nausea, 151
necrosis, viii, 29, 35, 48, 50, 116, 119, 126, 129, 199
neovascularization, 39, 46, 52, 146
nephropathy, 74
nervous system, 156
neurodegenerative diseases, 156
neurodegenerative disorders, 146
neurons, 144, 147
neutropenia, viii, 89, 91
neutrophils, 116, 118, 119, 120, 124, 125, 127, 136, 143
New Zealand, 87, 88
nitric oxide, 75, 136
nitric oxide synthase, 136
NK cells, 128
NMR, 47, 58
normal distribution, vii, 1, 3, 211
nuclear magnetic resonance, 47
nucleotides, 144
nucleus, 144, 145, 146

## O

obesity, 5
obstruction, ix, 38, 41, 115, 117, 118, 121, 124, 125, 133, 187, 198, 199
occlusion, viii, xi, 89, 195, 198
octopus, 196
omeprazole, 6, 7, 23, 78
oral hypoglycemic agents, 74
organ, ix, 31, 115, 120, 131, 139, 150, 151
organism, 45, 122
oscillation, 219
osteoarthritis, 146
ovarian cancer, 32, 49
oxidation, 6, 47
oxidative stress, 37
oxygen, 75, 76, 197
oxygen consumption, 75

## P

p53, 145
pacing, 177, 208, 210
paclitaxel, 24
pain, xi, 7, 117, 133, 134, 188, 195, 197, 198
palpitations, 188, 204
pancreas, 143
pancreatic cancer, 57
paradigm, 198
Paraguay, 203
parallel, 16, 39, 101, 112, 125
parameter, 215
parenchymal cell, 119
pathogenesis, 2, 36, 52, 105, 127, 131, 133, 136, 141, 146, 148, 150, 151, 156, 158
pathology, 47, 128, 129, 133
pathophysiology, ix, 52, 115, 116, 120, 121, 122, 123, 125, 133, 135, 165, 169, 204
pathways, 5, 8, 18, 31, 38, 103, 126, 128, 129, 210
PBMC, 36, 47

peptides, 33, 36, 42, 44, 56, 150, 157
performance, ix, 115, 132
perfusion, 55, 76, 98, 116, 117, 119, 125, 127, 134, 188, 192, 198
perinatal, 154
peripheral blood, 39, 54
peripheral blood mononuclear cell, 39
permeability, x, 140, 146, 151, 152
permission, iv, 161
PET, 198
pH, 38, 42, 144, 150, 155
phagocytosis, 145
pharmacokinetics, 6, 15, 27, 68, 90, 102, 108, 110, 113
pharmacological treatment, 218
pharmacotherapy, 119
phenotype, 39, 40, 130, 133, 143, 147, 172, 182, 183, 220
phosphorylation, 6, 26, 43, 54, 55, 78, 98, 141, 142, 145
physiology, 105, 137
pigs, 128, 132, 136
pilot study, 98
placebo, 6, 7, 12, 18, 19, 20, 28, 65, 77, 78, 92, 95, 96, 98, 99, 102, 103, 104, 107, 113, 189, 191
plants, 141
plaque, ix, 2, 19, 31, 36, 37, 38, 42, 43, 46, 47, 51, 121, 123, 125, 128, 131, 139, 146, 152, 154
plasma levels, 32, 46, 100
plasma membrane, 143, 144, 145
plasma proteins, 31, 32, 35, 42
plasmapheresis, 154
plasmid, 133
platelet aggregation, 3, 4, 5, 10, 11, 12, 13, 14, 15, 18, 20, 21, 22, 25, 26, 75, 93, 95, 96, 100, 102, 103, 104, 108, 110, 111, 124
platelets, 2, 5, 8, 36, 38, 44, 51, 52, 56, 90, 91, 93, 94, 95, 96, 99, 100, 101, 102, 104, 105, 106, 111, 125, 143, 146, 149
platform, 34, 140
pneumonia, 135
pneumothorax, 186
polymerization, 142
polymers, 142
polymorphism, 6, 22, 98, 135
polymorphisms, 6, 22, 98, 125, 154
potassium, 173, 206, 211
precursor cells, 39
predictability, 10
pregnancy, 142
premature ventricular contractions, 204

prevention, vii, viii, 2, 3, 16, 18, 20, 89, 91, 92, 95, 97, 98, 101, 106, 107, 110, 111, 112, 113, 188, 190, 215, 216
primary biliary cirrhosis, 158
primary prophylaxis, 216
primary school, 189, 192
probability, vii, 1, 167
probands, 182
problem solving, 218
profit, 94
prognosis, xi, xii, 47, 53, 118, 135, 161, 169, 180, 182, 195, 199, 204, 205, 213
pro-inflammatory, ix, 115, 128, 131, 145
proliferation, viii, ix, xi, 29, 45, 129, 131, 139, 144, 145, 149, 151, 203, 205
promoter, 51
propagation, 180
properties, 96, 101, 108, 130, 132, 210, 220
prophylaxis, 106
prostate cancer, 147, 157
proteases, 124, 127, 142
protein analysis, 49
protein folding, 37
proteins, viii, 6, 29, 31, 32, 33, 34, 36, 37, 38, 40, 42, 43, 44, 45, 46, 49, 51, 52, 54, 55, 56, 57, 58, 128, 129, 141, 143, 145, 146, 147, 150, 152, 156
proteinuria, 74, 112
proteoglycans, 43, 55
proteolysis, 54, 141, 143, 147
proteolytic enzyme, 37
proteome, 31, 32, 35, 37, 38, 40, 41, 42, 43, 44, 46, 49, 50, 51, 52, 55, 56, 57, 58
proteomics, 31, 40, 43, 44, 45, 48, 49, 50, 51, 55, 56, 57, 58
prothrombin, 73
proton pump inhibitors, 6, 23, 78
psoriasis, 130, 131, 147
psoriatic arthritis, 146
pulmonary hypertension, 186
purification, 54
purity, 43
PVC, 179, 206, 208, 214
pyrimidine, 14

# Q

QRS complex, 161, 162, 164, 166, 167, 169, 173, 175, 176, 210, 212
QT interval, 173, 181, 187, 209, 211, 212, 214, 216, 219, 220
quality of life, 215
quartile, 121

## R

race, x, 159
Ramadan, 157
reaction rate, 144
reactions, 31, 47, 126, 127, 141, 148, 156, 158
reactivity, 3, 4, 5, 6, 8, 9, 10, 17, 21, 22, 24, 26, 27, 98, 111
reality, 130
reasoning, 210
receptors, 4, 5, 6, 19, 90, 91, 93, 100, 104, 105, 120, 122, 130, 132, 138
recognition, 189
recommendations, iv, 63
recruiting, 98
recurrence, x, xii, 3, 122, 135, 160, 162, 164, 171, 176, 181, 188, 198, 199, 203, 213, 214
red blood cells, 64, 68, 75
redundancy, 130
regeneration, 39, 40
Registry, 24, 64, 67, 68, 73, 80, 82, 84, 88, 200
regression, 19, 101
remodelling, 54, 126, 128, 131, 132, 137, 143, 149
renal dysfunction, 72
renal failure, 18, 79
renin, 199
repair, 39, 40, 53
replacement, 45, 53
repression, 131
requirements, 77, 96, 99
residues, 144, 148, 150
resistance, vii, 1, 3, 4, 5, 9, 11, 13, 15, 20, 26, 27, 91, 94, 107, 133, 142, 148
resolution, 131, 183, 197
resources, 76
respect, 42, 44
respiration, 188
response time, 189, 196
responsiveness, 3, 11, 17, 20, 21, 93
restenosis, 38
resting potential, 180
reticulum, 144
retinoblastoma, 145
rheumatoid arthritis, 129, 130, 131, 137, 146, 150, 157
rhythm, xi, 36, 185, 188, 196, 210
right ventricle, xi, 172, 181, 208
rights, iv
risk factors, vii, 2, 12, 39, 53, 65, 125, 187, 188, 218
risk profile, 142, 189
RNA, 38, 90, 146
rodents, 147, 149

## S

saliva, 36, 50, 145, 155
saturation, 43, 55, 197
saving lives, 62
scar tissue, 126
sclerosis, 128
screening, 6, 36, 155, 167
secondary prophylaxis, 199
secrete, 119
secretion, viii, 29, 46, 130, 146, 147, 156
semen, 147
seminal vesicle, 156
sensing, 38
sensitivity, 9, 31, 68, 105, 162, 218
sepsis, 120, 132, 135
serotonin, 104
serum, 31, 34, 35, 36, 44, 46, 49, 50, 57, 58, 90, 97, 130, 131, 135, 143, 145, 148, 151, 214
sex, 69, 120, 173
shape, 148
shear, 9, 10, 100, 101, 102
shock, xi, 72, 122, 135, 188, 189, 195, 197, 199, 214, 215, 220
shortness of breath, 204
sick sinus syndrome, 180
side effects, viii, 89, 91, 97, 107
signal peptide, 45
signal transduction, 38
signaling pathway, ix, 139, 144, 145
signalling, 131, 132
signals, 36, 129, 166, 173
signs, vii, xi, 195, 197, 204, 210
silver, 54, 176
sinus rhythm, 166, 188, 206, 207, 208, 210, 219
skeletal muscle, 57
skin, 141, 143, 147, 149, 155, 157
small intestine, ix, 139, 150
smoking, 39
smooth muscle, 39, 46, 51, 58, 121, 143
smooth muscle cells, 46, 58, 121, 143
sodium, x, 77, 162, 171, 173, 180, 181, 182, 183, 206, 209, 212, 213
solid phase, 151
solubility, 42
space, 119
Spain, 1, 12, 29, 115, 195
species, 40
spherocytosis, 149
spleen, 131
stabilization, ix, 140, 146, 149, 152, 153
stable angina, 10, 14, 20, 35, 123, 132
statin, 37, 132

statistics, 105
stem cells, 39, 40, 46, 54, 58
stenosis, 35, 39, 53, 101, 197, 198
stent, vii, viii, 1, 2, 6, 7, 10, 11, 13, 14, 15, 17, 18, 19, 20, 21, 24, 25, 27, 78, 89, 94, 96, 99, 100, 107, 111
stimulus, ix, 115, 119, 122, 125, 145, 205
storage, 75
storms, 161, 164, 205, 209, 213, 214
strategy, 12, 17, 28, 30, 44, 76, 77, 134, 188, 189, 190
stratification, 63, 151, 164, 165, 167, 169, 181, 182, 183, 191
streptokinase, 106, 107
stroke, vii, viii, 2, 7, 12, 15, 16, 17, 29, 31, 32, 33, 34, 49, 53, 75, 76, 78, 91, 92, 93, 94, 97, 99, 101, 103, 104, 105, 106, 111, 112, 133
structural changes, 75
structural protein, 141, 142, 143
subacute, 10, 198
subdural hematoma, 64
subgroups, 15
substrates, 6, 142, 143, 144, 145, 147, 148
sucrose, 43
suppression, 12, 130
supraventricular tachycardia, 186, 220
surface area, 176
surgical intervention, 63, 64
surveillance, 37
survey, 44, 49, 56
survival, 7, 40, 120, 121, 129, 145, 161, 188, 189, 190, 192, 196, 213
survival rate, 189, 190, 196
survivors, 120, 160, 163, 168, 190, 196, 204, 210, 213, 214, 217, 220
Sweden, 24
Switzerland, 8
sympathetic nervous system, 76
symptoms, vii, 97, 148, 150, 151, 172, 188, 198, 204, 205, 213, 215, 220
synovial fluid, 145
synthesis, 37, 38, 74, 90, 91, 106, 131, 145, 148, 157

# T

T cell, 124, 128, 129, 131, 132, 135, 137, 138, 148, 155
T lymphocytes, ix, 115, 116, 123, 132, 135, 150
tachycardia, 76, 186, 187, 197, 220, 221
target organs, 123
T-cell receptor, 129
TCR, 129
technician, 8, 9
territory, 189

testing, 6, 14, 23, 209, 211, 212, 217
TGF, 104, 123, 124, 130, 131, 137, 145, 146, 152
Th cells, 130
Th1 polarization, 121
therapeutic approaches, ix, 115, 123, 128, 132
therapeutic interventions, 158
therapeutic targets, 44, 49, 56, 138
therapeutics, 105, 128
thinning, 125, 200
thrombin, viii, 5, 38, 56, 62, 77, 89, 90, 103, 104, 105, 142, 146
thrombocytopenic purpura, 102, 113
thrombolytic agents, 62, 66
thrombolytic therapy, 95
thrombosis, vii, viii, 1, 2, 4, 6, 10, 11, 13, 14, 15, 17, 18, 19, 24, 25, 29, 37, 43, 49, 52, 54, 56, 63, 72, 74, 76, 78, 90, 94, 95, 96, 98, 99, 100, 101, 102, 106, 107, 109, 110, 111, 112, 124, 142
thrombus, viii, 2, 35, 38, 41, 44, 46, 62, 89, 90, 95, 101, 106, 111, 151, 152, 198
time frame, 44
tissue, ix, x, xi, 31, 39, 40, 42, 43, 44, 45, 46, 55, 56, 57, 75, 95, 107, 109, 119, 122, 127, 139, 141, 143, 145, 148, 149, 150, 151, 153, 155, 156, 157, 158, 171, 172, 176, 178, 179, 181, 182, 183, 185, 187, 196, 207
tissue perfusion, 95, 109
TLR, 132
TLR4, 132
TNF, ix, 35, 37, 48, 115, 127, 128, 129, 130, 137
TNF-alpha, 137
TNF-α, 37
tones, 188
toxic effect, 196
toxic products, 119
toxicity, 214
training, 8, 189, 190, 192
transcription, 122, 145
transduction, 38, 149
transferrin, 31
transforming growth factor, 104, 123, 124, 152
transfusion, 63, 64, 75, 77, 79, 96, 99
transient ischemic attack, 15, 101, 103, 112
translation, 37, 38, 52, 127
translocation, 145
transplant recipients, 121, 135
transplantation, 46, 74, 131
transport, 56
transthoracic echocardiography, 197
trauma, 116
trial, 6, 7, 12, 13, 15, 16, 17, 19, 20, 22, 25, 26, 27, 28, 63, 65, 68, 69, 70, 71, 72, 73, 76, 77, 78, 92,

93, 95, 96, 97, 98, 101, 103, 104, 106, 107, 109, 110, 111, 113, 127, 136, 190, 192, 193, 214, 221
triggers, 157, 180, 182, 187
tryptophan, 122, 141
tumor, 35, 37, 44, 56, 121, 127, 146
tumor necrosis factor, 121, 127
tumors, 156
type 2 diabetes, 35, 50, 146, 156
tyrosine, 38, 52, 54

## U

UK, 62, 89
ulcerative colitis, 146
ultrasound, 198, 199, 200
United Kingdom, 62
unmasking, 217
unstable angina, viii, 2, 16, 22, 29, 39, 51, 62, 63, 67, 91, 95, 106, 107, 109, 125, 132, 151
unstable patients, 121, 123
updating, 26, 133
uric acid, 17, 97
urine, 31, 36, 47, 50, 58, 98

## V

Valencia, 26, 115
validation, 30, 31, 44, 45, 55, 162, 167
valvular heart disease, ix, 139, 146, 151
variations, 20, 35, 40, 95, 110, 142, 196
vascular diseases, 33, 113, 138, 155
vascular endothelial growth factor (VEGF), 133
vascular system, viii, 29
vasculature, 38, 39
vasoconstriction, 75, 198
vasodilation, 100
vasodilator, 6, 26
vasopressin, 76
vasospasm, 124, 198
vasovagal syncope, 209, 221

VCAM, 129
ventilation, 72
ventricle, 162, 197, 205, 207
ventricular arrhythmias, xi, xii, 160, 164, 167, 172, 179, 181, 182, 187, 191, 192, 199, 203, 205, 206, 207, 208, 210, 211, 212, 214, 216, 217, 218, 219, 221
ventricular fibrillation, vii, x, xi, 159, 161, 162, 163, 165, 168, 169, 171, 172, 181, 183, 186, 195, 196, 200, 203, 204, 208, 209, 212, 216, 217, 218, 219, 220, 221
ventricular septum, 208
ventricular tachycardia, xi, 169, 172, 173, 179, 186, 187, 191, 196, 203, 216, 217, 218, 219, 221
venules, 119
versatility, 133
very late activation, 129
vessels, ix, 35, 44, 58, 139, 152
victims, 189, 192, 196
viral infection, 198
viral myocarditis, 196
vision, 64
vitamin D, 197
VLA, 128, 129
vulnerability, 36, 220

## W

weakness, 37, 204
western blot, 151
white blood cell count, 134
white blood cells, 116
withdrawal, 11, 148
wound healing, ix, 38, 126, 139, 142, 144, 145, 153

## Y

yes/no, 64
young adults, x, 159, 167